D0491492

K07766

a textbook of
GENERAL PRACTICE

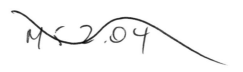M 2.04

a textbook of
GENERAL PRACTICE

2nd edition

Edited by

Anne Stephenson MB ChB, PhD (Medicine), ILTM
Senior Lecturer and Head of Undergraduate Teaching,
Department of General Practice and Primary Care,
Guy's, King's and St Thomas' School of Medicine,
King's College, London, UK

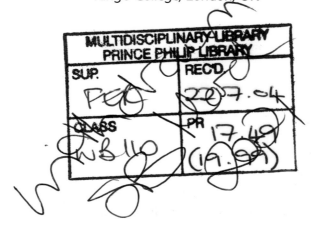

MULTIDISCIPLINARY LIBRARY PRINCE PHILIP LIBRARY	
SUP. PEO	REC'D 22.7.04
CLASS WB 110	PR 17.49 (19.99)

ARNOLD

A member of the Hodder Headline Group
LONDON

First published in Great Britain in 1998
Second edition published in 2004 by
Arnold, a member of the Hodder Headline Group,
338 Euston Road, London NW1 3BH

http://www.arnoldpublishers.com

Distributed in the United States of America by
Oxford University Press Inc.,
198 Madison Avenue, New York, NY 10016
Oxford is a registered trademark of Oxford University Press

© 2004 Arnold

All rights reserved. No part of this publication may be reproduced or transmitted
in any form or by any means, electronically or mechanically, including
photocopying, recording or any information storage or retrieval system, without
either prior permission in writing from the publisher or a licence permitting
restricted copying. In the United Kingdom such licences are issued by the
Copyright Licensing Agency: 90 Tottenham Court Road, London W1T 4LP.

Whilst the advice and information in this book are believed to be true and accurate
at the date of going to press, neither the author[s] nor the publisher can accept any legal
responsibility or liability for any errors or omissions that may be made. In particular
(but without limiting the generality of the preceding disclaimer) every effort has been
made to check drug dosages; however, it is still possible that errors have been missed.
Furthermore, dosage schedules are constantly being revised and new side-effects recognized.
For these reasons the reader is strongly urged to consult the drug companies' printed
instructions before administering any of the drugs recommended in this book.

British Library Cataloguing in Publication Data
A catalogue record for this book is available from the British Library

Library of Congress Cataloging-in-Publication Data
A catalog record for this book is available from the Library of Congress

ISBN 0 340 810521

1 2 3 4 5 6 7 8 9 10

Commissioning Editor: Georgina Bentliff
Development Editor: Heather Smith
Project Editor: Wendy Rooke
Production Controller: Lindsay Smith
Cover Design: Amina Dudhia

Typeset in 9.5/12 RotisSerif by Charon Tec Pvt. Ltd, India
Printed and bound in Spain.

Hodder Headline's policy is to use papers that are natural, renewable and recyclable
products and made from wood grown in sustainable forests. The logging and manufacturing
processes are expected to conform to the environmental regulations of the country of origin.

What do you think about this book? Or any other Arnold title?
Please send your comments to **feedback.arnold@hodder.co.uk**

CONTENTS

CONTRIBUTORS

Paul Booton BSc (Hons) MB BS MRCP MRCGP
Senior Lecturer, Head of Final Year, General Practitioner, Guy's, King's and St Thomas' School of Medicine, Clinical Skills Laboratory, London, UK

Joanna Collerton BM BCh MRCP MRCGP
Senior Research Fellow, The Institute for Ageing and Health, University of Newcastle, Newcastle upon Tyne, UK

Brian Fine MA MB BChir DRCOG
General Practitioner and Honorary Senior Lecturer, Department of General Practice and Primary Care, Guy's, King's and St Thomas' School of Medicine, King's College London, London, UK

Sue Fish BA (Hons) Cantab
Primary Care Service Manager, Lambeth Primary Care Trust, London, UK

Helen J. Graham DCH FRCGP ILTM
Senior Lecturer, General Practice and Primary Care, Guy's, King's and St Thomas' School of Medicine, King's College London, London, UK

Graham Hewett MSc BA (Hons)
Clinical Governance Development Manager, South East London Shared Services Partnership, London, UK

Roger Higgs MBE MA FRCP FRCGP
General Practitioner and Professor of General Practice and Primary Care, Department of General Practice and Primary Care, King's College London, London, UK

Mary Lawson BSc (Hons)
Senior Lecturer in Medical Education, Centre for Medical and Health Sciences Education, Monash University, Melbourne, Victoria 3800, Australia

Cath Miskin MB BS MRCGP DRCOG DipMedEd
Clinical Lecturer, Department of General Practice and Primary Care, Guy's, King's and St Thomas' School of Medicine, King's College London, London, UK; GP Principal, South London, UK

Richard Phillips MA MRCP ILTM
Senior Lecturer, Department of General Practice and Primary Care, Guy's, King's and St Thomas' School of Medicine, King's College London, London, UK

Mary Seabrook BEd DMS PhD (Education)
Freelance Education and Training Consultant, and Professional Life Coach, London, UK

Steven Smith MB BS MRCGP DRCOG BSc (Hons)
Clinical Adviser, South East London Shared Services Partnership, London, UK

Anne Stephenson MB ChB, PhD (Medicine) ILTM
Senior Lecturer and Head of Undergraduate Teaching, Department of General Practice and Primary Care, Guy's, King's and St Thomas' School of Medicine, King's College London, London, UK

Patrick White MB ChB BAO MRCP FRCGP
Senior Lecturer, Department of General Practice and Primary Care, Guy's, King's and St Thomas' School of Medicine, King's College London, London, UK

Ann Wylie MA (Health Education) ILTM
Senior Tutor, Associate Lecturer (Open University) and Senior Health Promotion Specialist (Berkshire), Department of General Practice and Primary Care, Guy's, King's and St Thomas' School of Medicine, King's College London, London, UK

PREFACE

This second edition has extended its range from being primarily intended for undergraduate medical students to include pre-registration house officers (PRHOs). New doctors, general practitioners (especially teachers) and other health professionals will find it useful. As a medical student 30 years ago, I was very keen to meet patients and experience the full range of conditions that I would face as a medical practitioner. I was also aware that my time as an undergraduate was limited. It was therefore important for me to gather a kernel of knowledge, skills and appropriate attitudes that would take me through my final examinations into my house officer years with sufficient substance to allow me to be a good and safe-enough doctor. However, at that time, either in the way that I perceived it or in the way that it was presented to me, general practice seemed to be such a vast and loosely determined discipline as to be too difficult to be used in this process. On the other hand, it also appeared to have all the dimensions and potential that I needed to explore the realms of health, illness and healing to my heart's content. Now, as a teacher and practitioner of general practice, I have been able to revisit the discipline from a new perspective and in a much more productive way.

Over the past 30 years the discipline of general practice has been greatly developed and refined so that departments of general practice are now in the forefront of medical education. The broad base of knowledge and wide range of skills that general practitioners hold and the opportunities that primary care affords in terms of an understanding of health and illness, together with the great organizational advancements that have occurred in primary care, are now widely recognized to offer a rich learning resource for budding clinicians. Undergraduate education, generally, also continues to be in a phase of rapid development. In Britain this is being promoted by the General Medical Council, which has outlined recommendations most recently revised in 2003 in *Tomorrow's doctors*. It sees the development of appropriate attitudes, in relation to both the provision of care of individuals and populations and to the student's personal development, as being as important as the acquisition of knowledge, understanding and skills. It encourages learner-centred, problem-orientated learning systems and the promotion of small-group and self-directed learning. Departments of general practice have been prime movers in these new directions.

This book reflects this development. It is a distillation of what is necessary for a medical student and a PRHO to know and understand about general practice and being a general practitioner. The second edition includes new chapters on healthcare ethics and law, prescribing and preparing to practise. All the original chapters have been updated, some quite substantially. The book is designed to encourage deep learning – a clearly presented and interesting text with a core of important information, and opportunities to reflect and experiment with the ideas in order to integrate and commit them to memory. It is left to your general practice teachers and other specialists to provide the detail with which you can build on what is presented here.

The book ends with two chapters about your intended life as a doctor, included to emphasize the fact that all the clinical knowledge and skills in the world do not, on their own, lead to a healthy and fulfilling life. In the competitive and demanding world of medicine, this can be easily forgotten. It is with this sentiment that I present this book, as well as with the wish that, as lifelong learners, we continue to experience the excitement and compassion that a life in medicine can provide.

Anne Stephenson

ACKNOWLEDGEMENTS

Editing the second edition of this book has again been a good process. My thanks go to the contributors and the publishers for their patience and hard work.

I also acknowledge and value the help the following people gave to me and the contributors in writing this book.

- The undergraduate tutors at what was the King's College School of Medicine and Dentistry and United Medical and Dental School and is now, after merger, the Guy's, King's and St Thomas' School of Medicine. They have, over the years, developed the teaching philosophy and skills that are reflected in this text.
- The students who, through their feedback, encourage us to provide the best learning environment possible.
- The patients who were patient with us when we were student learners and who show us when we are effective and when we are less effective.

In particular I would like to thank:
- Professor Roger Higgs, whose ideas and enthusiasm continue to be an inspiration.
- Doctors Sarah Bruml, Maria Elliot, Brian Fine, Tony Glanville, Helen Graham, Simon Shepherd, Kishor Vasant and Patrick White, senior general practitioners and teachers, who spent time talking with me about teaching experiences, some of which are included in this book.
- Ms Karen Fuchs, who took the photographs, and the medical students, general practice staff and patients who allowed the photographs to be taken.
- The various authors and publishers for permission to reproduce material.

I am grateful to Amadis and Meera for being so generous in their support.

Finally, I dedicate this book to Mum and Dad.

Anne Stephenson, 2004

INTRODUCTION

General practice is an important site for the education and training of medical students. Not only does it offer a large number of training opportunities in which medical knowledge can be applied, basic clinical skills acquired and attitudinal and ethical concerns explored, it also provides a wide variety of learning situations in which sound management decisions can only be made when this knowledge and skill are integrated with the experience and understanding of the practitioner and the patient. This textbook seeks to support and reflect this process.

The information that this textbook provides is largely generic in that it can be applied to all areas of medicine. In fact, general practice is a good teacher of the basic principles without which the more in-depth information provided by other specialisms cannot be understood. Although the book is largely based on the British experience, it is recognized that readers will be drawn from other countries and so the contents are relevant to any medical system.

The learning style of the book is based on experiential and reflective principles, cornerstones of modern educative theory and practice. Most medical teachers are now aware of the 'experiential learning cycle' (Fig. I.1) and use it in their teaching. Students learn by doing: active learning experiences are provided for the student; time is given for reflection on what actually happened. The student is then encouraged to think about and make sense of the experience, identifying principles and generalizations that can be taken forward into new situations and research-presenting topics. Other experiences can then be planned to support and further explore insights around these topics. Although this approach appears obvious, it is not always followed or valued. However, experiential and reflective learning is profound. Students who are encouraged to learn in this way have the potential to understand that every patient encounter is unique and that their education cannot provide definite answers to every question, only ways of approaching patients and clinical situations. In this process, the individual student's experiences and insights are valued and can be developed through self-directed learning, essential for ongoing professional development.

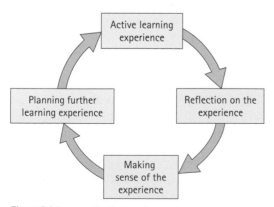

Figure I.1 The experiential learning cycle.

Active learning experience

Reflection on the experience

Making sense of the experience

Planning further learning experience

Tutor quote

I shall tell you about these American students. I think it is about my own hang-up about using certain new words and trying new skills. You have got to try them and this applies to other tutors. This situation was after the course that we attended. The homework was to try to use reflection in your practice when you are teaching. I had these American students who had been with me all day and there were two of them and maybe it was because there were two of them I didn't particularly talk with them. It seemed quite difficult to do and I was sitting in the car with them after the surgery and I wondered whether I should use the word 'reflection' or should I say, 'Can you first remember what happened and then can you

*remember what was in it that you learnt?' ...
something like that. Then I debated that briefly
and then I thought, 'No, let us just throw it in',
and I said, 'Could you reflect on what we did
today?', and that was it, and for the whole
journey there was all this information coming
through. I was amazed at the detail and the
maturity and that that word was enough. There
was no need to dress it up, no need to assume
that they wouldn't understand. We sometimes
do not give them the credit they deserve. So I
think for me what there is to learn is to try
new things, techniques; some might fail, some
might succeed spectacularly and that one was a
very good one. I enjoyed that.*

(It should be noted that the tutor quotes that
appear throughout the book have not been
quoted from the authors of the chapters.)

WAYS OF USING THIS BOOK

For the reasons explained above, this book is a
mixture of textbook and workbook. It is not
necessary to work through the book from the
first to the last page. Rather, we encourage you
to work with the chapters that are relevant to
your course and stage of development and of
interest to you and your tutor. However, as each
chapter works as a unit, it may be of greatest
use to you if you read the chapter as a whole
before you decide how to use it to structure
your learning experiences.

HINTS FOR CONDUCTING
THE EXERCISES

The exercises are of two main types: **thinking
and discussion points** and **practical exercises.**

The thinking and discussion points encourage
you, on your own or with your tutor and colleagues, to reflect on your knowledge and experiences around a particular topic. Examples are:
'What has influenced your views on general
practice?' or 'What questions would you like to
ask a patient before you decide whether or not
to visit them at home?' This type of exercise is
generally used to introduce a topic. It values
your personal insights and past experience as

highly relevant to your understanding of the
topic and to how you might approach further
learning around the topic. The text often gives
you pointers to help you in your thinking.

The practical exercises give you a structure
with which to investigate further a particular
topic. Examples here are: 'A way of evaluating
the effectiveness of a consultation' or 'How to
find out more about a particular medical condition'. These need to be carried out in tandem with
your tutor, and some exercises have extra guidance for your tutor so that they can run more
smoothly. Once again, the text often gives extra
help in what you might get out of the exercise.

CASE STUDIES

Case studies have been included to make the
information more real. All of these are based on
real experiences or an amalgam of real experiences. Where the stories are about people, many
identifying characteristics have been changed
to protect confidentiality.

REFERENCES AND FURTHER
READING

As mentioned previously, the factual content of
the book has been kept to a minimum. The
focus has been placed on you experiencing and
researching relevant clinical areas. To this end,
references and further reading have been placed
at the end of each chapter. We strongly encourage you to spend time capitalizing on your
practical learning by reading around the topics
that have been thrown up by clinical situations.

As with other medical teaching, there are
times when your tutor is unable to take much of
an active role in your learning. You may sometimes feel at a loss to know how to use your
session in general practice most wisely. If this
happens, flick through the book and pick out an
area that interests you. Read through the chapter and the exercises. You may be able to go to
the practice library and research a subject,
interview a member of the practice staff about a
topic that interests you, discuss one of the
thinking points with a colleague, prepare a presentation for your next seminar, or just have a

cup of tea and keep cool until your tutor returns. We hope that this book can be a companion to you in such situations.

This book celebrates the differences and variety in the way that general practitioners (GPs) and general practices work. Thus every chapter, although structured along the same lines, is presented in a slightly different way, dependent on the topic and the writers' approach. Chapters are of different lengths and some are more discursive and philosophical, others more practical and factual. The writers have met frequently and shared their ideas on what each chapter might contain, so we hope that the book appears cohesive and that links between chapters are evident.

The book opens with a chapter on learning in general practice that is a useful starting point for all readers as it outlines the learning opportunities that may be offered in the general practice setting as well as some of the challenges that may present. The work of a GP can only be understood in the context of the wider healthcare system. To be effective, a GP must link closely with other healthcare services in providing care for patients. Chapter 2 provides a brief overview of the primary healthcare system, particularly with reference to Britain, but with some reference to other countries. Chapter 3 introduces the central activity of a GP, the consultation. To have some understanding of what happens when a patient and a doctor meet is essential to an effective outcome. The earlier a student can understand the basic principles behind such professional communications, the easier it will be to develop this most important skill. The information and exercises contained in this chapter can be generalized to any clinical consultation and so have relevance to other medical disciplines.

One of the commonest questions that students ask when they enter general practice is how the presentation of illness differs from that of hospital medicine. Undergraduate medical curricula have often omitted teaching around illnesses that are perceived as not important by virtue of being either minor or self-limiting. However, the bulk of illnesses presenting to the healthcare system are of these types. Chapter 4 describes the common illnesses that people present to general practice, many of which will never need hospital care and yet are important for any doctor to know about. This chapter also gives guidance to students on how to access information on these illnesses. Psychological issues are given a special chapter, Chapter 5, as they are of particular relevance in a general practice setting where knowledge of patients and their inner and outer environment can provide insights into the nature of such presentations. The most frequent practical skills required of a GP and useful for any doctor are described, in detail, in Chapter 6. These descriptions are often missed out of medical texts and should provide a helpful introduction to the supervised practice of these skills. Chapter 7 explores the diagnostic and acute management processes on which a GP's work is based. The topic of prescribing, being that it is such an important area in terms of patient well-being and economic burden, is added as the prescribing chapter, Chapter 8.

Chapter 9 addresses the management of the chronically ill. This essential clinical subject is often not specifically addressed in a medical course and yet it is a major component of every doctor's work. It may be seen as not as exciting or as fulfilling as areas of acute medicine, and the mention of long-term illness may even lead to a feeling of hopelessness or failure on the part of the clinician. However, chronic illness has a profound effect on the lives of patients and their families. Structured care in such situations is now being seen to provide great advantage, and general practice is at the forefront of these developments. Treating people at home can provide unique insights into their illness and treatment. This kind of experience can be of great benefit to patient and clinician. General practice can provide such opportunities and Chapter 10 gives an introduction to how a medical student can best benefit from such an experience. Health promotion in general practice is discussed in Chapter 11. This is an area of clinical work – logically more important than treating illness once it has occurred – often cited as important by medical teachers and yet very often, in practice, ignored or approached badly with poor outcomes. This completely revised chapter explores some of the reasons why this is a challenging area as well as presenting some possible positive approaches. Chapter 12, 'Healthcare ethics and law', is a new chapter, included because the 'broader questions about what is best for patients or staff, what it is right to do, or whether we are acting within the law commonly arise in practice for anyone who reflects on their work'. This chapter suggests ways of approaching these issues and reaching conclusions that are satisfactory for all concerned.

Medical knowledge is increasing at a rapid rate and, looking from the outside, it must sometimes seem to medical students that the task of becoming a competent doctor in a few short years is impossible. Where does one begin? We hope, in this textbook, not to alarm you further. We have deliberately kept facts to a minimum and concentrated on important principles rather than dazzle you (or frighten you) with detail. Actually, you *will* get there, and much more easily if you start with the basics, fully understand them and have carefully structured experiences on which to hang them. But how do we keep up with research evidence and relating this to improvements in patient care? Chapter 13 examines ways in which you can cope with change and the acquisition of relevant knowledge and skills. The business side of medicine has long been seen as perhaps necessary but not relevant to a medical student's education.

With the recent increase in the complexity of health service delivery, a working knowledge of medical management is no longer an option but an essential part of every medical student's training. Chapter 14 provides an introduction to this subject using 'the general practice' as a manageable unit with which to explore this area. Chapter 15, 'Preparing to practise', is a new chapter aimed at the later years of a medical student's progression to a pre-registration house officer. Nine learning objectives around clinical reasoning, written communication skills, teamwork, organizational skills, uncertainty and personal limitation, constructive criticism, professional conduct and lifelong learning explore areas of professional development that are essential for the safety of a new doctor.

Finally, whether or not you are an aspiring GP, Chapter 16 talks about the life of a GP to remind us that a personal and a professional life are inextricably intertwined and to concentrate on one without regard for the other will only lead to discontent. Whatever branch of medicine you enter, we hope that, by reading this chapter, you will be encouraged to consider how you live your life so that you experience fulfilment both professionally and personally.

A glossary has been added at the end of the book to help with the definitions of terms common to the work of GPs.

LEARNING IN GENERAL PRACTICE: WHY AND HOW?

The structure, culture, atmosphere and pace of general practice are different from those of other healthcare settings. General practice provides an opportunity to learn new things and to compare different approaches to health care. This chapter will help you to plan how to get the most out of general practice.

LEARNING OBJECTIVES

By the end of this chapter, you will be able to:

- identify what can best, or only, be learnt in general practice;
- compare the hospital and general practice settings from the perspective of doctors, patients and students;
- plan ways of learning effectively in general practice.

INTRODUCTION

Students often have preconceptions about what they are going to learn in general practice. The following expectations were expressed by students preparing for their attachments.

Student quotes

It will be nice to see a broader spectrum of the community – in hospital it's mostly older people. I'm looking forward to seeing children and babies.

Seeing a wide spectrum of people and problems, not knowing what sort of problem is going to present next. Being able to use all your medical knowledge.

Improving my interviewing and diagnostic skills.

Experience to observe some more 'social skills', e.g. breaking bad or unwelcome news.

Seeing what a GP's life is like. Good to check out career options.

Others commented on aspects of the learning process they thought they would enjoy.

Student quotes

It will be good to have a bit of independence rather than six or so students stood around one patient and being questioned.

Patients may actually like to talk to us. In hospital they get a bit sick of seeing students.

Being involved at a more personal level with the patients, e.g. many GPs seem to know their patients and families very well and the GP is someone seen as a friend too.

Students can also have concerns about learning in general practice. The following are some of the common concerns.

Student quotes

I might get a GP who's not keen on teaching and just leaves you sitting there.

Dealing with ailments that are mundane and medically uninspiring.

Feeling isolated or not liking the GP with whom I am spending my time.

The fact that the problem presenting can be almost anything – how do you come to a diagnosis in such a short amount of time?

I am worried about the level of knowledge that is required and the degree of autonomy given.

Difficulty in getting to the place as I don't have any transport.

To address these points, we include below a list of frequently asked questions.

Frequently asked questions about learning in general practice

Why learn in general practice?

In recent years, major components of health care have been transferred out of the hospital and are now only found in the community. For example, community rehabilitation has increased enormously as patients often leave hospital shortly after their operations or treatment. Chronic or long-term diseases such as hypertension, asthma and diabetes are managed primarily in the community, as is much terminal care. Hospitals are offering increasingly specialized care, and patients are often only in hospital during particular, critical stages of their illness. Without community experience, students would see little of many common conditions and snapshots of disease and treatment rather than natural progression and long-term management. General practice also provides a good context for learning particular skills and aspects of medicine (see 'What will I learn in general practice?').

Is general practice relevant for those going into hospital careers?

About 50 per cent of UK medical graduates enter general practice. Some decide early that they

want to take this option; others plan a career in hospital medicine but find, for various reasons, that they switch to general practice at a later stage. Before deciding on a career path, it is important to explore all the options, and general practice attachments will give insight into this branch of medicine.

Whatever your choice of specialty, it will be important that you have a good understanding of all the services available in primary care and how to access them. Without a detailed knowledge of what is available within your area, you will not be able to refer patients appropriately, and thus provide the best care for them.

How will it help when I start work?

It is becoming increasingly common to include a block of general practice experience in the pre-registration year. Studies of general practice teaching suggest that it promotes a patient-centred approach to medicine which will be useful in hospital medicine too. It should help doctors to acquire knowledge of primary and community services, enabling patients to be discharged effectively and receive the appropriate care in the community, and should reduce unnecessary readmission.

How will it help to pass exams?

This depends on individual medical schools and the nature of their assessments. General practice provides the opportunity to experience a lot of common illnesses. These will be central to the core curricula which most medical schools have developed and assess. In addition, general practice commonly provides one-to-one or very small group teaching, which allows for the possibility of teaching tailored to particular learning needs. Thus it is a good opportunity to ask for help and experience in the areas you find most difficult. It is also a good environment in which to get supervised practice of the sort of clinical skills that are tested in Objective Structured Clinical Examinations (OSCEs) and other clinical examinations.

What will I learn in general practice?

Key areas for learning in general practice include the following.

1. The range of statutory and voluntary services which contribute to health and well-being, and how to access them:
   - the structure, functioning and funding of community health and social services,
   - when, how and to whom to refer patients, and who can refer to whom,
   - understanding of what voluntary sector services offer patients and how this contributes to health.
2. The effects of beliefs and lifestyle factors on health:
   - how patients' beliefs, understanding and attitudes towards health affect their use of services, e.g. why people don't take medication, the impact of religious and cultural beliefs, attitudes towards complementary therapies,
   - how to involve patients in decision making, e.g. healthy lifestyle choices,
   - health promotion and disease prevention skills and strategies.
3. Environmental, social and psychological factors affecting health:
   - reasons for the differential morbidity and mortality rates in different geographical areas,
   - causes of health inequalities between different groups of people, e.g. reasons for differential rates of mental illness diagnoses among different cultural/gender groups,
   - learning to recognize and explore the impact of psychological as well as physical causes of illness, e.g. social isolation, stress in the workplace, unemployment and family dynamics.
4. The management of common conditions:
   - diagnosis and ongoing management of common conditions, e.g. depression, hypertension, diabetes,
   - detecting and preventing long-term complications,
   - experience of the progression of illness and its impact on the lives of patients and their families,
   - the differing roles of the general practitioner (GP) and other members of the practice team, hospital team and social services,
   - practical ways of supporting patients and carers,
   - ongoing monitoring and screening of patients.
5. Specific skills:
   - the skills required to distinguish between serious and non-serious conditions, e.g. whether a depressed patient is at risk of suicide or self-harm, whether a methadone patient is at risk of relapse, monitoring a pregnancy for signs of risk such as pre-eclampsia, deciding whether a rash on a child is due to measles, meningitis or an allergy,
   - practical skills, such as measuring blood pressure, giving an injection, examining an ear and immunization regimes.
6. A different model of healthcare practice:
   - a different approach to patients and their healthcare needs,
   - a different model of inter-professional working,
   - a different organizational structure,
   - learning to function in a primary care team.

Below, students describe some of the things they have learned in general practice.

> ### Student quotes
>
> *You got more of a view of the whole patient – the GP tends to know the whole family.*
>
> *You learn to rely less on investigations.*
>
> *They let you go and clerk and examine and they come in and you present, and that was excellent because it gets your clerking and examining skills up to scratch and it's a different type of clerking than in the hospital. It's got to be done in about a minute or two. It makes you learn hopefully to home-in on something. You learn to sort what is most important.*
>
> *Dealing with a wide variety of cases and a wide range of patient groups.*

In general then, we suggest that general practice is the best place to learn about:
- the range of primary care services and how to access them,
- the effects of patient beliefs and lifestyle factors on health,

- environmental, social and psychological factors affecting health,
- the management of common conditions,
- the skills required to distinguish between serious and non-serious conditions.

Why can't I stick to 'real' medicine?

By *real* medicine, students usually mean patients with good signs and symptoms, with an acute illness that can be cured by the doctor, often by some 'high-tech' intervention. In fact, only a tiny proportion of health care actually takes place in the hospital, and teaching hospitals in particular are very specialized, often taking very rare cases. Despite advances in technology and treatment, many conditions cannot be *cured*, and the doctor's role is often one of providing long-term *care*, support and symptomatic relief. Spending time in general practice provides a more realistic picture of the health care required to manage conditions with high mortality and morbidity rates. It is also a myth that there is no acute medicine in general practice. For example, most heart attacks and acute psychiatric crises occur outside the hospital.

Traditionally, medical education was based almost exclusively in hospitals. This is changing to reflect current patterns of care, and to provide a better balance of experience.

What will I do in general practice?

General practice attachments at different stages of the medical course may be designed to fulfil different purposes, for example learning about general practice as a potential career, learning specific skills, accessing a wide range of patients or facilitating the long-term follow-up of an individual patient or family. The purpose of the attachment will dictate to a large extent whether you spend your time observing practice, practising skills, interviewing patients, collecting information for a project (e.g. audit data) or doing other activities.

The quotes below reflect the variety of learning a student may experience at different times within the medical course in general practice.

Student quotes

It was good for learning a lot of specific procedures like taking blood pressure, looking in ears and eyes, giving injections.

You can see how the team work, how they interact. It gives you more understanding of their role and what actually the patients go through. You get time with the practice nurse, with the administrator of the GP practice and with the receptionist. You see what a hard time they have because often the patients, if they're in a bad mood, don't complain to the doctor, they complain to the receptionist, and it's good to know that and perhaps know how to save your receptionist some grief.

I saw a suspected case of meningitis, and I'm not sure if it was or not, but that was interesting.

The best thing was going to visit patients in their own homes. Patients behave differently in their own homes than in surgery.

I saw a patient at home with classic signs of asthma attack.

How can I make the most of my time in general practice?

In most jobs, you become more proficient with experience. Many students enjoy learning in general practice because they get more direct supervision (often one-to-one teaching), which can be more closely tailored to their individual learning requirements.

Students in general practice have to accept the limitations of the clinical environment, and recognize that their learning cannot always be a priority. For example, teachers may be called away at short notice or there may be no diabetic patients available on the day students plan to examine or interview them. Students have to find ways to gain the experience they need within the existing structures. This section looks at what you can do to make the most of your time in general practice and to cope with any problems that may arise.

SUGGESTED PREPARATION/EARLY ORIENTATION

Before the placement starts, you will need to consider practical issues such as transport, access, security and personal safety, particularly if you are on an individual placement. There are many resources on which you can draw within a general practice. At the start of your attachment, we suggest that you undertake the following.

- *Introductions.* Introduce yourself to everyone for courtesy and security reasons, and so that you can return when you need help. Remember to include part-time and non-clinical staff, such as visiting or associated counsellors, health visitors, midwives, hospital consultants providing outreach clinics, child psychologists, complementary therapists, behavioural therapists, community pharmacists or community psychiatric nurses.

- *Staff in the practice.* Find out what their roles and responsibilities are, when they work and what training and experience they have.

- *Patient notes.* Find out where these are stored, in what format (paper or electronic) and how to access specific sorts of information. Remember to consider issues of confidentiality. Check whether the practice has guidelines on this.

- *Patients.* There are opportunities for meeting patients outside the actual consultation, e.g. in the waiting room, patients coming in to collect prescriptions, make appointments or see other members of the practice team. Be careful not to upset the appointments system, so make sure that the relevant staff know what you are doing, where you will be and how long it will take. Some practices may have a spare room. Remember to consider issues of confidentiality, informed consent and privacy.

- *Relatives and friends.* A patient's relative or friend may also provide useful opportunities for finding out about the impact of illness, use of services, etc.

- *Clinics and other activities.* Find out what else happens in your general practice and when. For example, there may be special health promotion or disease-related clinics, meetings of patients' or carers' support groups, staff meetings or voluntary groups which you can ask to attend.

- *Other resources.* Find out what other resources are available. These may include health education leaflets for patients, clinical books and journals for staff, videos or computer programs and postgraduate learning events.

TEN TIPS FOR LEARNING IN GENERAL PRACTICE

In general practice, as in many other situations, how people present and conduct themselves will affect how they are treated. Below are listed ten tips for having a successful attachment in general practice; these have been devised by teachers and students. Most will also be applicable in other clinical settings.

1. *Attend.* There is, unsurprisingly, a high correlation between students who attend regularly and those who do well in finals and other exams.

2. *Set yourself clear and realistic goals.* Try to identify some specific objectives for your time in general practice, and keep these under review. Mark off items you have achieved and add new ideas as you go along. Let your tutor know what you want to achieve.

3. *Clarify at the beginning what you should have achieved by the end.* This needs to be done in consultation with your GP and the medical school.

4. *Say hello to everyone every day.* This may sound silly, but a little goodwill goes a long way and will help you to fit in. Also think about how you present yourself, e.g. dressing in a way that patients and GPs will find acceptable.

5. *Ask questions.* Teachers often say that they wish students would ask more questions as it helps them to teach at the right level. It also shows that you are interested and enthusiastic.

6. *Ask for teaching, supervision and feedback.* In the rush to get things done, teachers may overlook opportunities for you to practise skills or learn about something new. If you see such opportunities, ask if you can gain experience and then ask for feedback on how you did.

7. *Choose your timing and don't react personally.* Most people are willing to help and will often go out of their way to do so. However,

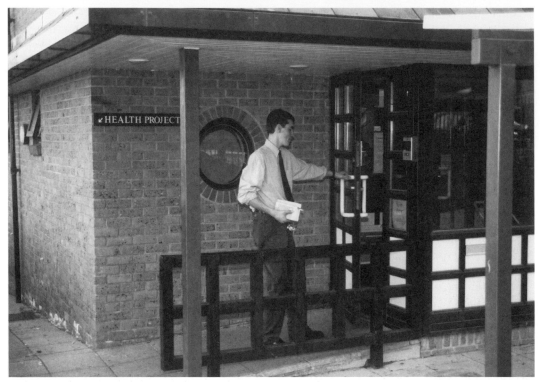

Figure 1.1 The student's first day: making an entrance.

certain times are better than others. Don't ask for things when people are obviously rushed off their feet. Try to help out wherever possible. If someone appears unhelpful, it may be because they are under stress, so don't take it personally. Choose your timing and, if there is someone who always seems busy, ask when would be the best time for you to talk to them.

8. *Recognize the potential of those around you to teach.* The GP is an obvious source of help, but many other people have expertise which may not be immediately obvious. Look on everyone you meet in the practice as a potential teacher. Receptionists, for example, may be skilled in communicating with angry patients. Patients and their relatives may be enormously knowledgeable about their particular conditions and the local services available.

9. *Thank people when they devote their time to teaching you.*

10. *See the wood and the trees.* During your time in general practice, you will probably meet many patients and hear lots of individual stories. Whilst it is important to see and respect each person as an individual, you also need to try to relate back to more general principles and concepts you have learnt in other parts of the course. Try to think about how the basic science, sociology, psychology, communication, public health medicine, ethics and law etc. which you have covered apply to each patient you meet. Base your reading on the patients you have seen.

COMMON PROBLEMS AND DILEMMAS FOR STUDENTS IN GENERAL PRACTICE

General practices vary greatly, for example in size, style, provision, ethos and staffing. There is probably no such thing as a 'typical' general practice. Equally, undergraduate courses vary in terms of the amount of time you will spend in general practice, what you are expected to learn, who teaches you and how well it integrates with the rest of your studies.

In this section we look at some difficulties encountered by students in general practice and how you could deal with them if they happened to you.

Student quote

The patient refused to see me so I had to leave.

In general practice, patients often feel able to say 'no' to things which they might not in hospital. Don't take it personally. Make sure your GP knows if you need experience in a particular area so that s/he can try to identify another opportunity.

Student quote

The worst thing was meeting angry patients. One patient was really annoyed by my presence out of no reason.

Some patients may feel inhibited or embarrassed or unwilling to have a student present, particularly for personal worries or intimate examinations. You should think carefully about issues of access and informed consent in both contexts.

Student quote

It was the same patients every time with trivial complaints, much less exciting than in hospital.

Learning to distinguish the genuinely trivial from early signs of something more serious is an important skill to develop, as described above. Is a headache a sign of stress, period pains, or an incipient brain tumour? Sometimes patients present with a seemingly trivial symptom as a cover for something that is really worrying them.

Student quote

The GP couldn't be bothered. I just had to sit in the corner and listen.

In these situations, it is a good idea to have some activities in mind which you

can use to fill this time. Observation can be a useful way to learn, but sometimes you need to be more actively involved. Throughout this book there are various exercises that you could use in this way, or you may think of your own. However, your tutor should also guide and facilitate your learning. If you are not satisfied, you should first make an attempt to improve things for yourself. For example you could:

- ask questions of the GP following the consultations,
- tell your GP that you're not clear what you should be getting out of the sessions and ask for clarification,
- ask the GP how s/he feels you are getting on,
- tell the GP you're worried that you're not learning enough and ask if s/he can suggest what you should do,
- ask if you can clerk and present some patients to your GP,
- ask if you could gain some practical experience as you feel you learn better that way,
- read up about certain areas the previous evening and then look out for these in the consultations,
- approach another member of the practice team and ask for help.

If you have made efforts to improve the situation and are still feeling unhappy, you should probably now approach the course organizer for help. You are entitled to expect a certain minimum standard of teaching from your GP.

Student quote

You didn't know if another student's GP was better and you were missing out.

General practices, like hospital clerkships, vary in their quality and student-friendliness. You need to do your best to fit in and try to make the placement work. However, if you feel that your teaching is really sub-standard, you should discuss this with someone in the medical school.

SUMMARY POINTS

To conclude, the most important messages of this chapter are as follows.

- General practice provides an opportunity to see a large volume of undifferentiated patient problems, which will give you a realistic picture of illness patterns and allow you to develop your diagnostic and 'sifting' skills. About half of medical students eventually practise as a GP.
- General practice provides the best opportunity to see the progression and management of disease, to study common illnesses and to practise many clinical skills. It provides insight into environmental, social and psychological factors which contribute to ill-health, and represents a different model of care from that of hospital medicine.
- Students can take steps to make their time in general practice productive.

2

GENERAL PRACTICE AND ITS PLACE IN PRIMARY HEALTH CARE

The work of the general practitioner and the general practice team takes place within the context of the primary healthcare setting. To make sense of general practice, the student needs to understand something of its relationship to the primary healthcare system. The central figure in regard to care within the system must be the patient.

LEARNING OBJECTIVES

By the end of this chapter, you will be able to:

■ define primary health care and list what it is broadly aiming to achieve;

■ name a few of the principal members of the primary healthcare team and briefly describe their roles and training;

■ place general practice in the context of the primary care service;

■ describe the role of the general practitioner in the functioning of general practice;

■ list the kinds of things that a patient requires of general practice and the primary care service in order to receive most benefit from it;

■ consider the possible future of general practice and primary care.

WHAT IS PRIMARY HEALTH CARE AND WHAT IS IT AIMING TO ACHIEVE?

Primary health care – that which provides health care in the first instance – is present in one form or another for all peoples in the world. Whether it be for someone who needs antenatal care, an immunization, a dressing for a minor injury, a blood pressure check or an immediate assessment and referral for suspected appendicitis, primary care systems are an essential part of any health service. In some countries primary healthcare systems look after the great majority of most people's health issues. In other, more affluent, countries, secondary and tertiary services play a larger part in the delivery of health care. However, it is widely recognized that a substantial and effective primary healthcare service is the cornerstone of a healthy population and that, without this, the provision of health care is an expensive and ineffectual exercise.

Thinking and Discussion Point

Think about experiences that you or someone else you know has had when obtaining health care in situations other than in general practice or hospitals. List the places in which this care was received.

WHAT IS THE DEFINITION OF PRIMARY CARE?

It is not something that is done in one place or by one type of health professional. It is a network of community-based healthcare services, supported by a network of social services that provides over 90 per cent of health care in the UK (Fry, 1993). In its most restricted sense, it means 'first contact care' and this can be provided by any number of different healthcare workers. However, primary health services have a much wider role than this. Their role includes health maintenance, illness prevention, diagnosis, treatment and management of acute and chronic illness, rehabilitation, the support of those who are frail or disabled, pastoral care and terminal care.

Thinking and Discussion Point

Carrying on from the previous thinking and discussion point, select one situation that you remember well.
❑ Why does this event stick in your memory?
❑ What were the factors that made this either a positive or a negative experience for you?
❑ How specific or general is this experience?

Extend your thinking and list some of the attributes that a primary healthcare service should have in order to make it most acceptable to patients and professionals. What attributes should it have in order to make the most of limited resources?

WHAT IS PRIMARY HEALTH CARE AIMING TO ACHIEVE?

There are four main objectives of a primary healthcare service (Marson et al., 1973).
1. It must be *accessible* to the whole population.
2. It must be *acceptable* to the population.
3. It must be able to *identify* the health needs of a population.
4. It must make the most *cost-effective* use of its resources.

Obviously, given that resources are limited, all these objectives cannot be perfectly met. However, these are goals that we can aim towards.

People need to be able to see their doctor (or another health professional) when necessary without having to wait unduly for an appointment. The distance between the patient's home and the healthcare centre should be as small as possible. Where the patient has difficulty in getting to the healthcare centre, a home-visiting service should be provided. All efforts should be made to enable the patient and professional staff to communicate effectively.

In terms of acceptability, regular reviews of services must include a measure of patient and professional satisfaction. The rights and responsibilities of both patient and health professional need to be considered and made clear to both parties. This process is a constant and developing one.

In setting up mechanisms to identify a population's health needs, we get away from just responding to demand to a position where we can start properly to distinguish priorities in the services we provide. Strategic planning based on need rather than demand will make the best use of limited resources.

Given that we (as provider and user) have decided on the minimum standards we wish to uphold and the priorities for service provision and development, we then need to determine the resources that are available for health care and decide how to apportion them. To provide all desirable services would be impossible, so judgements need to be made as to the most cost-effective use of limited person-power, money and effort. This kind of decision is bound to be made partly on guesswork, as it is rare that all the information required to make such decisions is available.

WHO ARE THE PRINCIPAL MEMBERS OF THE PRIMARY HEALTHCARE TEAM?

In the UK National Health Service (NHS), there are two main providers of primary care, *general practice* and *community health services.* Other providers, such as accident and emergency departments, dentists, pharmacists, opticians and optometrists, will not be mentioned here. In addition, UK NHS Direct, which opened in 1998, offers 24-hour advice about personal health care, and NHS walk-in-centres, the first of which opened in 2000, offer free health advice and treatment for minor injuries and illnesses and are open and available for anyone.

General practice (family practice) provides first contact, patient-centred, comprehensive and continuing care to a patient population. The general practice tasks are to promote health and well-being and to treat illness in the context of the patient's life, belief systems and community and work with other healthcare professionals to co-ordinate care and make efficient use of health resources. It has responsibility for a population of people and is activated by patient choice.

Community health services are provided by a variety of generalist and specialist staff who have particular functions, such as the multidisciplinary care of the long-term ill, continuing care for those discharged from hospital, services for well people (including school health, child health and sexual health/family planning), care for particular groups of the population at risk (for example the homeless, refugees) and the provision of such things as training or equipment on a wide scale. They also provide support to general practices with all these activities, as well as providing staff such as health visitors, district nurses, community midwives and community psychiatric nurses who work with general practices.

PRINCIPAL MEMBERS: WHO THEY ARE AND WHAT THEY DO

Members of the primary healthcare team are many and various (Fig. 2.1). Table 2.1 lists some of the more well-known UK professionals, particularly those who work with general

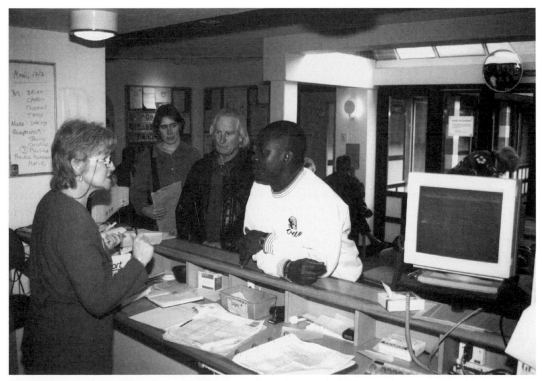

Figure 2.1 The practice receptionist at work: 'Would you mind seeing a student...?'

Table 2.1 A selection of the members of the UK general practice team

Name	Employed by	Role includes	Training
Receptionist	General practice	Reception and telephone duties, filing	Various
Practice manager	General practice	Planning, organizing, managing a general practice	Various
Practice nurse	General practice	Assessment, diagnosis, treatments, health promotion, special extended roles	Registered General Nurse (RGN), nursing experience
District nurse	Primary care trust	Assessment, dressings, stoma care, arranging services, support	RGN, nursing experience, specialist training
Health visitor	Primary care trust	Antenatal, 'under 5' care, sometimes elderly care	RGN, nursing experience, specialist training
Community psychiatric nurse	Primary care trust	Assessment, management, support of the mentally ill	RGN, nursing experience, specialist training

practice. The role of the general practitioner (GP) is discussed later in this chapter.

BOUNDARIES

In the UK, as in many other countries, increased importance (and thus resource) is being placed on the primary care sector of the health service. With this has come the realization that we must become much clearer about the responsibilities of each of its professional groups. Within the primary care service there are many health professions, often with very different ways of working. Their connection with secondary health services may also become troublesome if communication is not very clear. A 'seamless service' is a concept often mentioned, but we are in danger of ever-increasing fragmentation if we do not *respect and know about each other's skills*, and *work together in developing and delivering services*.

CASE STUDY 2.1

Mrs C, an 89-year-old woman, lives with her **daughter**. She wakes one morning and finds herself unable to talk properly or move her right arm. Her daughter, on finding her like this, rings their general practice and speaks to the **receptionist**, who arranges for their GP to visit. The GP visits and finds Mrs C peaceful and adamant that she does not want to be hospitalized. The daughter agrees with this and is willing, with support, to care for her mother at home.

The GP contacts the **district nurse** for an assessment of the nursing needs.

Many situations like this occur in general practice and require the co-operation of patients, their informal carers and several members of the healthcare team.

CASE STUDY 2.2

Ms F, a 28-year-old woman on medication for schizophrenia, presents to her **GP** pregnant. She wishes to keep the baby. With the woman's consent, the GP contacts her **psychiatrist** and **community psychiatric team**, who make arrangements to see her, check her medication and arrange for close follow-up. The GP also makes an appointment for her with the **hospital antenatal services**. The woman offers to come back and see the GP the next week with her **partner**, the father of the baby, to talk about the pregnancy further.

Sometimes, the kind of care required can be very resource intensive. What do you think enabled this woman to obtain such integrated care so quickly and efficiently?

HOW DO GENERAL PRACTICE AND THE GENERAL PRACTITIONER CONTRIBUTE TO PRIMARY HEALTH CARE?

Traditionally, general practice, with its central figure, the GP, and its central activity, the consultation, has been the cornerstone of primary health care. Historically, this has developed from 'the doctor working alone' to 'the practice as an organization'. As this model of health care has been widened to include consideration of such things as population-based health promotion (as well as diagnosis and treatment) and care of populations (as well as individuals), the role of general practice has changed and that of the GP has become less clear. (See more in Chapter 16, 'Being a general practitioner'.)

Thinking and Discussion Point

❏ What do you see your GP doing?
❏ What connections does he or she make?
❏ What do you see as the advantages and disadvantages of your GP's role?

CORE VALUES OF GPs

The majority of GPs would see their central activity as the consultation in which doctor and patient meet and work together to make decisions regarding the patient's health and life plan (see Chapter 3). However, with the mounting complexity of health service provision, this role is increasingly in conflict with other administrative and population-based responsibilities. The same can be said of the role of other primary care practitioners, for example the practice nurse, the speech therapist or the audiologist.

Practical Exercise

Spend 10 minutes discussing with your GP tutor what areas of his or her work are most important and/or satisfying. Pick the top three and list them in order of priority.

CORE VALUES OF THE PRACTICE

The major responsibility of the general practice, on the other hand, is to its practice population as a whole, ensuring that its patient population obtains the best service possible and that the general practice is organized and managed to meet this responsibility (see Chapter 14).

Practical Exercise

Spend 10 minutes discussing with the practice manager what areas of his or her work are most important. Pick the top three and list them in order of priority.

IS PERSONAL CARE COMPATIBLE WITH TEAMWORK?

As GPs have traditionally been the leaders in their general practices, the new and more time-consuming responsibilities of running a practice have often resulted in confusion and dissatisfaction amongst GPs and other practice staff. Is the traditional role of a GP compatible with the more population-based role of 'new' general practice? Increasingly, other professionals, such as practice managers, are being brought in to complement the GP's work and deal with areas of work not directly connected with the consultation (see Chapter 14).

POWER, ETHICS, ACCOUNTABILITY

Difficulties in working relationships may arise because of the differences in power structures, ethical considerations and accountability between the practitioner and the practice. Practitioners usually see their major responsibility as being 'their' patients and, in theory at least, aim to empower patients as much as possible. They are mainly accountable to their patients and to their peers. The practice, on the other hand, is mainly responsible for the practice population and may need to have 'power over' the decisions of a few to benefit the whole. Accountability for the practice is to the practice population and, in Britain, nationally to the Secretary of State for Health for General Medical Services (GMS) practices and locally to the Primary Health Care Trusts for Personal Medical Services (PMS) practices. (See more about these arrangements in Chapters 14 and 16.)

Practical Exercise

It is a busy surgery on a Monday morning. A patient is demanding that the GP sees him immediately. The receptionist is very rushed and is hurriedly explaining that there are no appointments free for that morning but that she will speak with the doctor about seeing the patient urgently. The doctor, at that moment, comes into the waiting area and, without referring to the receptionist, warmly welcomes the patient and ushers him in to her consulting room.

❏ What do you think led the GP to this action?

❏ How do you think the receptionist felt as a result of this action?

❏ What measures could be taken to ensure that the receptionist and doctor support each other's work?

HOW DO WE ENSURE THAT THE PATIENT RECEIVES MOST BENEFIT FROM GENERAL PRACTICE AND THE PRIMARY HEALTHCARE SERVICE?

'PATIENTS AS EXPERTS'

Thinking and Discussion Point

❏ As a patient, what qualities do you most require of your GP?

❏ As a student doctor, what qualities do you most require of a patient?

For a consultation to work, doctors and patients need to see themselves as experts in their own right, meeting to share ideas and come to an understanding of what is happening and what needs to be done in a particular situation (more on this in Chapter 3). The patient comes to a consultation with knowledge of the nature of the presenting issue and the historical and psychosocial context in which it is embedded. The patient also has the power to decide, ultimately, what the outcome will be. The doctor, on the other hand, has access to specialist biomedical information and to services. Without a sharing of these pieces of information, the course of action that is best for the patient, and most cost effective, may not be followed.

THE IMPORTANCE OF COMMUNICATION

CASE STUDY 2.3

Mr S, a 69-year-old man, has been taken to hospital by ambulance, very frightened, after suffering a sudden attack of light-headedness. This clears before the doctor has seen him, enabling him to be sent home. He is later told that this symptom is a side effect of the anti-hypertensive drug on which he has recently been started. Once he knows this, he deals effectively with the symptom, which, after a little time, becomes much less of a problem.

An explanation of the possible side effects of his medication on initiation of treatment would have prevented unnecessary distress and an expensive trip to hospital for this man.

WHAT PATIENTS CAN TEACH PRACTITIONERS

It is important for doctors and students to listen and learn from patients and to understand illness as a human experience rather than just a cluster of symptoms and signs.

CASE STUDY 2.4

Mr G, an 84-year-old widower who lived alone, had mild non-insulin-dependent diabetes mellitus. His GP was constantly frustrated by the man's refusal to monitor his urine or adjust his diet. One day Mr G asked the GP to visit him at home. He spoke with the GP about his life and the few pleasures left to him, of which sweets and biscuits were one. The GP was able to see that the problem was her inability to accept the more limited but possible and reasonable goals of the patient.

CONSULTING THE PATIENT

An encouraging sign in the development of primary care services has been the inclusion of 'patients' in the development process. User and community participation at all levels of practice development has led to the setting up of patient-participation groups and dialogue between service providers and 'users'; self-help and community groups which provide information and support for those with particular conditions or in particular situations; and the Commission for Patient and Public Involvement in Health (CPPIH), set up in 2003 and sponsored by the Department of Health, replacing community health councils.

WHAT IS THE FUTURE FOR GENERAL PRACTICE AND PRIMARY HEALTH CARE?

THE BRITISH SITUATION

In Britain, since the beginning of the 1990s, the pace of primary care development has been extremely rapid and, since April 1996, the development of the NHS has been *led* by primary care. The central place of general practice in the provision of primary healthcare services has not been challenged. However, there has been an increasing reliance on general practice to continue to develop and provide free and equal access to health care in the face of greater restraints on resources. This has placed an enormous strain on general practice providers. In spite of this, a large range of primary care activities and organizations has been developed and introduced to meet the challenges and to support general practice. These have included a move towards integrating health and social services in primary care; primary care-led purchasing; a greater accountability of general practice to the NHS; general practice fund-holding; the development of paperless general practice systems, morbidity databases and audit; the development of general practice management; the introduction of the nurse practitioner; and experimentation with different types of integrated community care centres.

THE INTERNATIONAL SITUATION

It appears that primary care, internationally, is being increasingly recognized as central to a good health service and as needing to be supported by secondary and tertiary services rather than being dominated by them. The WHO–UNICEF meeting in Alma-Ata in 1978 (World Health Organization, 1978) underlined this principle, and the Alma-Ata declaration, in which many countries, including Britain, committed themselves to raising the profile of primary care, was an important catalyst in the development of primary care.

The international exchange of ideas in this field has been very active since then, and shared challenges and responses to these challenges are evident. Particular demographic developments are common shared problems internationally, such as an increasingly ageing population; escalating costs of health care, particularly with new technologies; greater restraints on spending; an over-supply and/or a maldistribution of doctors; a devaluing of the primary care generalist and a greater administrative burden on healthcare workers. The WHO 2003 International Conference on Primary Health Care in Alma-Ata, the twenty-fifth anniversary of the 1978 meeting at which the Alma-Ata Declaration was presented, requested member states to continue to work towards providing adequate resources for primary health care; tackling the rising burden of chronic conditions; supporting the active involvement of local communities and voluntary groups in primary health care; and supporting research in order to identify effective methods for strengthening primary health care and linking it to overall improvement of the healthcare system.

Of particular importance is whether or not the role of the primary care practitioner as gatekeeper is supported. In European countries such as Britain or Denmark where this is so, there is generally control of the geographical distribution of doctors, registration of patients, paying of GPs by capitation and salary, and essential 24-hour patient-care coverage. In European countries where the primary care doctor is not a gatekeeper, such as Germany and Sweden, these characteristics commonly do not exist, and the role of the primary care generalist is not as developed or valued. Outside Europe, for example in Canada or Australasia, these grouped correlations are not as evident. In the USA, a useful distinction exists between the gatekeeping role of the practitioner within a health maintenance organization (HMO) and the non-gatekeeping role of the private primary care practitioner. It has been shown that fee-for-service practitioners have a 40 per cent excess of hospital admissions over HMO practitioners. However, the relationship between different systems and quality of care is extremely difficult to measure past very crude parameters such as life expectation. Assessing quality is the present-day task.

SUMMARY POINTS

To conclude, the most important messages of this chapter are:

- a primary healthcare system provides health care in the first instance;
- a primary healthcare system aims to be accessible, acceptable, cost effective and responsive to health needs;
- the GP works as a member of a general practice and of the primary healthcare team that has responsibilities both to the individual and to the community as a whole;
- the patient and the health practitioner need to work together to ensure that health-related decisions are optimal.

REFERENCES

Fry, J. 1993: *General practice. The facts.* Oxford: Radcliffe Medical Press.

Marson, W.S., Morrell, D.C., Watkins, C.J. and Zander, L.J. 1973: Measuring the quality of general practice. *Journal of the Royal College of General Practitioners* 23, 23–31.

World Health Organization 1978: *Primary health care.* Geneva: WHO.

FURTHER READING

Meads, G. (ed.) 1996: *Future options for general practice.* Oxford: Radcliffe Medical Press.

Pratt, J. 1995: *Practitioners and practices – a conflict of values?* Oxford: Radcliffe Medical Press.

The above two books from the Primary Care Development Series, published in association with King's Fund, London, focus on the development of general practice within the British primary healthcare service. The discussions also include the international context.

With the constant development of primary care around the world, the following websites give some of the most up-to-date information:

http://www.nhshistory.com/

http://www.nhs.uk/

http://www.who.int/

The following references are also worth reading.

Mathers, N. and Hodgkin, P. 1989: The gatekeeper and the wizard: a fairy tale. *British Medical Journal* 298, 172–4.

WONCA EUROPE, 2002: *The European definition of general practice/family medicine.* http://www.globalfamilydoctor.com/publications/Euro–Def.pdf

3

THE GENERAL PRACTICE CONSULTATION

The central event in the general practitioner's professional life is the consultation. There are a number of perspectives and frameworks that you can employ to assess the effectiveness of consultations. From observing others' consultations, you can begin to reflect upon how to make your own consultations more effective.

LEARNING OBJECTIVES

By the end of this chapter, you will be able to:

- understand the qualities that set general practice consultations apart from other types of consultation;
- define and view the content and process of a consultation, the roles within it and the doctor-centred and patient-centred approaches to it;
- view, document and reflect upon the patient's and doctor's tasks in the consultation;
- formally stage a consultation by using three given frameworks;
- consider behaviours that help or hinder a consultation;
- consider the narrative approach to the consultation.

THE GENERAL PRACTICE CONSULTATION

About one million general practitioner (GP) consultations take place in the UK each working day. The meeting between a GP and a patient, at which health-related issues are presented and explored and management decisions made, provides the material with which general practice works.

Understanding what happens in a consultation is the key to understanding the role of the GP. To focus on the consultation is a valuable and manageable task from which further exploration of primary care medicine can follow.

The general practice consultation has a set of particular qualities that set it apart from other types of consultation.

■ The patient makes the decision to consult with the GP. This is an important difference from, for example, the hospital-based consultation, in which patient contact is generally initiated by referral from another doctor. Patients in primary care thus come with their own agenda, often unknown by their GPs until presentation. Effective communication between GP and patient is the key to accurate identification and discussion of the pertinent issues. The idea of the patient-centred consultation, in which the practitioner works with the person rather than the illness or the presenting issue, is further explored later in this chapter.

■ The general practice consultation is well situated for what is called 'whole-person medicine'. The GP is often the first and frequently the only medical port-of-call for the patient, who might present for a variety of reasons repeatedly and over a long period of time. The family, friends and community of the patient are also often known by the GP in a similar way. The GP can therefore often understand the patient and the presentation in the context of the fullness of the patient's life. A great understanding of who the patient is and the meaning of the presentations can thus be achieved.

■ GPs and their patients are readily accessible to one another, often over many years. This results in the opportunity for a kind of medicine that allows for a developing professional relationship between patient and doctor and provides for:
  – an extended type of patient and doctor observation, allowing the collection and processing of information over a period of time;
  – an extended type of diagnostic process which can be developed and altered over time and which can incorporate many levels of information, including physical, psychological and social aspects;
  – comprehensive care, which considers the physical, psychological and social needs of patient, family, carers and community;
  – continuing care, which can be initiated by the patient and flexibly adapt to unforeseen as well as foreseen needs;
  – preventive care, where every presentation is an opportunity for health promotion.

■ The general practice consultation is a central activity within the health service, as it is in the main through the GP that the patient gains access to the more specialized and usually more expensive health services. The GP thus has a central role in the proper use and containment of limited health resources.

It is important to recognize these qualities and to realize that to be party to a single consultation and fail to see this in the context of many such consultations over time leads to a limited understanding of the process of general practice.

Thinking and Discussion Point

Consider a type of consultation other than a general practice consultation (e.g. a hospital-based consultation).
❑ What are its particular qualities?
❑ How does it compare with the GP consultation?
❑ What are the perceived strengths and weaknesses of each type of consultation?

As part of your training, especially initially, you will do some 'sitting in' on GP consultations (although we encourage you also to 'sit in the doctor's chair' and interview patients under close supervision as early as possible). It is useful to have some frameworks with which to view and experience this event. In this way, you will become a more active observer and your observations will be of greater value to yourself, your tutor and, ultimately, the patient. Observing and reflecting upon your tutor's consultations will be a good introduction to your own consulting and provide a template for thinking about consultations you observe in other parts of your course.

There have been many frameworks set up for describing a consultation; a few of the major ones are outlined below.

Before we look at some observation frameworks, there are three concepts with which you need to be conversant in order to understand more fully what is going on.

1. The difference between content and process in the consultation.
2. Roles within the consultation.
3. The doctor-centred and the patient-centred approach to the consultation.

THE CONTENT AND PROCESS OF THE CONSULTATION

There is a basic distinction between the tasks that are focused upon in a consultation (the content) and the behaviours that go on in the consultation (the process). Obviously there are certain tasks that are accomplished within a consultation. Examples are defining the reason for the patient's attendance and arriving at a management plan. This is the content of the consultation. However, the way that the consultation is conducted (the process) is also very important and directly determines the effectiveness of the encounter. The process describes the way that the doctor and the patient behave towards each other, verbally and non-verbally.

Let me put it another way. The content and process have parallels in both music and theatre. In music the content would be the score and the process the dynamics. In theatre the content would be the script and the process the

stage directions. You will probably need to observe quite a few consultations and discuss with your tutor these concepts in the context of what happens before you fully understand the difference. Because you will find it useful to understand the concepts of process and content, the following exercise will help you in this task.

Practical Exercise

Sit in on two to four consultations. It would be useful if you could observe in pairs for this particular task so that you can take turns to record either process or content in successive consultations and put your findings together afterwards. Otherwise you will need to concentrate on content for one consultation (or part of a consultation) and process for another. Either way, compare notes with your tutor afterwards. You may wish to report on just part of a consultation, as reporting on the whole may prove to be too big a task. Figure 3.1 is a sample recording sheet and an example to help you in your task.

ROLES WITHIN THE CONSULTATION

Traditionally, society has assigned to doctors and patients certain roles or ways of behaving. Doctors have been given the power, authority

Content	Process
Doctor: Are you sure of your dates?	Patient: Pregnant, little anxious.
Patient: Yes, I am 26 weeks.	Doctor: Busy, but interested; trying to establish how many weeks pregnant the patient is. *(leans forward)*
Doctor: You can't be!	Patient: Very sure of dates.
Patient: Yes I am. Look at the ultrasound report.	Doctor: Querying dates.
Doctor: When was the last one done?	Patient: Slightly interested and tells doctor about ultrasound.
Patient: Today.	Doctor: Relieved, slightly embarrassed. *(sits back)*

Figure 3.1 What happens in a consultation: an example of a recording sheet.

and respect to attend to a patient's needs and make certain decisions on behalf of the patient. The patient has been encouraged to give this responsibility to the doctor and to enter into the 'sick' or 'dependent' role, at least temporarily or partially. The tendency is for doctors and patients to accept these behaviours and expectations and invite them from the other party. These assumptions are increasingly being challenged, with many doctors working towards becoming less autocratic and patients working towards retaining their autonomy. However, it is essential that we, when we are in the doctor role, become aware of these roles and tendencies and, for each patient encounter, determine how much they are in the best interests of patient well-being and when they are detrimental. At times, for example when a patient is very acutely and seriously ill, we may need to assume total responsibility for their care. However, in most situations, seeing the consultation as a meeting of two individuals, each with his or her own areas of expertise, and focusing the consultation on the patient's ideas, concerns and expectations, seems the healthiest option. Of course we are all, at times, patients, so it is also helpful to reflect upon any changes in behaviour that might occur when we are in the patient role and how this impacts on the satisfaction, process and outcome of the consultation.

However, conflicts may arise between doctors' and patients' values and the interests of patients and their partners or families or those of their community or 'the state'. When it is discovered, for example, that a patient is carrying the human immunodeficiency virus (HIV):

- How might this cause a conflict of values for some doctors and patients?
- What does a doctor do if a patient receives a positive HIV test and does not want their spouse to know?
- What is the situation when we have to decide whether to screen and treat a community with high HIV prevalence with expensive retroviral drugs?
- Should patients who are thinking of being tested for HIV be informed of any potential insurance problems?

THE DOCTOR AND PATIENT CENTREDNESS OF THE CONSULTATION

The degree to which a consultation is doctor centred or patient centred is related to the roles that the patient and doctor adopt in their interchange. It is measured by the extent to which the consultation agenda, process and outcome are determined by the doctor or the patient.

Obviously, the doctor has expert knowledge diagnostically and therapeutically. However, patients are also experts in that they bring with them the information and experience with which the consultation primarily works. At times, patients are, in fact, much more knowledgeable about their illness or presenting issue than their doctor, for example when they have a rare medical condition or a condition that requires ongoing self-management. For a consultation to be successful, the doctor and patient must work together to agree on the issues that they are dealing with and to share information about the issues and possible explanations and consequences (Fig. 3.2).

That the patient plays an active role in the consultation and that the patient and doctor have a dialogue and work together to come to a satisfactory conclusion are the aims of a consultation. Of most importance is the idea that the consultation is there to focus on patients and their ideas, concerns and expectations about what is happening to them. This is what is termed a **patient-centred consultation**.

> ### Tutor quote
> *I had a female student here a year ago and I had an unusual experience with her. She was sitting here in this chair and I asked her to interview this guy who was 60, 65 perhaps ... an alcoholic with TB ... very nice quiet man who had not been attending for his treatment. He was always drunk and if you looked at him, you would think what a waste ... you know ... you could see that he was trying to be a nice man but he came over as a bit of a funny sort of chap ... very sad case. I asked this student to take a history and I sat down there. She couldn't keep a straight face ... she was*

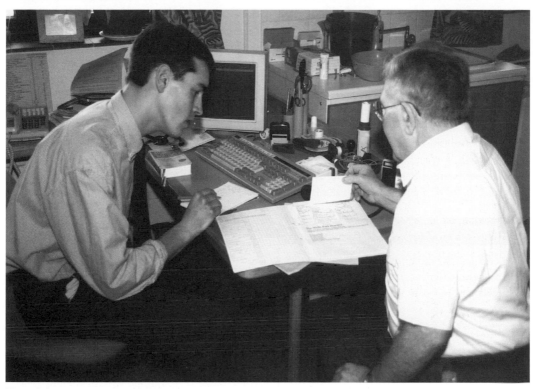

Figure 3.2 The consultation – but who's consulting whom?

actually laughing or smiling ... she couldn't concentrate on what she was asking this man ... it was really uncomfortable for me and for the patient. The patient suddenly stopped and said, 'Look young lady, you are laughing, you shouldn't laugh', and the odd thing was that I could see there was a problem and I couldn't cope with it, yet this man coped with it so well. Honestly it was so awkward. Then she said, 'I am not laughing', and then she became very serious because she realized there was something going on and there was a breakdown. He looked at me so all I could do was take over. I talked to him and I didn't know how I was going to take things forward and then, again, he saved us. He said, 'I am sorry young lady but I had to tell you. Somebody has to tell you. You can't laugh at patients. You have to be serious.' Then he carried on talking to her for a while and they had a conversation.

When he had finished, I mean, I was a bit shaken by the whole thing, I felt very angry, sorry for him. I felt sorry for her but I didn't know how to actually tackle her. So many issues. How do I tell her? Why was she laughing? Did I do that when I was young? That is where it is unresolved in my mind. I actually think she really did learn something from it and I definitely learnt something from it. I thought how graceful the patients are and how wonderful despite being alcoholic and how wise he was, you know, the way he dealt with it. I felt it was brilliant. She didn't really put herself in his shoes. Maybe if I could have told her that every time a patient comes in she needed to try to see if she could put herself in their shoes, she wouldn't actually have that problem, but it was too late.

The consultation in which the doctor interrogates the patient and determines diagnosis and further management without involving the patient in the process is a **doctor-centred consultation**. Most consultations lie somewhere on the continuum between doctor centredness and patient centredness. Research shows that patients do want patient-centred care where doctors take into account 'the patient's desire for information and for sharing decision making and responding appropriately' (Stewart, 2001).

Given this background, and that you now have a basic understanding of the concepts of content, process, roles and patient and doctor centredness within a consultation, let us move on and look at a few of the common ways of viewing, documenting, reflecting upon and learning from the tasks and stages of a particular consultation.

Practical Exercise

Read through the rest of this chapter and pick out the framework that most appeals to you to begin with. Perhaps talk with your tutor before you sit in on a surgery, and discuss how you might like to start to focus on the consultations. Once you have looked at what goes on using one perspective, you might like to try some different ways of looking at the consultation. There may well be others that you discover or that your tutor suggests you explore further.

We will first look at the patient's task in a consultation and compare this with the doctor's task in ensuring that the patient's needs, perceived and real, are met. Remember that, from both the patient's and the GP's perspective, the real and the perceived needs of the patient may not always be the same. From here we will go on to consider a way of looking at a more formal staging of a consultation. The final framework that will be presented combines both the tasks and the formal staging of a consultation.

THE PATIENT'S TASKS IN THE CONSULTATION

Cecil Helman (1981), a medical anthropologist, has suggested that patients come to the doctor to answer six questions.
1. What has happened?
2. Why has it happened?
3. Why to me?
4. Why now?

5. What would happen if nothing were done about it?
6. What should I do about it or whom should I consult for further help?

The patient may not always ask all of these questions in every case. For example, not everyone would consider 'why to me?' and 'why now?' after falling down stairs and spraining their ankle (although they might be useful questions in such cases). Also, some consultations are about health promotion issues, for example pregnancy, contraception, well-man or well-woman care or immunization. However, particularly with more serious or long-term illnesses or when illnesses or accidents happen at inconvenient times, such as just before a wedding or in the midst of an important time of work, they may well be asked. It is important that the doctor is aware that the patient may be considering them, as sometimes they loom large in a patient's mind but may need a bit of sensitive probing by the doctor to bring out into the open. On the other hand, the patient may prefer to discuss such issues with another person such as a close friend or mentor, and the doctor also needs to be sensitive to this option. Here is an example to illustrate the patient's task.

CASE STUDY 3.1

Mrs G, a 56-year-old woman, had come to see her GP 2 weeks earlier with a lump in her right breast which had been present for some time and which had been getting larger and more irregular. She had also noticed some similar, smaller lumps in her right axilla. It was obvious at this time that she was extremely worried, as both her mother and her sister had suffered from breast cancer. She was also just entering into a new and very promising relationship after being divorced 10 years previously, and her life otherwise was flourishing. Her GP referred her, urgently, to a specialist for assessment and it was discovered that she did indeed have breast cancer. Together, the GP and the patient made a long appointment to talk about what all this meant. Indeed, she did wish to talk around all of Helman's six questions. A very moving and intense consultation took place. Not all the questions could be answered by patient or doctor and some of the others could be answered only partially. However, the opportunity to air these most important issues with someone she trusted went a little way towards relieving some of the profound anger and fear that she was experiencing.

This is a rather extreme example, the like of which, I expect, your tutor will not ask you to consider at this stage of your training. However, it illustrates the depth into which consultations, at times, enter. An exercise will be suggested to explore this further, in a simpler way, after the doctor's task in the consultation has been considered.

THE DOCTOR'S TASKS IN THE CONSULTATION

Perhaps the simplest model, used in medical schools for all types of 'medical encounters', is the 'three function' model (Gask and Usherwood, 2002). The three parallel functions are to build the relationship (with the patient), collect data and agree a management plan.

Roger Neighbour (1987), a GP, has looked at the tasks of a consultation purely from a doctor's viewpoint and has listed them as follows.

1. To *connect* with the patient: does this consultation feel comfortable?
2. To *summarize and verbally check* with the patient that the reasons for the attendance are clear: my understanding is ...
3. To *hand over* and bring the consultation to a close, checking out with the patient: does that cover it?
4. To ensure that a *safety net* exists in that no serious possibilities have been missed: what if ...?
5. To deal with the *housekeeping* of recovery and reflection: am I okay to start another consultation?

Case study 3.2 is another example that illustrates this way of looking at a consultation.

CASE STUDY 3.2

Mr D went to see a GP with a 2-week history of lethargy, associated with an extremely sore throat and slight diarrhoea. The GP had not seen him before, although he had been a patient at the surgery for some time. Mr D's usual doctor was on holiday. He was anxious as he told the GP that his partner had similar symptoms that had been tentatively diagnosed as glandular fever. Mr D had also recently started an exciting new job and did not want to have to take time off.

It was important for the GP first to connect in some way with Mr D, as this was a first meeting and the patient was obviously worried about his condition and needed to trust that the GP was competent and had his best interests at heart. The patient talked a little about his new job and the good relationship that he had with the surgery and his usual doctor. The GP told him about other work that he was involved in at the hospital and how much time he spent doing sessions at the surgery. The GP then moved on to Mr D's reasons for coming to see him, first checking that he was clear about the presenting symptoms and anxieties. This checking out continued, at times, throughout the consultation.

As the consultation moved on, the GP discovered that Mr D was concerned about the slight possibility that he might have contracted HIV and they discussed this. Mr D also told the doctor that he and his partner were going through a rocky patch in their relationship. He needed some comforting at this stage. After examining him and discussing what should be done, the GP once again summarized and verbally checked that his understanding matched the patient's understanding about future management.

Throughout the consultation, at times, the GP was mentally checking that no serious possibilities were being missed, such as serious illness not considered or suicide risk. The GP brought the consultation to a close by checking out with Mr D that his concerns had been covered and by arranging to see him again once some initial investigations had been carried out. Finally, the GP took a few minutes out to have a cup of tea, as this consultation had been quite exhausting. He then felt okay to start another consultation.

This sounds rather an ideal consultation and, in reality, few consultations run so smoothly or cover such ground so successfully, especially on a first meeting. However, it serves to illustrate the stages that Roger Neighbour lists in his model of the consultation from the doctor's perspective.

Below is an exercise that you can use to examine how a consultation addresses *the experience of both patient and doctor*. It is composed of a number of stages, which means that your tutor will need to organize things quite carefully beforehand.

Practical Exercise

For this exercise, your tutor will need to organize the following:
❏ 45 minutes of lightly booked surgery;
❏ a space for you to interview patient(s) before and after the consultation(s);
❏ time to discuss the process and the consultation(s) with you;
❏ receptionists to understand and explain the process to patients and to seek patient consent;
❏ one or two patients who would be suitable for the exercise;

This exercise requires you (the student) to:
❏ interview a patient briefly before they see the doctor about why they have come for a consultation;
❏ accompany the patient into the consultation and observe what happens;
❏ talk with the patient afterwards about what happened: find out whether they think their questions were answered and whether they got what they wanted from the consultation;
❏ talk about the consultation with the doctor in terms of his or her perception of what happened;
❏ discuss your findings with your tutor (who will probably be the consulting doctor as well in this case).

Carry out this exercise with one or two patients.

THE FORMAL STAGING OF A CONSULTATION

We have so far looked at the behaviours that occur and the tasks that patients and doctors hope to address (to a greater or lesser extent) in consultations. Let us now examine the stages of a consultation. By this is meant the route that the consultation takes in order to meet the tasks that are set by patient and doctor. The simplest framework with which to stage consultations is that produced by Byrne and Long in 1976 after they analysed more than 2000 tape recordings of over 100 doctors' consultations. They came up with the following six stages, rarely strictly in this order.

■ Phase I: the doctor establishes a relationship with the patient.
■ Phase II: the doctor either attempts to discover or actually discovers the reason for the patient's attendance.
■ Phase III: the doctor conducts a verbal or physical examination, or both.
■ Phase IV: the doctor, or the doctor and the patient (in that order of probability), considers the condition.
■ Phase V: the doctor, and occasionally the patient, details further treatment or further investigation.
■ Phase VI: the consultation is terminated, usually by the doctor.

Practical Exercise

Try looking at some consultations to see if these stages are in fact dealt with and, if so, in what order. Discuss this first with your tutor. You may also like to discuss whether and to what extent this order is ideal and how and why stages may be missed out or dealt with in a different order in different situations. You may also like to observe and reflect with your tutor how patient centred or doctor centred the different stages of the consultation are.

A rather more comprehensive framework that combines both the tasks and the staging of a consultation was produced by Pendleton et al. in 1984 and updated in 2003. It details seven aims of the consultation, from the doctor's and patient's viewpoints, which it puts together in a logical, although not necessarily always appropriate, order. It also talks about the patient's problem. It is worth stressing here that consultations are not just about problems or illnesses. Some are about health rather than illness issues such as a wanted pregnancy or health care for travelling. However, this model is included because it is comprehensive and you might be interested in looking at consultations, in whatever situation, in a more detailed manner.

Task 1. To understand the reasons for the patient's attendance, including:

1. the patient's problem:
   - the nature and history of the problem
   - its aetiology
   - its effects.
2. the patient's perspective:
   - their personal and social circumstances
   - their ideas and values about health
   - their ideas about the problem, its causes and its management
   - their concerns about the problem and its implications
   - their expectations for information, involvement and care.

Task 2. Taking into account the patient's perspective, to achieve a shared understanding:

1. about the problem
2. about the evidence and options for management.

Task 3. To enable the patient to choose an appropriate action for each problem:

1. consider options and implications
2. choose the most appropriate course of action.

Task 4. To enable the patient to manage the problem:

1. discuss the patient's ability to take appropriate actions
2. agree doctor's and patient's actions and responsibilities
3. agree targets, monitoring and follow-up.

Task 5. To consider other problems:

1. not yet presented
2. continuing problems
3. at risk factors.

Task 6. To use time appropriately:

1. in the consultation
2. in the longer term.

Practical Exercise

Pick out one of these aims (for example 'how time or resources were used' or 'involving the patient in management decisions') as a focus for a surgery session. Discuss with your tutor the extent to which you both thought this aim had been achieved in a variety of consultations.

Task 7. To establish or maintain a relationship with the patient that helps to achieve the other tasks.

Finally, there is a Danish model (Larsen et al., 1997) that is also focused on a patient presenting with an illness. This model brings together the patient's views of illness ('voice of the lifeworld') and the doctor's view of illness ('voice of medicine'). A nine-stage model, with the mnemonic P-R-A-C-T-I-C-A-L, is as follows.

- Prior to the consultation, the patient has prepared for the visit and comes with his or her own story.
- Relationship: let the patient talk. The doctor needs to let the patient take the lead in telling his or her story.
- Anxieties: what does the patient want? Allow the patient to divulge his or her ideas, concerns and expectations.
- Common language: the GP's summary. This ensures that the doctor and the patient are speaking the same language and have the same understanding about the reasons for the consultation.
- Translating: from lifeworld to the world of medicine. Here the doctor can complete necessary clinical history taking and examination, bearing in mind the biopsychosocial model.
- Interaction: negotiation on what to do. The two models of the patient and the doctor might need to be reconciled in the development of the management plan.
- Converting insight into action: from consultation to everyday life. The doctor and patient look at factors that may impede or facilitate the management plan in order to come to a plan that is achievable.
- Agreement check, safety netting: The doctor and the patient check their understanding of the consultation and seek to agree their plan. They also discuss what to do if the plan does not work out.
- Leave from consultation, time for reflection: The doctor and patient say goodbye and the doctor, before s/he moves to the next consultation or activity, either takes a little time to reflect on what went on or makes a note to do so at a later stage.

Practical Exercise

Together with your tutor, choose a consultation in which the patient appears to have good insight into the process. Speak with your tutor and the patient after the consultation. How well do they think that these stages were achieved?

BEHAVIOURS THAT HELP OR HINDER A CONSULTATION

A number of different ways have been given to assist you in observing consultations in a focused, structured and, it is hoped, helpful way. To complete this chapter on 'the consultation', what you might observe as behaviour that helps or hinders a consultation is briefly summarized and discussed.

Consultations frequently go wrong when the doctor fails to determine the patient's reason for attending, when the doctor fails to grasp the ramifications of the patient's condition, or when the doctor fails to discuss and communicate the options for diagnosis and therapy properly. The patient goes out of the surgery feeling misunderstood and frustrated. The doctor is totally unaware of this, is left with an uneasy feeling that the consultation did not go well, or is left dissatisfied knowing that the consultation was not as effective as it might have been.

Three major skills which will assist a consultation are:

1. listening
2. getting to the real reason for presentation
3. recognizing and understanding cultural differences.

Listening carefully and respectfully to a patient's story, verbal and non-verbal, seems easy, but appears difficult for many of us. Attentive listening will, in the long term, identify and deal with problems more effectively than a hurried interrogation of the patient.

We all know that what the patient presents initially at a consultation is not always the principal problem or issue. For example, somatic problems are often easier to present than psychosocial problems and, in fact, the patient may use a somatic symptom in the initial presentation as a 'ticket of entry'. It has been shown that where a psychosocial issue is initially presented, this is the principal issue in nearly all cases. However, where a somatic problem is initially presented, this is the principal problem in only 53 per cent of cases (Burack and Carpenter, 1983). A more sensitive problem may be presented only indirectly or left until last, even until the patient is at the door. GPs usually become quite adept at picking up these indirect messages. However, sometimes, in fact quite frequently, the real reason or one of the reasons for consultation, if it does emerge, can surprise the doctor, often at the end of a lengthy consultation in the middle of a busy surgery.

CASE STUDY 3.3

Mr H, a 45-year-old man, opened the consultation by asking for the result of a full blood count ordered by my partner because he had a very prolonged sore throat. The lymphocyte count was just below normal and I spent a long time discussing its significance. I was immensely relieved that he was happy to do nothing and just put up with the nuisance of his sore throat. Then, just as I was about to say 'Is there anything else?', he flattened me with the observation, 'Actually my main reason for coming is that I have a discharge from my penis.' No wonder he wasn't bothered about his lymphopenia!

Practical Exercise

Note the presenting symptoms and the principal problems identified during some consultations. How often do they correlate? Can you detect any indirect presentations? You may detect what your tutor misses.

A common cause of poor communication is cultural misunderstanding. If we consider the term 'culture' in its broadest sense, this includes differences in the doctor's and patient's experience and understanding in terms of such things as age, gender, sexual orientation, physical difference, learning ability, educational background, ethnicity, socio-economic background and prior health experiences and values. Often such behaviours and beliefs, on the part of both the doctor and the patient, are not explicit and we are not consciously aware of them. For other consultations, for example when the patient and doctor do not share the same language, the differences are obvious (see the 'Special communication skills' sections of Chapter 6). It is important that we, as doctors, are aware of difference, valuing diversity and finding pleasure in learning from those of other cultural backgrounds. Valuing diversity also requires a heightened sensitivity to issues of stereotyping and prejudice.

Tutor quote

There is a guy with an Italian second name, nice guy, and he was a student here, ages ago. There was this woman came in, he was sitting in, and she was an elderly Italian woman who I knew pretty well. She was always miserable and I said to the student 'Look, why don't you take her off into the room for half an hour'. So he said 'Yes', and so he did, and later on in the morning I had sort of half forgotten about it and I said absentmindedly, 'Well, did you crack it then?' and he said 'Oh yeah'. 'Well what is the scam?' and he said 'Oh, it is because she is from Venice and her husband is from one of the neighbouring rural villages and therefore this wasn't acceptable in the villagers' eyes, so it was all to do with the sort of class system relating to, you know, the village life in the Venice area'. This was the basis of her disgruntlement with her husband, which had been lifelong, and that was why she was always disgruntled and it was worse here.

Practical Exercise

Take every opportunity to share with your fellow students and tutors your own beliefs and cultural experiences, especially in the health-related area. As tutors, particularly, we need to provide situations in which such information can be discussed in a respectful atmosphere.

Very early on in your training, you will be encouraged to be with patients and to listen to

Practical Exercise

A useful way of reflecting on consultations is to write your experiences down and then discuss them with fellow students and tutors. What we have found helpful with our students is to create what we call a log diary of, say, four consultations, each of one side of A4 paper (no more than 500 words). We suggest the following framework:

❑ brief description of presentation, content and process of the consultation (one paragraph),
❑ brief discussion of the outcome of the consultation (one paragraph),
❑ your own response to the consultation (one paragraph),
❑ what you learnt from the consultation (one paragraph).

In this exercise, the description of your response to the consultation and what you learnt from the consultation are as important as your description of patient presentation and outcome.

The following headings are suggestions for topics you can use to describe your experience of different consultations.

❑ Common self-limiting condition.
❑ Long-term condition.
❑ Disability.
❑ Screening/prevention or health promotion.
❑ Life event.
❑ Health beliefs.
❑ Prescribing.
❑ Conflict.
❑ Other.

It is also a good exercise to think of a caption that encapsulates your sense of the consultation, for example 'Nothing to fall back on – the physical injury mirrors the emotional difficulty'.

We have found it useful to discuss one or more of these case studies in seminar groups, in order to make the task of completing the remaining case studies more enjoyable and rewarding. The resultant log diary can be used for assessment purposes.

their stories. As you get more skilled, you will be able to start consulting formally. At this stage, you will be looking at your own consultations in these ways and getting feedback from your tutor to assist this process. You may also be given the opportunity to use video recordings and audiotapes to record your consultations. Take every opportunity to sit and talk with patients, and discuss with your tutor how to accomplish this in the safest and most appropriate and effective way for both you and the patient. Remember that to be a doctor or to be a patient are just two of the many roles that you have. Doctors are not exempt from being patients at times.

THE NARRATIVE APPROACH TO THE CONSULTATION

The 'stuff' of the consultation is the story, in fact the intersection of stories – those of the patient and the patient's family and community, the doctor and society. Over the last 30 years generally and the last 5 years in the medical world, there has been an increasing interest in the idea of narrative. This 'study of story telling' explores how we construct our stories as individuals and communities, how we tell them to each other, and how stories change over time. The narrative approach challenges ideas that we might have regarding reality and the authoritative voice of Western medicine in defining reality. Could even scientific reality be just a set of stories that a group of people happen to believe for a period of time? The narrative approach invites us as doctors to hold dual respect and an open mind for the worth of both the medical story and the patient's story, the scientific *and* the patient's explanation of reality and of the meaning of health and illness.

All our talk of the patient's and doctor's tasks and the formal staging of consultations does perhaps give us a sense of order and control –

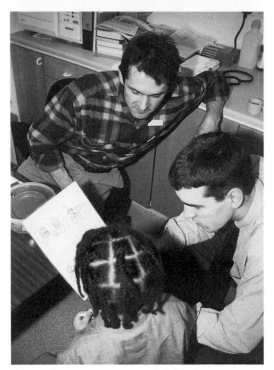

Figure 3.3 Learning from the patient.

of a process that can be understood and measured – and knowledge is power. However, is a more open-ended approach to the consultation, with a resultant relinquishing of some of the power that we hold as doctors, more valuable in making sense of health and illness? We, as doctors, may feel safer following the rules of history taking or the staging of a consultation, but what if this differs from what the patient wants to reveal to us? At times, simply witnessing the patient telling their story is all that is required (Fig. 3.3). At other times, the stages of the consultation may be reached after many consultations. Even more widely, the story that is told and the actions that follow may belong to a family or a community. The narrative approach broadens our understanding of the consultation.

SUMMARY POINTS

To conclude, the most important messages of this chapter are:

- the consultation is the central activity of a GP;
- it is important to be able to distinguish between the content and process of a consultation;
- the roles that the patient and doctor adopt in the consultation are related to the degree of doctor or patient centredness in that consultation;
- the tasks of the doctor and patient in a consultation have different emphases and, for a consultation to be effective, the doctor and patient need to meet as experts;
- listening, getting to the real reason for presentation and understanding cultural differences are three key areas which contribute to an effective consultation;
- valuing the stories that we hear helps us all to make sense of the patient's journey.

REFERENCES

Burack, R.C. and Carpenter, R.R. 1983: The predictive value of the presenting complaint. *Journal of Family Practice* 16(4), 749–54.

Byrne, P.S. and Long, B.E.L. 1976: *Doctors talking to patients.* London: HMSO.

Fry, J. 1993: *General practice. The facts.* Abingdon: Radcliffe Medical Press.

Gask, L. and Usherwood, T. 2002: ABC of psychological medicine. The consultation. *British Medical Journal* 324, 1567–9.

Helman, C.G. 1981: Disease versus illness in general practice. *The Journal of the Royal College of General Practitioners* 31, 548–52.

Larsen, J.-H., Risor, O. and Putnam, S. 1997: P-R-A-C-T-I-C-A-L: A step-by-step model for conducting the consultation in general practice. *Family Practice* 14(4), 295–301.

Neighbour, R. 1987: *The inner consultation.* London: Kluwer Academic Publications.

Pendleton, D., Schofield, T., Tate, P. and Havelock, P. 2003: *The new consultation.* Oxford: Oxford University Press.

Stewart, M. 2001: Towards a global definition of patient centred care. *British Medical Journal* 322, 444–5.

FURTHER READING

Byrne, P.S. and Long, B.E.L. 1976: *Doctors talking to patients.* London: HMSO.

This is one of the 'classics' in general practice research and is well worth reading if you are interested in the general practice consultation.

Fraser, R.C. 1992: *Clinical method. A general practice approach*, 2nd edn. Oxford: Butterworth Heinemann.

This is a very useful and succinct British text of general practice that has two good chapters on the consultation and the doctor–patient relationship.

Kai, J. 2003: *Ethnicity, health and primary care.* Oxford: Oxford University Press.

This is a concise and practical introduction to ethnicity and health care. The general principles outlined in this book are readily transferable to other healthcare settings and issues of diversity.

Launer, J. 2002: *Narrative-based primary care.* Abingdon: Radcliffe Medical Press.

Both philosophical and practical, this is a good introduction to the narrative approach, challenging our understanding of the consultation.

McWhinney, I.R. 1989: *A textbook of family medicine.* Oxford: Oxford University Press.

This is a larger text than that of Fraser. It is based on the North American and British experiences and is more philosophical in nature. It has some wonderful reading on all aspects of general practice, including the consultation.

Morgan, M. 2003: The doctor–patient relationship. In: Scambler, G. (ed): *Sociology as applied to medicine,* 5th edn. Edinburgh: WB Saunders.

An up-to-date summary of sociological thinking around the doctor–patient relationship.

Neighbour, R. 1987: *The inner consultation.* London: Kluwer Academic Publications.

This is an enjoyable book to read, perhaps more for postgraduate students of general practice. It explores the art of consulting.

Pendleton, D., Schofield, T., Tate, P. and Havelock, P. 2003: *The consultation.* Oxford: Oxford University Press.

This is an update of another of the classic general practice texts on the consultation.

Tate, P. 1994: *The doctor's communication handbook.* Abingdon: Radcliffe Medical Press.

This concentrates on how to communicate with patients in whatever setting you meet them. It is easy and fun to read.

Tuckett, D., Boulton, M., Olson, C. and Williams, A. 1985: *Meetings between experts.* London: Tavistock Publications.

This thought-provoking book makes for useful reading for all clinicians and aspiring clinicians. From a study of more than 1000 primary care consultations, questions about the objectives of such meetings are asked and discussed.

COMMON ILLNESSES IN GENERAL PRACTICE

Only 20 per cent of symptoms experienced by the general population are presented to a healthcare practitioner. This chapter considers the factors that influence the decision to consult and the types of conditions seen in general practice. A framework for aiding learning about medical conditions is presented.

LEARNING OBJECTIVES

By the end of this chapter you will be able to:

- understand the reasons why patients bring problems to their general practitioner;
- list the types of conditions that present to general practice in the UK;
- list the key general practice conditions for student learning;
- seek further information about a particular condition and know how best to structure that information to aid learning.

WHAT DO PEOPLE DO WHEN THEY FEEL UNWELL?

Members of the general population experience symptoms very commonly. A study by Wadsworth et al. (1971) found that 95 per cent of a randomly selected sample of 2153 London adults experienced symptoms in a 14-day period. Figure 4.1 shows the proportion of the general population who suffer from a selection of common problems in a year. As you can see, the majority of the population experience such problems each year. Fortunately, not all of these are brought to general practice!

When an individual feels unwell, they may choose to:
- ignore the symptoms;
- 'self-care', i.e. to cope with the symptoms themselves or to seek help from friends or relatives (the lay referral system); self-care may take the form of no action, home remedies (e.g. honey and lemon for a cough) or 'over-the-counter' remedies (e.g. cough linctus);
- consult a traditional healthcare professional such as a GP or practice nurse;
- consult a practitioner of alternative medicine such as an aromatherapist or osteopath.
(Armstrong, 1995).

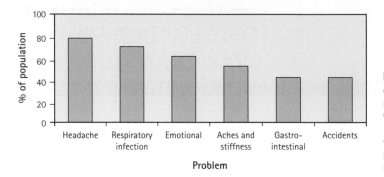

Figure 4.1 The annual occurrence of common problems in the general population. From Fry, J. and Sandler, G. 1993: *Common diseases: their nature, prevalence, and care*, 5th edition. Newbury: Petroc Press, p. 7. Reproduced with kind permission from Petroc Press.

Practical Exercise

The objectives of this exercise are to look at the actions people take when they experience common symptoms and to consider the factors that influence the decision to seek medical advice.

❏ Choose a common symptom, e.g. headache, cough, nausea, indigestion.

❏ Design a short questionnaire aiming to explore the objectives above.

❏ Arrange with your GP tutor to interview a sample of subjects. The easiest way to do this is to interview patients in the doctor's waiting room.

❏ Introduce yourself to each patient and obtain their permission for a short interview. If possible, find a room where you can have a confidential conversation. Patients will be worried about missing their turn with the doctor, so make arrangements with the receptionist to ensure this does not happen; if necessary, complete your interview after their appointment.

❏ Pilot your questionnaire and make any necessary adaptations.

❏ Interview at least ten people.

❏ Review their responses.

❏ Discuss your findings with your GP tutor.

(After Graham and Seabrook, 1995).

The ways in which people react when they experience symptoms form part of their *illness behaviour*. This can be defined as 'the ways in which given symptoms may be differentially perceived, evaluated and acted upon (or not acted upon) by different kinds of persons' (Mechanic, 1962).

A helpful way of understanding an individual's illness behaviour is to consider the Health Belief Model (Rosenstock, 1966; Becker and Maiman, 1975). This proposes that individuals differ in the way they perceive:

■ their susceptibility and vulnerability to illness: those who believe themselves to be more vulnerable are more likely to seek medical attention;

■ the severity of their symptoms: in general, symptoms more likely to be perceived as serious include unusual symptoms, those with an acute onset and those associated with visible

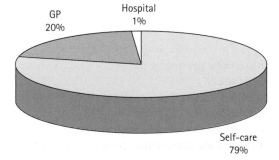

Figure 4.2 Common symptoms experienced by the general population: proportions cared for at self-care, general practice and hospital levels. From Fry, J., Brooks, D. and McColl, I. 1984: Utilisation of resources and content of work. In: *NHS data book*. Dordrecht: Kluwer Academic Publishers, p. 129. Reproduced by kind permission from Kluwer Academic Publishers. Copyright 1984 John Fry, David Brooks and Ian McColl.

In the majority of cases, people self-care. In the UK, only 20 per cent of symptoms reach general practice, 79 per cent are dealt with by self-care, and the remaining 1 per cent present directly to hospital (Fry et al., 1984). This is illustrated by a pie chart in Figure 4.2. The term *the clinical iceberg* refers to the high proportion of symptoms dealt with outside formal health care.

signs, although there is great variation amongst individuals; symptoms perceived as serious are more likely to be brought to the attention of a healthcare professional;

- the costs of health-seeking behaviour: possible costs include the inconvenience of attending surgery, a potential lack of sympathy from the doctor and the financial cost of a prescription;
- the benefits of health-seeking behaviour: possible benefits include obtaining therapy to cure symptoms and legitimization of an illness by obtaining a sick certificate.

Certain triggers to the timing of consultations with healthcare professionals have been identified (Zola, 1973):

- the occurrence of an interpersonal crisis;
- the perceived interference with social or personal relations;
- sanctioning or pressure from family or friends;
- the perceived interference with vocational or physical activity;
- the setting of a deadline ('If I'm not better by Monday...').

In any consultation, it is important to consider not only why that person has presented, but also why at that particular time. Zola (1973) found that if doctors paid insufficient attention to the specific triggers prompting an individual to seek help, that person was less likely to comply with treatment. (More about this in Chapter 5, 'Psychological issues in general practice'.)

CASE STUDY 4.1

Mr J, a 45-year-old business man, develops acute back pain following a long car journey. He is usually fit and well and does not like to think of himself as ill. Initially, he tries to ignore the pain, but when it starts to affect his sleep he takes some paracetamol. However, the pain persists and begins to interfere with his work. He mentions it to a friend who has had similar problems in the past. His friend recalls that his GP was unable to cure his symptoms, so he went to an osteopath instead. Although expensive, this proved very effective. Mr J decides to follow his friend's example and consults an osteopath.

Thinking and Discussion Point

Reflect on Case study 4.1; can you identify any aspects of the Health Belief Model or Zola's triggers in Mr J's behaviour?

Seventy-eight per cent of individuals registered with a GP will consult a GP or practice nurse at least once a year. Each person who consults a doctor does so, on average, 3.8 times a year, giving an average doctor consultation rate of 2.9 per person registered (McCormick et al., 1995). Factors affecting consultation rates include the following (Campbell and Roland, 1996).

- Age: the elderly and children are more likely to consult than young adults or the middle aged.
- Sex: women are more likely to consult than men, partly because of their use of obstetric and contraception services and partly because they have higher rates of illness.
- Social class: individuals in lower social classes have higher morbidity and mortality than those in middle and upper classes and consult more frequently. However, such individuals still make less use of health services than would be expected on the basis of their poorer health.
- Ethnicity: in the UK, consultation rates vary amongst different ethnic groups, e.g. Asians and Afro-Caribbeans consult more frequently than Caucasians. This is thought to be due partly to increased morbidity and partly to differences in illness behaviour.
- Social networks: the existence of a good social support network is associated with a lower consultation rate. This appears to be due a combination of improved health and a better ability to cope with problems in those who are well supported.
- Accessibility of health care: an individual is more likely to consult if the surgery is nearby and appointments are easy to obtain.

In summary, the presence of a symptom is not the only determinant of whether an individual decides to consult. The way in which the person evaluates that symptom affects the action he or she takes, and this is profoundly affected by psychosocial factors, including cultural and family influences. There seems to be little correlation between a person's decision to consult and either the true seriousness of the condition or the doctor's perception of the need to consult. There are people who fail to present despite suffering from serious disease (Last, 1963), and many people consult with what GPs consider to be trivial or minor complaints (Cartwright and Anderson, 1981).

> ## Thinking and Discussion Point
>
> Consider your interview sample; what actions did your interviewees take when they experienced symptoms and what factors influenced their decisions to seek medical advice? Can you identify any of the factors mentioned in this section?

WHICH TYPES OF ILLNESSES PRESENT TO GENERAL PRACTICE IN THE UK?

The illnesses seen in general practice differ in severity and type from those seen in hospitals. Data on the disease groups and the specific minor, chronic and major conditions commonly presenting to general practice in the UK are summarized in this section. The source of much of this data is the Fourth National Study of Morbidity Statistics from General Practice 1991–1992 (McCormick et al., 1995), in which consultations in 60 general practices across England and Wales were analysed, representing a 1 per cent sample of the population.

Tables 4.1–4.4 summarize two key statistics for a range of conditions commonly seen in general practice:

1. the percentage of a practice population who consult at least once a year with each condition,
2. the number of cases an average GP (list size 2000) would expect to see in 1 year.

Table 4.1 shows the *disease groups* that commonly present to general practice: respiratory, nervous system, skin, musculoskeletal, injury and poisoning, and infections.

In addition to considering the disease groups that present to general practice, it is also useful to classify conditions as *minor*, *chronic* or *major*. Minor conditions are defined as self-limiting, chronic as lasting more than 6 months, and major as acute and potentially life threatening. Figure 4.3 shows the proportions of illnesses

Table 4.1 Common disease groups presenting to general practice

Disease group	Percentage of practice population consulting in 1 year	Number of cases seen by average GP in 1 year
Respiratory	30	600
Nervous system (including eyes and ears)	17	340
Skin	15	300
Musculoskeletal	15	300
Injury/poisoning	15	300
Infections	14	280
Genitourinary (excluding obstetric)	11	220
Gastrointestinal	9	180
Cardiovascular	9	180
Psychiatric	7	140
Endocrine/metabolic	4	80
Non-specific symptoms and signs	15	300

From McCormick, A., Fleming, D. and Charlton, J. 1995: *Morbidity statistics from general practice: fourth national study 1991–1992.* Crown copyright 1995. National Statistics Crown copyright material is reproduced with the permission of the Controller of HMSO.

presenting to general practice classified in this way, and illustrates that the majority of conditions are minor or chronic, with a smaller proportion of major conditions.

Fifty-two per cent of all illness presenting to general practice can be classified as *minor* or self-limiting. Table 4.2 shows the most common minor conditions.

Thirty-three per cent of illnesses presenting to general practice may be classified as *chronic*.

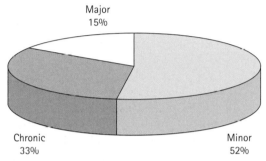

Major
15%

Chronic
33%

Minor
52%

Figure 4.3 Grades of disease presenting to general practice. From Fry, J. and Sandler, G. 1993: *Common diseases: their nature, prevalence, and care*, 5th edition. Newbury: Petroc Press, p. 27. Reproduced by kind permission from Petroc Press.

Table 4.3 shows the most common chronic conditions. (See more in Chapter 9, 'Chronic illness and its management in general practice'.)

Fifteen per cent of conditions presenting to general practice may be classified as *major*. Table 4.4 shows the most common major conditions.

The National Morbidity Studies provide valuable information concerning those conditions presenting to general practice. However, it is important to remember that the data refer only to those patients who consulted either a GP or a practice nurse. They give no indication of disease rates among individuals who do not attend general practice because they are not registered with a practice or they self-care or go direct to hospital. The data cannot, therefore, be used to estimate the true incidence or prevalence of diseases in the community as a whole.

Data have been presented on the specific *diseases* seen in general practice. However, many consultations involve a confusing mass of physical or psychological symptoms which students (and GPs) find difficult to classify as a particular disease. In addition, many general practice

Table 4.2 Specific minor conditions presenting to general practice

Condition	Percentage of practice population consulting in 1 year	Number of cases seen by average GP in 1 year
Acute throat infections	8	160
Psycho-emotional	7	140
Backache	6	120
Eczema	5	100
Acute otitis media	5	100
External ear problems (mainly wax and otitis externa)	4	80
Hay fever	3	60
Dyspepsia	2	40
Headache	2	40
Dizzy spells	1.5	30
Constipation	1	20
Piles	1	20
Varicose veins	0.9	18

From McCormick, A., Fleming, D. and Charlton, J. 1995: *Morbidity statistics from general practice: fourth national study 1991–1992*. Crown copyright 1995. National Statistics Crown copyright material is reproduced with the permission of the Controller of HMSO. Also from Fry, J. 1993: *General practice: the facts*. Oxford: Radcliffe Medical Press, p. 25. Reproduced with kind permission of Radcliffe Medical Press.

Table 4.3 Specific chronic conditions presenting to general practice

Condition	Percentage of practice population consulting in 1 year	Number of cases seen by average GP in 1 year
Respiratory		
Asthma	4.3	86
Chronic obstructive airways disease	1.2	24
Cardiovascular		
Hypertension	4.2	84
Ischaemic heart disease	1.7	34
Musculoskeletal		
Backache	4	80
Osteoarthritis	3	60
Endocrine		
Diabetes mellitus	1.1	22
Thyroid disorders	0.7	14
Gastrointestinal		
Irritable bowel syndrome	1	20
Peptic ulcer	0.5	10
Inflammatory bowel disease	0.3	6
Diverticular disease	0.2	4
Neurological		
Cerebrovascular disease (after-effects)	1	20
Epilepsy	0.4	8
Parkinson's disease	0.2	4
Multiple sclerosis	0.1	2

From McCormick, A., Fleming, D. and Charlton, J. 1995: *Morbidity statistics from general practice: fourth national study 1991–1992.* Crown copyright 1995. National Statistics Crown copyright material is reproduced with the permission of the Controller of HMSO. Also from Fry, J. 1993: *General practice: the facts.* Oxford: Radcliffe Medical Press, p. 26. Reproduced with kind permission of Radcliffe Medical Press.

Table 4.4 Specific major conditions presenting to general practice

Condition	Percentage of practice population consulting in 1 year	Number of cases seen by average GP in 1 year
Acute chest infection	7.5	150
Severe depression	0.6	12
Acute myocardial infarction	0.3	6
Acute cerebrovascular accident	0.3	6
Acute abdomen	0.3	6

From McCormick, A., Fleming, D. and Charlton, J. 1995: *Morbidity statistics from general practice: fourth national study 1991–1992.* Crown copyright 1995. National Statistics Crown copyright material is reproduced with the permission of the Controller of HMSO. Also from Fry, J. 1993: *General practice: the facts.* Oxford: Radcliffe Medical Press, p. 27. Reproduced with kind permission of Radcliffe Medical Press.

consultations do not deal with disease alone. Social issues such as poverty, unemployment, homelessness and divorce influence the health of a population, and it has been estimated that one-third of general practice consultations involve such social issues (Fry and Sandler, 1993). Twenty per cent of consultations deal with preventative and health promotion activities such as cervical smears, immunizations and travel advice (Fry and Sandler, 1993).

Practical Exercises

The following exercises may be carried out within a routine surgery. Discuss the issues involved with your GP tutor in advance and decide on the best way of recording and interpreting the information you obtain.

❏ Interview a selection of patients prior to their consultation with the doctor. Attempt to identify the reason why each patient has come to the GP and what they hope to gain from their consultation (this may not be as straightforward as it sounds).

❏ Sit in on these patients' consultations with the doctor. Observe the consultation; does the GP obtain the same information as you did?

❏ Following each consultation, discuss the issues raised with the GP. Compare your analysis of the perceived reasons for each consultation with those of the GP tutor.

Not infrequently, there is a discrepancy between the reason a doctor thinks a patient has consulted and why the patient has actually consulted. What influences may this have on patient care?

❏ Classify the conditions presenting into minor, chronic or major. Compare your results with the figures given in this chapter.

❏ Consider how many consultations have a social agenda.

KEY GENERAL PRACTICE PRESENTATIONS FOR MEDICAL STUDENTS

As you will have realized, any disease may present to general practice, and it can be difficult for students to know which conditions to focus on during their general practice module. As a guide, you should read up about those conditions you come across during your GP attachment; it is easier to recall information about a condition if you can relate it to a particular patient. In particular, reflect on how the presentation, diagnosis and management of each condition differ between the general practice and hospital settings. Check whether your medical school has defined a core curriculum of general practice conditions. When the author was working in the Department of Primary Care at Oxford University, the GP tutors developed a core curriculum of conditions for students to focus on, which is presented below as a starting point for your own learning.

■ Sore throat (extend to include coughs and colds)
■ Earache
■ Low back pain
■ Dysuria
■ Dyspepsia
■ Acute chest pain
■ Depression
■ Asthma
■ Hypertension
■ Ischaemic heart disease.

Note that most of these conditions are *symptoms* rather than specific diseases, reflecting the way in which patients present in primary care.

HOW TO FIND OUT MORE ABOUT PARTICULAR ILLNESSES

A full description of common general practice conditions is beyond the scope of this book, so where should you look for further information? A good starting point is to identify the subject matter, for example general medicine, obstetrics or paediatrics, and then consult the standard student textbook on that subject recommended by your medical school. However, many minor conditions are poorly covered in standard medical books, so you will also need access to a specialized general practice text; this will provide information on the presentation and management of key conditions with a specific primary care focus (see examples in the further reading list at the end of this chapter). Note, however, that the information contained in textbooks is frequently out of date, especially with regard to up-to-date therapy, and you may need to consult the current research literature on the topic. The section on evidence-based medicine in Chapter 7 provides guidance on how to do this.

Most medical students are overwhelmed by the amount of information they are expected to remember about a bewildering array of different conditions. It is helpful to structure this information under various subheadings, to aid learning and recall, both in exam settings and when practising as a doctor. The following scheme is a starting point for you to adapt for your own use.

1. Definition.
2. Epidemiology (incidence and prevalence; age, gender, geographical, social class variations).
3. Aetiology and risk factors.
4. Basic science (what aspects of pathology, physiology, anatomy etc. are relevant?).
5. Clinical features (typical symptoms and signs).
6. Investigations (which to request and what results to expect).
7. Differential diagnosis (what other conditions may present in a similar way and how can you differentiate between them).
8. Management (remember to think more widely than drug therapy).
9. Prognosis.

Now consider how this scheme can be applied to acute otitis media.

1. *Definition*: acute inflammation of the middle ear.
2. *Epidemiology*: very common – 5 per cent of a practice population will consult in 1 year (30 per cent of children under 3 years) and 50 per cent of children under the age of 10 are affected at some time; rare in adults. The average GP will see 100 cases per year (equates to 1.5 million cases annually in England and Wales).
3. *Aetiology*: most commonly follows an upper respiratory tract infection. The commonest bacterial pathogens are *Haemophilus influenzae*, *Streptococcus pneumoniae* and *Moraxella catarrhalis*, but many cases are viral in aetiology.
4. *Risk factors*: eustachian tube dysfunction, e.g. short tube (children), obstructed tube (adenoids, allergy) and unresolved middle ear effusions.
5. *Basic science*: further detail not necessary in this case.
6. *Clinical features*: symptoms include earache, fever, irritability, aural discharge and deafness; signs include pyrexia, a red, bulging tympanic membrane and discharge. Common presentations include an infant with fever and irritability and a young child with earache, fever and deafness.
7. *Investigations*: seldom performed; culture of aural discharge, where present, in refractory cases.
8. *Differential diagnosis*: other causes of otalgia (e.g. eustachian tube dysfunction, glue ear, otitis externa, dental pain) and other childhood infections.
9. *Management*: education (as to the nature of the condition and its natural course) and reassurance of parents and child, together with analgesia and temperature control are the main aims of care. The role of antibiotics is a subject of much debate. Antibiotic use for acute otitis media varies from 31 per cent of cases in the Netherlands to 98 per cent of cases in the USA and Australia. A recent Cochrane Review (Glasziou et al., 2003) confirmed the effects of antibiotics to be modest and their use not without problems in terms of side effects, antibiotic resistance and financial cost. A more appropriate approach might be to use antibiotics, at first presentation, only in those at risk of poor outcome, and in the majority of cases to assume a policy of 'watchful waiting', using antibiotics only for those cases which fail to settle. If antibiotics are prescribed, the usual choice is amoxycillin (5-day course). Patients should be instructed to return if symptoms persist, and all cases of perforation should be followed up to ensure healing occurs.
10. *Prognosis*: resolution over 2–3 days is usual (80 per cent of cases). The drum may remain dull red or pink and deafness may persist for 2–3 weeks. In some cases, the tympanic membrane perforates, leading to discharge

and resolution of the pain; the perforation will heal spontaneously in the majority of cases. The most important risk factors for poor outcome are young age and attendance at a day-care facility. Other risk factors include white race, male sex and a history of enlarged adenoids, tonsillitis or asthma. The role of environmental tobacco smoke is controversial. Forty per cent of cases will recur within 12 months; those with unresolved middle ear infections are particularly prone. Recurrences tend to cease after the age of 8 years. Complications such as mastoiditis and cerebral abscess are very rare in developed countries.

There is more about the diagnosis and management of acute illnesses in general practice in Chapter 7.

Practical Exercise

Use the suggested scheme to learn more about a particular medical condition.

❑ Choose a condition about which you know little or nothing, based on a patient encounter during your general practice attachment.

❑ Research this topic and try to organize your learning using the scheme detailed above.

❑ Consider how the information you gain applies to the patient you saw.

❑ Arrange a time when you can present the information to your GP tutor and, perhaps, an audience of practice staff.

❑ The next time you see a patient with this condition, consider how you can apply your knowledge to understand his or her problems better.

SUMMARY POINTS

To conclude, the most important messages of this chapter are as follows.

- Only 20 per cent of symptoms experienced by the general population are presented to a GP; the majority are dealt with by sufferers or their families. The presence of a symptom is not the only determinant of whether an individual decides to seek medical help. The way in which they evaluate that symptom affects the action they take and is profoundly affected by psychosocial factors, including cultural and family influences.
- Seventy-eight per cent of a practice population will consult a GP or practice nurse at least once a year, with an average doctor consultation rate of 2.9 per person registered.
- The illnesses seen in general practice differ in severity and type from those seen in hospital. In general practice, most conditions are minor or chronic: 52 per cent of all illness presenting to general practice can be classified as minor, 33 per cent as chronic and 15 per cent as major.
- The most common minor conditions are acute throat infection, psycho-emotional disorder, backache, eczema and ear disorders.
- The most common chronic conditions are asthma, chronic obstructive airways disease, hypertension, backache, osteoarthritis, ischaemic heart disease and diabetes mellitus.
- The most common major conditions are acute chest infection, depression, myocardial infarction, cerebrovascular accident and acute abdomen.
- Social factors influence the health of the population and play a role in 33 per cent of consultations. Health promotion and preventative activities take place in 20 per cent of consultations.
- Knowing where to seek further information about a particular condition and how best to structure that information are important aids to learning.

(UK data)

REFERENCES

Armstrong, D. 2002: *Outline of sociology as applied to medicine*, 5th edn. London: Arnold.
Becker, M. and Maiman, L. 1975: Sociobehavioural determinants of compliance with health and medical care recommendations. *Medical Care* 13, 10–24.

Campbell, S. and Roland, M. 1996: Why do people consult the doctor? *Family Practice* 13, 75–83.

Cartwright, A. and Anderson, R. 1981: *General practice revisited: a second study of patients and their doctors.* London: Tavistock.

Fry, J. 1993: *General practice: the facts.* Oxford: Radcliffe Medical Press.

Fry, J., Brooks, D. and McColl, I. 1984: *NHS data book.* Dordrecht: Kluwer Academic Publishers.

Fry, J. and Sandler, G. 1993: *Common diseases: their nature, prevalence, and care.* Newbury: Petroc Press.

Glasziou, P., Del Mar, C., Sanders, S. and Hayem, M. Antibiotics for acute otitis media in children (Cochrane Review). In: *The Cochrane Library*, Issue 2, 2003. Oxford: Update Software. The Cochrane Library can be accessed free of charge through the National Electronic Library for Health at http://www.nelh.nhs.uk

Graham, H. and Seabrook, M. 1995: Structured learning packs for independent learning in the community. *Medical Education* 29, 61–5.

Last, J. 1963: The clinical iceberg: completing the clinical picture in general practice. *Lancet* 2, 28–30.

McCormick, A., Fleming, D. and Charlton, J. 1995: *Morbidity statistics from general practice: Fourth National Study 1991–1992.* London: HMSO.

Mechanic, D. 1962: The concept of illness behaviour. *Journal of Chronic Diseases* 15, 189–94.

Rosenstock, I. 1966: Why people use health services. *Milbank Memorial Fund Quarterly* 44(3), Suppl., 94–127.

Wadsworth, M., Butterfield, W. and Blaney, R. 1971: *Health and sickness: the choice of treatment: perception of illness and choice of treatment in an urban community.* London: Tavistock.

Zola, I. 1973: Pathways to the doctor: from person to patient. *Social Science and Medicine* 7, 677–89.

FURTHER READING

Armstrong, D. 1995: *An outline of sociology as applied to medicine*, 4th edn. London: Arnold.
    A good introduction to medical sociology that contains further information concerning illness behaviour.

Campbell, S. and Roland, M. 1996: Why do people consult the doctor? *Family Practice* 13, 75–83.
    A helpful review article that summarizes the reasons why people seek professional medical help.

Fry, J. and Sandler, G. 1993: *Common diseases: their nature, prevalence, and care.* Newbury: Petroc Press.
    A useful book that contains fairly detailed information about diseases commonly seen in general practice, including those poorly covered in standard medical texts.

Jones, R. (ed.). 2003: *Oxford textbook of primary medical care.* Oxford: Oxford University Press.
    A two-volume text, the second of which, the clinical volume, covers in depth all the medical problems commonly seen in general practice worldwide.

Mead, M. and Patterson, H. 1999: *Tutorials in general practice*, 3rd edn. Edinburgh: Churchill Livingstone.
    An illuminating selection of case studies focusing on problems commonly seen in general practice.

Murtagh, J. 1999: *General practice*, 2nd edn. Australia: McGraw-Hill Health Professions Division.
    A useful reference source that presents a systematic review of patient assessment and management strategies for common conditions in general practice.

Taylor, R.J., McAvoy, B.R. and O'Dowd, T. 2003: *General practice medicine.* Edinburgh: Churchill Livingstone.
    An illustrated text that outlines common illnesses seen in general practice.

PSYCHOLOGICAL ISSUES IN GENERAL PRACTICE

Psychological issues are important in all encounters between a doctor and a patient, and the ability to comprehend, assess and manage these, in partnership with the patient, is a basic medical skill. This is particularly so in general practice, where many of the necessary skills can be learnt and insight obtained.

LEARNING OBJECTIVES

By the end of this chapter, you will be able to:

- describe the importance of psychological issues in primary medical care;
- describe the ways in which patients may present with these issues, and how they can be assessed;
- list the overall classifications of such concerns currently used in primary medical care;
- outline the possible responses that can be offered, and by whom;
- give an account of the way in which doctors and other members of the team may be affected by this work, and how it can be managed;
- outline the common ways in which personal and family developments may influence these issues;
- describe the possible impact of social and cultural factors on presentation and their management by professionals and the team;
- outline appropriate models of management based on dynamic and systemic thinking;
- outline the common ethical concerns raised by the above.

WHY ARE PSYCHOLOGICAL ISSUES SO IMPORTANT?

A common and now outmoded model of medical care assumed that a *patient* has a *physical* *disease* and comes to a *doctor* for it to be *cured*. We can only begin to address the questions if we understand the importance of the *new* model of medical care which your patients, your teachers, the medical school and society expect you to understand. This group, unfortunately, also includes examiners!

Thinking and Discussion Point

Look at the opening statement of the paragraph above and see how many of the ideas in it you would consider 'outmoded' in general practice and primary medical care.

You may be interested to know that this idea that every patient has a physical disease and comes to the doctor for it to be cured is not just a problem for you, but for everyone who is involved in planning and delivering health care. The following are some of the ways in which we all have to bring ourselves up to date. Each will be followed by a case study, which you will want to explore further later, but you should read with an eye to the psychological issues you think are important, and a view of how you might have handled the case yourself.

BECOMING A 'PATIENT'

The first point at which a person meets the health service is primary care, and this is often (but not exclusively) in general practice. However, people may not see themselves as patients, or accept the idea (even if the doctor or others see it as necessary), and may wish to think long and hard about the consequences of this new 'role'.

CASE STUDY 5.1

A young couple presented to the general practitioner (GP) in evening surgery. The woman explained that she had brought her partner in because she had become very upset and depressed on their holiday together. She had thought she was pregnant, but had had a period while they were away. They had been trying to have a baby for 2 years. When the doctor talked about both their backgrounds, the man looked alarmed: 'Don't bring me into this doctor – there's nothing wrong with *me*.'

Thinking and Discussion Point

❑ Make a note of your reactions to Case study 5.1
❑ Taking each of the three people involved in turn, what would they be feeling and what would they want to achieve? If the feeling is standing in the way of their reaching their goals, what can be done to change things?

'PHYSICAL'

Although doctors are often distinguished by their concerns for bodies, the mind is also part of that body. The split between mind and body (represented, to be fair, by our title) may have been a common way of looking at things but now seems increasingly unhelpful. We recognize the existence and state of our own body by using our senses, and these are collected and co-ordinated by the brain or mind. For instance, a pain cannot be seen: however physical its origin, it is perceived and responded to initially by the mind. Equally, many of the ways in which we establish mental states are expressed by the body, such as weight loss, sweating, crying, shouting. One of the influential philosophers who wrote about things in this split way was the French thinker Descartes. He was influential at the beginning of the scientific revolution, and this form of divided thinking is often called 'Cartesian' after him (although the label does not do justice to his excellent and careful approach in his philosophy).

CASE STUDY 5.2

A middle-aged executive presented to her doctor feeling tired, but not prepared to say much else about herself. Her doctor checked her and found nothing physically wrong. He reassured her, but a week later the patient committed suicide with paracetamol.

Thinking and Discussion Point

With reference to Case study 5.2:
❑ what are your reactions to this alarming case?
❑ what surprises you about it and about your reactions?
❑ could the doctor have done anything to prevent the patient's death and, if so, what and how?

'DISEASE'

This is one of the words that many people (including doctors, surprisingly) use imprecisely. It is usually used for an objectively recognizable condition, often in contrast to an *illness*, which is a set of feelings which someone recognizes (subjectively) and can tell the doctor about, but which usually cannot be defined objectively by examinations or tests. In general practice, feelings or symptoms usually bring people to consult a health professional, and so it is initially the subjective concerns about illness (which, of course, are detected and acted on by the mind) that primary care physicians must understand and work with.

CASE STUDY 5.3

A young man came in on Saturday morning with a headache. He was a large man, and looked extremely tough. He said he had not been drinking much the night before, but said he was a bouncer at a nightclub. In the silence that the doctor allowed to develop after this, the patient explained that he was going to court on Monday to defend himself on an assault charge, and was unable to think clearly because of the headache.

Thinking and Discussion Point

Does the man in Case study 5.3 have a disease or an illness and, if so, what? If not, what else might be wrong which a doctor could help with?

'DOCTOR'

By now, there should be no need to say that many people other than doctors make contact with patients in primary care, and share the processes of assessment and management.

CASE STUDY 5.4

The receptionist in a single-handed practice came in to explain to the doctor how he had been talking to the next patient due to see her and that the patient was extremely upset about her son, who was going through a difficult time. The receptionist felt this knowledge would help the doctor to get to the point of the patient's visit. When the patient came in, the doctor mentioned that she knew something about the family problems. 'Oh thank you, doctor, but I've talked to that nice man on the front desk all about that. I've come to see you about these horrible varicose veins ...'

Thinking and Discussion Point

Consider for a moment the skills that might be needed to deal with the different case studies you have read in this chapter. Which of these skills particularly should a doctor have, and do you feel confident that you are already or could be skilled in this way? If not, who in your learning environment would help you?

'CURED'

Maybe we all wanted to be doctors in order to offer cures. The cynic might say that medical work seems really to be divided into coping with problems such as viral illnesses, which mostly get better by themselves (provided the patients do not react too badly to any medicines they use), and following conditions such as heart disease and diabetes, which come on gradually and cannot be got rid of, only managed. Even if that is too harsh, do you agree with Case study 5.5?

CASE STUDY 5.5

A student was asked to see the Head of Department for General Practice because he had not attended enough of his general practice sessions. He said in explanation that though he liked the GP and the surgery, he 'really wanted to see patients who could be cured'. 'Such as?' 'Oh, like a myocardial infarct ...' 'Excuse my ignorance, but could you tell me how you cure a myocardial infarct?' An uncomfortable silence followed.

The modern concept of medical work embraces all sides of illness and disease, which include the social and psychological as well as the physical (the holistic or biopsychosocial model); takes as much notice of what the patient says as of what the professional observes;

considers factors which influence professional judgement as well as the sick person's presentation; considers prevention and long-term care even in acute situations; and sees medical work as a team game. Focusing on psychological issues means that we shall want to know about feelings and emotional issues as much as about madness, and that we should be prepared to look at ourselves as professionals (how we view our work, our relationship with our patients, the effect we have on them and they have on us, and so on) and as members of a group. Before focusing on psychological issues specifically in *primary care*, it would be worth thinking through the implications of what you have just read for yourself.

Thinking and Discussion Point

❑ Do you agree that the above describes medical work? If not, why not?

❑ What are the dangers of doctors having too wide a role, and what limits have to be set to doctors' responsibilities?

❑ If you are already aiming for a particular type of doctoring (if you want to be a neurosurgeon or a parasitologist, for example), what are the implications of this discussion for your chosen area of work?

WHY ARE PSYCHOLOGICAL ISSUES SO IMPORTANT IN PRIMARY CARE?

The answers we offer to this question do not make sense without the previous section, but we need now to get down to clinical details.

■ *Preventing preventable deaths* is one of the prime tasks of all doctors. An important cause of death in many societies is serious depression that may result in suicide. Other causes of death include violence and road traffic accidents. Alcoholism enters this list both in its own right and as a risk factor in precipitating any of the above three. Although doctors have potential duties alongside many other agencies in this respect, Case study 5.2 demonstrates that some desperately distressed

people first visit their GP – some studies have suggested this is a common pattern (Matthews et al., 1994). So intervention at this time might be considered important, even if only a small percentage of people at risk were influenced, or even if the work was not completely effective.

■ *Time off work* is another measure of illness, and reducing it might be a marker of an important contribution. Probably as many days off work are due to psychologically related conditions as physical illness in modern societies.

CASE STUDY 5.6

Although he could not go abroad himself for family reasons, the young GP took up a part-time job with an overseas charity, and was astounded to find that most people who had to come back from their overseas posts because of illness came back with a psychiatric diagnosis.

Studies show that the *main* or *most important diagnosis* in general practice is a psychological one (anxiety, depression etc.) in at least 10 per cent of cases that present to the professionals. The figures vary, because what patients choose to offer to their doctors is influenced by many things – such as the social conditions locally, the availability of other forms of help, whether they think the doctor can help – but

Practical Exercise

Make a note of the main issues relevant to each patient you see with your GP, especially:

❑ the main diagnosis or diagnoses made by you and the GP;

❑ the reason the patient came to the doctor;

❑ how the patient behaved in the consultation;

❑ whether you felt, or the patient exhibited, any obvious emotions during that time, and what they were.

Do you note any difference between these four headings when you use them? Do they fit with the statistics above and, if not, in what way and why? Do you think using these ideas expands the importance of psychological issues in general practice?

perhaps most particularly by how they expect to be received by the doctor when they introduce this topic. Many people still feel shy of discussing their feelings with doctors, because they think they will be seen as 'not really ill', 'making a fuss', or perhaps that the doctor will make a mistake and will think they are upset when in reality they have a serious condition. Cultures vary, but in many groups there is still a stigma attached to mental illness of all kinds.

Some people might claim that almost *everybody who comes to the doctor is anxious* in some way, otherwise they would not come! Even if this argument seems a bit circular, it logically makes the handling of that anxiety part of the requirements for every consultation.

CASE STUDY 5.7

It was the second time that the medical student had been to the doctor with chest pain. He had been told he was as 'fit as a fiddle' but that had not reassured him. 'What was he worried about? Had he seen something which upset him?' He told the doctor about the post mortem on a lung cancer patient he had seen, and how he could not get out of his mind how like his Dad the patient had looked.

Thinking and Discussion Point

Think of four situations in which you have experience of being anxious. How were you helped to cope with that anxiety, and what else would you have liked to see done or provided at the time?

At the other end of the spectrum, the serious *distress of madness*, which is perhaps best classed in medicine as 'psychosis', makes some people reluctant to come to doctors, either because they are suspicious that they will come to harm or because their pattern of thinking makes doctors irrelevant. Family or friends who might otherwise bring them to the surgery may not be perceived by the distressed individual as being 'on my side' either. However, although specialist psychiatry is particularly concerned with these problems, there are many reasons why hospital is not the best environment for

people who are seriously distressed, so primary care staff have a significant role in detecting and helping to manage serious distress.

Thinking and Discussion Point

❑ Does this category (madness/psychosis/serious distress) make sense to you? How is it helpful and how unhelpful?
❑ What do you think the main needs of people who are going through such an experience are? Who might answer these needs?
(You might like to read some more – see the Further reading list at the end of this chapter.)

Thinking and Discussion Point

If you have met someone who seems to you to be in this category, what did you feel about the situation, for yourself, for the ill person, and for the professional? Did you understand anything of what the patient was going through? Did you feel safe?

If your answers to the last two questions are positive, or if you meet someone who was seriously distressed but now seems 'better' and your GP thinks it is all right for you to do so, see if you can find time and a suitable place to ask the patient if he or she would help you to understand the background by telling you about the experience and what it felt like, as far as both the illness and the treatment were concerned. Make it very clear that the patient is absolutely free to refuse and that this is only for your education.

Patient quote

Have I ever had any psychiatric help over the years? Well, I suppose I have, rather in the sense that someone adrift at sea might shout 'Help!' to a passing supertanker, be thrown a lifebelt, and the tanker go on its way.

In between the (almost) 'normal' anxiety of every patient who comes to a doctor and the deep distress of a suicidal or psychotic patient, most thoughtful doctors detect a group of people who seem particularly drawn to seeking help about a medical condition when they are also *going through a difficult or turbulent phase in their lives*. It could be said that it would be possible to detect issues like this in the lives of most people who are seeing the doctor: is this part of the cause of their illness, or does it come as a result of their medical condition and its handling? All of these aspects need to be taken into account.

Thinking and Discussion Point

❑ Have you noted people coming in with this sort of background problem to your GP?

❑ Do you have experience in your own life, or the lives of your family or friends, when a circumstance seemed to make you ill or drive you to see a doctor?

There are many different words to describe this interaction between social circumstances and health. 'Life events' are the experiences which people have that seem particularly associated with increased illness or increased attendance at doctors. Clear associations are found with moving house or losing someone who was loved. 'Life transitions' or 'adjustment disorders' may be another name for a similar phenomenon, and this suggests, rather than things happening to us, that there are phases which everyone experiences as they go through life, and there are times of particular vulnerability, such as adolescence or retirement. Particular 'crisis points' are now widely recognized, for instance the 'mid-life crisis' of late middle age. We shall return to these ideas when we look at 'depression'.

CASE STUDY 5.8

Julie was 11, and had been brought by her mother to see the doctor four times in 6 weeks with minor complaints. 'Are you having a difficult time at the moment Julie? You look as if life at the moment is a bit tough.' In the silence that followed, she looked at her mother: 'Doctor, I think you're quite right. Julie's just gone to big school, and is finding it quite hard as all her friends are at the other one. We do talk about it, but it is affecting her.'

Psychosomatic is the name given to those illnesses or diseases for which there seems to be a clear connection, even a causal one, between stress and physical illness. The conditions that used to be quoted classically were ulcerative colitis, asthma and rheumatoid arthritis. The idea that there is a particular group is now questioned: most physical conditions are influenced by state of mind and reactions to circumstances, and many patients now ask 'Could this be stress-related?'.

THE DEBATE ABOUT MENTAL HEALTH

You may have noticed that this chapter often refers to different or changing ways of looking at things. This may be uncomfortable or unsettling, but it is to help you recognize that the area of psychological issues/psychiatry/mental health is a 'contested' field. There are different ways not just of describing what we all observe, but also of *thinking* about and explaining these observations ('discourses'), and these ideas are themselves still changing or developing. In this respect it is probably no different from the rest of your medical studies, but the arguments seem sharper in mental health in general. There are debates about the use of drugs, diagnoses, ways of managing distress or compulsory treatment that start from completely different points of view.

Thinking and Discussion Point

❑ Do you agree with what has just been said about different discourses? If so, what do you think creates these differences of opinion?

❑ What are the important things you need to be aware of when practising as a doctor in the wider community?

Some of these changes may be due to the way in which society in general seems to think. For instance, in the lifetime of the author of this chapter, consensual homosexual acts between adult men have ceased to be considered as crimes in the UK, and being gay has stopped being a recognized condition in psychiatry, for which people are 'treated'. (We are still not at the point at which everybody agrees that adults are free to express their sexuality as they wish, provided they do not harm other people, so some forms of sexual desire or behaviour still cause distress, and people will come to doctors to be helped.)

Some of the issues that seem particularly important in mental health debates at the moment are:

- power, control and respect for autonomy,
- danger and safety,
- depersonalization and stigma,
- dependency and relationships.

CASE STUDY 5.9

The old man had always been eccentric, and the doctor regularly had to deal with neighbours who did not like his singing or the plastic flowers planted in his front garden. The doctor secretly admired odd behaviour, but it was when the rubbish began to accumulate outside, and the old man shouted abuse through the letterbox at anyone who called, that he realized he had to take a new view of what was going on. In the words of the immediate neighbour, 'something must be done'.

Practical Exercise

- ❏ As you see patients in your current attachment, listen to what other members of the team or relatives and neighbours have got to say, and to how the patient describes his or her own conditions.
- ❏ Do these suggest different ways of looking at the problem and, if so, do these differences help you to see different solutions, or do they make things even more difficult?
- ❏ If people disagree on what approach should be used, and there is conflict, whose ideas should win?

CLASSIFICATION AND ASSESSMENT: HOW DO WE MAKE SENSE OF IT ALL?

Different people approach even this problem in different ways. Classical medical teaching is that diagnosis must precede treatment, but this is not always possible. When physical specialists are often perplexed by the lack of physical signs in psychiatry, psychiatrists, by using questionnaire 'instruments' of various sorts, claim that their classifications are as clear and objective as any. But even within that branch of the profession, opinions differ. The psychodynamic school might look at what has to be worked with, the behavioural at what life problems need to be worked on, and so on. There is a radical mode of thought that rejects all labelling as stigmatic: labels are seen as traps for overworked or under-involved people, who just follow someone else's thinking and do not listen carefully to what the patient is really saying. A helpful way of combining different approaches in general practice is through the concept of narrative – the story a person is trying to tell. We shall come back to that concept later in this chapter.

One thing we can be sure about: distressed people often get physically ill, and people with a physical illness often find this very distressing. We are dealing not with 'either/or', but with 'both/and'. Our classifications must be inclusive, not exclusive, and allow us to keep open minds.

CASE STUDY 5.10

The new young GP had a special interest in depression. His patient, aged 55, had just lost his mother, and was tired and listless. At the third session, when there seemed no improvement, the patient muttered, 'I don't know, everything seems to be psychological these days – but I feel *ill*.' The doctor quickly remembered that he had not done a physical assessment. The erythrocyte sedimentation rate (ESR) was raised and the patient had multiple myeloma, as well as a difficult bereavement reaction.

Thinking and Discussion Point

Before going further, think of the important classification ideas that you might have already.

QUESTIONS IN CLASSIFICATION

Some people say that questions are more useful than answers. In the area of mental health classification in primary care, you might think some of the following questions were useful.

- Is the condition *dangerous*, in the sense of a threat to life or offering the possibility of serious harm to self or others?
- Does the condition seem to be triggered mainly by *outside events*?
- Is there something that can be *usefully done* and, if so, is it to be done by the health service or by other agencies?
- Does addressing the problem mainly depend on what the patient does for *himself* or *herself*?
- Is it a *long-term* condition, or has there been a *recent change*?
- Does it seem mostly related to a *physical illness*, which needs treatment too?
- Is there a *pattern* in the person's behaviour that seems to cause much of the difficulty or offer important clues?
- Does the person seem to be thinking in a way we understand, or is their *thought in some form of disorder*?
- Is the person's *age* or *gender* crucial?
- Does the condition seem to have been initiated, or made worse, by some *psychoactive substance*?
- Even if we understand the distress and the reaction seems normal, do we need to help because of the *degree of distress*?

Psychiatric classification will look quite different: consult your recommended reading in this field, as there is not scope to cover it all here. You will notice that most of these classifications are also a mixture, and that in the individual case people often recommend looking at a psychiatric assessment from several different points of view – a 'multi-axial' approach, which also underlies the international classification (Tylee et al., 1995).

Grouping might depend on:

- symptoms,
- behaviour,
- a recognized pattern or syndrome,
- probable cause,
- society's judgement of what is acceptable,

- what the patient will agree to,
- what treatment is available.

As you read down this list, some of the headings may have become uncomfortable to use and may raise *moral questions* for you that must be faced and may need to be revisited. Certainly, outcome will depend on resources for treatment, for instance, but *diagnostic assessment* also might do so.

CASE STUDY 5.11

The patient was 39, and sat impassively clasping and unclasping her hands as the tears ran down her face. 'How long have you felt like this?' A pause. 'It all started about 12 years ago, when I had my son. I was terribly depressed, and only stopped myself killing him and myself by thinking about the horror of the consequences. It was a daily struggle, and in that I succeeded; I suppose that's something to be quite proud of.

Thinking and Discussion Point

Try looking at some of the people you have met, or cases you have come across, who might be in the following jumbled categories in relation to the questions at the start of the 'Questions in classification' section:

- ❏ learning difficulties
- ❏ child abuse
- ❏ suicidal threat
- ❏ phobias
- ❏ alcoholism
- ❏ bereavement
- ❏ anorexia nervosa
- ❏ Alzheimer's disease
- ❏ panic disorder
- ❏ post-natal depression
- ❏ retirement crisis
- ❏ psychopathy
- ❏ hypochondriasis
- ❏ school refusal
- ❏ delirium
- ❏ post-traumatic stress disorder
- ❏ mania
- ❏ obsessive–compulsive behaviour
- ❏ schizophrenia
- ❏ divorce.

Every now and again I would make up my mind to tell my doctor, but she never had time to listen. I don't really blame her; she had her hands pretty full without my misery to add to it. But now I just can't go on ...'.

Whatever groupings seem to be most helpful (and it is likely that, like other areas in medicine, there will continue to be changes), medicine is a subject for which practical skill is needed, and you might like to match some of these conditions with the questions above, and with your own. You will notice that sometimes this necessitates putting together two conditions that do not have a common or similar cause. You might also like to write down the words which ordinary people would use to describe them in your particular community.

DANGEROUSNESS

In doing the exercise on the previous page you might find something odd. For instance, when dealing with the first question (about dangerousness), you may pick out suicidal depression, anorexia nervosa, delirium, drunkenness, acute schizophrenia, child abuse and psychopathic behaviour. But the way of approaching it will have to depend on some of the same sort of questions, such as the following.

- What sort of threat is there, and to whom?
- Is it acute, in the sense of needing immediate action, or will it wait for a different sort of assessment?
- What are my duties, and how far will the law allow me to go?
- Should other people be informed?
- What sort of resources can we muster to cope?
- Do I need help and, if so, of what sort?

CASE STUDY 5.12

At the end of a Saturday morning surgery, the doctor received a message that one of his male patients 'was not very well – would he call round?' The receptionist had been unable to find anything else out, and said that the wife had seemed very 'cagey' on the phone. Irritated, but in a hurry to get to his son's football match, the doctor decided just to call in quickly on his way home. He left his main bag in the surgery

and just took a stethoscope and a prescription pad. When he arrived, he found the husband was in an acute and violent paranoid state. Trapped in the bedroom, with no emergency drugs, the doctor took over an hour to fight his way to the phone to ring the police. When six officers arrived, the patient was clearly overwhelmed and immediately settled down; he was admitted to an acute psychiatric ward, and recovered in 3 weeks without a final diagnosis being made. The doctor missed the football match.

This case, a rare occurrence it needs to be said, illustrates some issues that are obvious but worth emphasizing:

- the doctor was himself one of the people at most risk;
- asking for help is not a sign of weakness but ...
- thoughtless rushing about is not likely to be helpful so ...
- think ahead and consider safety issues as well;
- most acutely psychotic people will give in to a show of numbers;
- doctors' irritation is one of the major causes of poor management.

Thinking and Discussion Point

- ❑ What might have improved the outcome?
- ❑ What problems does the doctor face in his future care of this couple?

SYMPTOMS AND CIRCUMSTANCES

If dangerous, mad behaviour is (fortunately) rare and containable (and in many cases, as above, just one episode in a life which afterwards may well return to normal), the usual presentations of distress in our society are very different, and often much less easy to typify or describe. One of the reasons, as we have seen, is that unhappiness and illness go hand in hand. Being ill makes us anxious; worrying can make us ill. So it is much more difficult to sift out from all those with symptoms which concern them enough to bring them to a doctor, the particular individuals whose main issue is psychological distress. Community surveys have suggested psychiatric morbidity rates from as little as 3.7 per cent to 65 per cent. It all depends how it is defined. What is clear is that at least one in ten consultations are overtly about psychological problems in most practices, and that the more a professional looks, the more is likely to be found. We can say with certainty what sort of symptoms should alert the doctor to psychological distress, but we cannot ever say that certain symptoms are always excluded. In other words, we could be sure that in some cases a person is distressed, but it is hard to be sure that they are not, given all the ways in which most cultures try to inhibit open expression of distress in general.

Symptoms have usually arisen from feelings, emotional states of one sort or another that medicine classes as **anxiety** or **depression**. Although these could be seen as increased or reduced arousal, in practice these states are often mixed and one may progress to the other: acute worries may produce long-term tension, which looks more and more like depression as the days pass and the feelings or circumstances persist (Fig. 5.1).

Anxiety may be easier to detect. It is usually episodic, and we are all aware of the likelihood of headaches (as in Case study 5.3) being possible signs – tension headaches – and of the symptoms of panic: a pounding heart, dry mouth, breathlessness, waves of nausea, sleeplessness or diarrhoea are all symptoms commonly associated with anxiety. Management of

the symptoms is half of the battle here, as their very presence is part of a vicious cycle which makes the person even more anxious because of secondary concerns – the dry mouth which makes public speaking impossible, the disgrace of public sickness or dashing to the lavatory, and so on. These help to persuade sufferers that there is something seriously amiss, adding further to anxiety levels. The second half of the battle is to get to the root of the anxiety.

CASE STUDY 5.13

A young woman presented with recurrent chest pain and wheezing which she insisted were due to a physical illness undetected by the doctors. Negative tests were initially of no avail in unravelling the problem, until she began to talk about her mother's illness from breast cancer, and she and the doctor were able to make the connection between her physical feelings and the unresolved grief she felt after having lost the person she had seen as both her greatest challenger and her greatest supporter. Once she was prepared to make the link and work on it, she abandoned her demands for further specialist referrals and agreed to work with a counsellor.

Thinking and Discussion Point

The challenge in Case study 5.13 was the patient's own decision that anxiety and grief were not 'real' symptoms, and that because she did have real symptoms the doctors must be missing something.

In observing other health professionals at work, note how they re-educate as well as diagnose. You should collect phrases and approaches that seem to you to help doctor and patient to reach an understanding. In dysfunctional or difficult consultations, what seems to make things go wrong?

The long-term management of people who tend to become anxious, are constitutionally 'highly strung' or who worry constantly about their health is perhaps less easy now than two or three decades ago, because of the current understanding of the hazards of most long-term

Symptom peaks

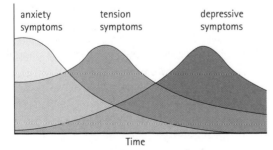

Figure 5.1 A typical symptom series for distress in primary care.

anxiolytic treatment. The psychopharmacology and physiology of anxiety make it very unlikely that a medication will be developed in the near future that reduces anxiety without in the long term running the risk of dependency, and of seriously disabling symptoms on withdrawal. This is one of the areas in which the prescriber runs great risk of doing more harm than good: it is not uncommon to find that the symptoms of an anxious person who has become dependent on tranquillizers and then withdraws remain permanently worse than the original symptoms.

CASE STUDY 5.14

A woman in her 40s who became sleepless and overwhelmingly anxious during the break-up of a violent marriage was put on benzodiazepine tranquillizers by her GP, which she used for several years until her life changed and she wanted to come off them. To her alarm, even the smallest reduction in dosage precipitated limb pains, chest pain and surges of panic. The psychological features eventually settled, but 3 years later she still suffers from persistent limb and chest pains.

Practical Exercise

❑ Review the psychoactive side effects of medications you see being prescribed regularly.
❑ Take every opportunity to ask patients whether they feel differently on medications, and whether they feel worse when they have come off them.

Dependency is the link between the relief obtained by socially accepted and available drugs such as nicotine or alcohol and medical or 'dangerous' street drugs such as barbiturates, tranquillizers and heroin. Although each may have a particular pattern, the withdrawal syndrome is often much the worst feature for the patient, and (as with barbiturates, for which tolerance levels are all-important) is potentially lethal.

The message for those treating anxiety is not to be pressed into unwise prescribing, even in the short term, and to look wherever possible

towards behavioural or lifestyle management methods which empower patients to deal with their own anxiety. Examples include relaxation tapes, yoga classes, behavioural treatment of phobias, exercise regimes etc.

Practical Exercise

Discover what treatment methods are available in your current clinical attachments, how they are administered and by whom. What can you learn from the patients you meet?

Depression is more difficult to detect but has more clear-cut treatment schedules, even if the best methods are disputed and outcomes still open to question. Like anxiety, headache and appetite loss may be pointers, but sleeplessness is classically described as waking early (whereas people who are anxious often have difficulty getting to sleep). Overwhelmingly the best way of making the diagnosis initially is simply to *think of it*. Doctors differ in their abilities to detect it, but this can be changed, at least in the short term, by training (Tylee et al., 1995). It seems that a lot of patients meet doctors who prefer to turn a blind eye, or are too busy, or who in some way cannot cope with what they see as being a painful or difficult assessment. This is perhaps excusable if the doctor is overworked, or even depressed: it is difficult to deal with a problem in someone else that one cannot cope with oneself. But much of this points to the failures in detection being due to failures in the detection instrument – the clinician.

Once the diagnosis has been made and accepted, the attitudes and aims of patient and clinician may determine how the illness is seen and treated: as a disease to be eradicated, at one extreme, or as an opportunity for reflection and change, at the other. Perhaps best results combine different approaches.

CASE STUDY 5.15

A young music publisher presented to a doctor about heavy drinking, but in assessment revealed that the drinking was happening to cover increasingly bleak moods and feelings of disappointment and disgust. After a programme of abstinence, he began on high levels of anti-depressant treatment with weekly counselling, and was able to confront the experiences of a bleak and intellectual childhood, and the way in which he 'set up relationships to fail'.

A different model for the causes and management of depression derives from the work of Professor George Brown and colleagues (Brown and Harris, 1978), examining the social origins of depression in women. A pattern emerges of a model in which a potentially vulnerable person, faced with a current crisis and losing or failing to gain a proper support system, may be unable to cope. The characteristics of the urban women in Brown's original studies that seemed associated with depression were:

■ poverty,
■ no job or outside interest,
■ low self-esteem,
■ no extended family,
■ no close confidante,
■ poor communication with spouse,
■ more than three young children at home,
■ death of mother in childhood,
■ death of a close relative or friend in the previous few months.

The interplay of personality, experience and relationships with lack of support or recent crisis has not been explored in every context, or with men, but rings true with clinical experience in primary care. Many patients describe a 'last straw' that makes life apparently intolerable or distress overwhelming, and such experiences, although important, often seem too minor to create the disturbance that has resulted unless attention is paid to the other issues that affect the patient. The aspect of current support at home or being in control of one's work in the working environment is insufficiently emphasized in some approaches. What the social model does is to reveal the interplay of factors, and this may be helpful to the observer in general practice when the patient appears more disturbed by a physical symptom than is appropriate or understandable. Figure 5.2 illustrates typical components that lead to major symptoms.

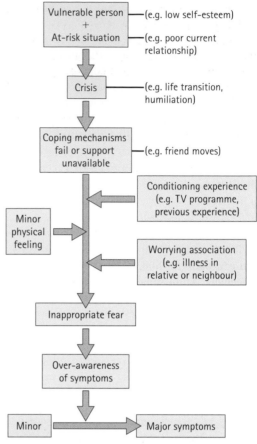

Figure 5.2 Typical components leading to major symptoms.

A recent review by Brown (1996) also suggests that severe events which seem to lead to depression may also include some of these other characteristics, such as a strong commitment by the person to the role involved in the event, an element of devaluation in one's own or someone else's eyes, the experience of defeat, a feeling of being trapped and a lack of sense of control. These are all part of changes or crises in interpersonal relationships, even if the precipitating event does not initially seem to be expressed in that way.

Severe depression used to be divided into these cases, called 'reactive', and an endogenous group of melancholic patients whose illness arises without obvious precipitant cause. Community studies show that these are in the minority (perhaps about 10 per cent), whereas they are over-represented in hospital settings.

In community epidemiological studies, the majority of patients who are depressed become so because of unpleasant events, which find them in a vulnerable state without support, and deprive them of important life goals.

CASE STUDY 5.16

Andrea was 42, and had been a single parent since her partner left her when their son was aged two. A capable and ambitious woman, she had juggled an administrative career with detailed care of her son's education. In the late primary school stage, it became clear that his poor performance was due to severe dyslexia, hitherto unrecognized. She fought the local education department for 18 months to obtain special education for him, and won a rare boarding placement. At the same time as he began his new school and left home for the first time, her work underwent reorganization and she was effectively demoted and placed in a position which appeared to be a career cul-de-sac. She became deeply depressed and was unable to return to work for 9 months.

WHO CAN HELP PROVIDE HELP AND HOW?

These different models suggest ways in which psychological disturbance can be managed in primary care. Prescribing issues are dealt with in detail elsewhere, but, particularly in depression, there is now agreement as to what constitutes good and safe prescribing, and this does not mean the use of medication without other approaches to reinforce positive and neutralize negative aspects of the situation. It also opens up the area for the work of those members of the team who have little or no ability to prescribe, but who nevertheless can be vital in management. A health visitor with a young family, a district nurse with an elderly couple, counsellors, groups and even reception staff all have a part to play, whether formal or informal.

The activities which may help the patient within the frameworks set out above include being able to explain and talk about the problem (ventilation), being given time to identify and clarify the main issues, being given 'permission' to express the distress (by crying, being angry etc.), and then being provided with a frame of reference, in terms of support or interpretation, to show the patient a new way of coping with apparently insurmountable problems or distress. There is dispute about the best forms of intervention here, and their effectiveness; but what can never be in dispute is that a human response as well as a pharmacological one is a moral and therapeutic necessity.

Transitions have been noted as points of particular vulnerability, and this seems easiest to understand because such change involves a life event or *loss*. The loss may be obvious, such as when a bereavement has occurred, or when a person becomes redundant, retires or gets divorced. However, even apparently happy events, such as the birth of the first baby or moving to a new home, may contain loss of freedom or intimacy between a couple in the first situation, and of familiar patterns, environment and friendships in the second. In addition, humiliation or a feeling of defeat or being trapped adds strongly to the experience of loss if the event or loss is severe.

Fears (anticipation of loss) may underlie and underline such losses. Everyone at some time has to confront fears of isolation or annihilation, but illness or depression can swiftly strip away the barriers people put up against such thoughts, even if the condition itself may be apparently minor. The simple question 'What are you most afraid of now?' may be what is needed to allow people the chance to express (and so confront and gain support in facing) a fear that is causing symptoms (Table 5.1).

SYSTEMS AND FRAMEWORKS

A way of thinking about personal development and its pitfalls which takes account of the way in which people interact with each other and their environment as part of normal human life may seem a long way from the idea of depression as a *disease*. Yet we accept the processes of ageing in arteries or in joints as medical conditions, even though it is the fortunate few who survive to old age without suffering from their effects. The boundary between the ill and the well is not so sharp. If this model suggests that

Table 5.1 Milestones and millstones of different age groups

Milestone problems in the under 5s
Parental anxieties
Rate of development of child (e.g. slow to speak, to walk, to grow)
Abnormalities in development or illness (e.g. clumsiness, sight/hearing problems, poor co-ordination, epileptic seizures, idiosyncratic talk)

Individual patient problems
Eating problems (food fads and refusal)
Sleep problems (disturbed sleep, insistence on sleeping with parents, nightmares)
Behaviour problems (over-clinging, dependent, shy child; tantrums when not getting own way; sibling jealousy)
Separation reactions such as after hospitalization
Fears (of the dark, of being left alone, of strangers, of large animals)
Difficulty in learning to share things, with friends and siblings, to wait one's turn

Milestone problems in children (6–12 years)
Parental separation (e.g. starting school)
School refusal
Enuresis
Encopresis
Social relationships: problems in making friends, shy, withdrawn, bullying or child abuse
Competitive problems: winning, losing, co-operating

Milestone problems of adolescence (12–20 years)

Personal problems	*Social problems*
Problems of sexual development (development earlier or later than peers, periods, sexual behaviour, promiscuity, 'bravado')	Problems adjusting to larger secondary school
Feelings of being different from others, an outsider, 'lost'	Influence of peers, desire to be like others and accepted by peers
Worries about the future (job, career etc.)	Smoking, drinking, glue sniffing, illegal drugs
Unplanned pregnancy, contraception	School refusal and truancy
Conflicts between wanting to be seen as an adult (and behave as such) and anxiety about whether capable of behaving as an adult	Antagonism with authority, parents, teachers, police
Crisis in self-confidence, wavering self-esteem, identity questions	Trying out new things, getting out of depth
Feelings of boredom, 'depression', restlessness, listlessness	Upsets with boyfriends/girlfriends
Expression of emotion by acting out (minor overdoses)	

Settling down: milestone problems of young adults (20–30 years)
Personal relationships
Problems with forming stable relationships
Adjustment to living away from home, setting up own home, reconciling ideals with reality
Anxieties about being left 'on the shelf'
Trying out different types of relationships, trying to find the 'right' person
Coping with over-protective or interfering parents

Table 5.1 (Continued)

Family relationships
Anxieties about birth of first child, being a parent and adjusting life to these responsibilities
Concerns about competence as parent
Financial and housing problems as family increases
Concerns about children and adjustment to permanent problems, e.g. child with learning difficulties
Post-natal reactions
Sexual problems, marital problems
Anxieties about fidelity
Fertility problems

The fourth decade: milestone problems of maturity
Coping with adolescent children, adjusting to their growing independence
Housewife's blues, 'tea and tranquillizers', disenchantment and boredom with mother role
Husbands feeling bored and trapped by responsibilities, job etc.
Problems of childlessness
Single-parent problems, practical and emotional problems, stress, loneliness, feeling rejected and unlovable
Women returning to work after long break

Milestone problems in middle age (40–60 years)
Mid-life crisis: 'What have I achieved? How many years have I left?'
Adjustment to menopause, anxieties about attractiveness
Illness anxieties, breast lumps, arthritis, heart attacks
Feelings of loss of role and purpose in life for mothers whose children have left home
Concern about ageing parents
Redundancy, fear of being useless, unable to find new work

Letting go: milestone problems of the elderly
Retirement
Failing physical health
Death of spouse and friends
Concerns about being dependent on others
Concerns about death – wish to die or fear of dying
Loneliness
Practical problems with financial problems, reduction of mobility
Fear of outside world, being attacked, robbed
Problems in understanding a rapidly changing outside world

Higgs (1983).

we are all potentially patients, then that may be a good reminder for doctors. But it also suggests the reverse: that apparent breakdown, or intense distress, may be a pathway to development or new understanding. Certain patterns of thought or behaviour may be signposts within a family group or a culture. Systemic thinking sees the way in which individuals are part of a structured group with particular ways of doing things or thinking, and suggests that these ways, usually supportive, can on occasions be unhelpful, or may help the doctor and patient to see why something is so much of a problem to an individual. Questions such as 'What would your mother have made of this?', 'What would your father have wanted you to do?', 'How would your relationship with X change if you got better?' may help someone to see the framework of their emotional life and begin to help them to challenge the destructive parts and be supported by the aspects which will enable them to make progress.

THE NARRATIVE APPROACH

All doctors in training are taught how to *take a history* from patients (see Chapters 3 and 7), but this may differ from the *story* a patient may want to tell. What has happened to patients, what they have done, thought about, wanted or planned, and how they react to the crises, excitements or disappointments in their lives so far may all be crucially important to their own mental or emotional state. It may be difficult for the doctor to make sense of the patient's presentation (and so even harder to provide an adequate response) without an understanding of some of these parts of a patient's story. Yet in all healthcare encounters time is short, so with the best will in the world doctors often find themselves firing questions at a patient when it is not clear what is going on. This may be because the doctor is afraid of losing control of the consultation if the patient heads off on a personal track, but in reality what the resort to closed questions often loses is just these details and insights that will help that doctor make sense of the presentation, and so help the patient to make sense of the problems in the context of his or her individual life. If the patient is frightened, confused or chaotic, a measure of control of the discussion may be vital, if offered in a sensitive and kind way, but getting the balance right is a key skill for professional practice. In most situations outside medicine when we are not sure what is going on, we keep quiet until we are, and that may be a more helpful way forward in primary care too. We have two obvious choices if we wish to do that: to give the patient the time he or she needs right now and accept the problems of running late, or to arrange a suitable time (and possibly longer) in the near future. There are advantages and disadvantages of each, but either way this work must to be done properly. Access and continuity in primary care are key issues. As stories unfold, it may become clear that others (such as partners or family members) may have another side to tell. The assessment and management of mental health care in general practice are often

provisional, iterative and on the move – more like driving a car through a big city than painting a picture. Also, we may not be the only drivers available. If it is clear that there is a long, deep and significant story that has to be told, it may be appropriate to refer to someone else in the primary care team – a counsellor, psychiatric nurse or other mental health specialist – or to the relevant agency in secondary care.

Learning about possible narratives will require us to think more broadly than just about medicine. In training, it will usually be very helpful to give yourself time to make a full assessment of some people. In our own lives, it will mean, too, that the things we enjoy in our spare time – soap operas, novels, plays, films or reading newspapers – will not only be a source of pleasure (although that's important enough) but also of insight into how people 'tick', and what sorts of things can cause distress or can help people to move on. In the process, it is crucial we understand our ownselves better.

EFFECTS ON THE PROFESSIONS: THE WAY FORWARD

So, in sum, several things can undeniably be said about clinical practice in primary care. One is that it is hard to limit demand, and to work to time, so that there may be few opportunities for a doctor to work as much at length or at depth with a patient as either would wish. The clinician has to develop ways of working at speed, of making assessments rapidly and taking imaginative shortcuts. The available resources to be expanded are the patient's own enthusiasm, skill and time (so that helping people to help themselves is a key aim of this type of medical practice), and the clinician's own intuitive understanding.

Most medical work turns a blind eye to the emotional aspects of the condition or its treatment. Primary care is largely where such feelings demand to be expressed, and where people will often bring distress or dread. A practitioner can either try to avoid recognizing the feeling that it is being brought, or can help to give it expression and shape. Either way, the emotion is there, and will affect the doctor as well. Every practitioner working in this field must develop ways of being able to deal with the effect of distressing emotions on himself or herself, within the doctor–patient relationship immediately, with colleagues, or outside the surgery (Higgs, 1994).

This can work the other way. As doctors, we can also be affected by the delight of a situation.

Tutor quote

Sometimes students do get emotionally affected by seeing patients. I was thinking of the pregnant mother. Often it is the first time that students have examined a pregnant woman. I think we underestimate the impact that has and I certainly have had one student who, after examining an abdomen, was in tears at the end of the couch. She said, 'I just thought it was so wonderful'. I was like that when I first delivered a baby.

Finally, few things point as clearly to the moral position we take, or values we hold, as our own and our profession's approach to psychological issues. We can reduce the people we meet to biomechanics, or defend ourselves from involvement with real life by prescribing medicines at every turn. But if we sincerely intend to do the best for our patients, to minimize harm to them, to increase their autonomy and their own control over their minds, bodies and lives, to help them become whole again, then we need to become skilled in detecting and managing distress in a way that expresses human values and recognizes potential as well as pathology in the people we meet.

SUMMARY POINTS

To conclude, the most important messages of this chapter are:

- in sorting and responding to psychological distress in primary care, account must be taken of all the issues that may influence the situation, relating to physical conditions, social circumstances, relationships, goals and values of both the patient and the system in which he or she lives and works;
- appropriate management of patients and of their presentation should include an understanding of what the professional brings, as well as what the patient brings;
- medication is only one aspect of management, and team care and self-care are vital to progress, recovery and prevention of future distress;
- listen to the story the patient may be trying to tell.

REFERENCES

Brown, G. 1996: Life events, loss and depressive disorders. In: Heller, T., Reynolds, J., Gomm, R., Muston, R. and Pattison, S. (eds). *Mental health matters: a reader*. Basingstoke: Macmillan/Open University, 1996, 36–45.

Brown, G. and Harris, T. 1978: *Social origins of depression*. London: Tavistock.

Higgs, R. 1983: *Psychosocial problems 1–4*. Modern Medicine Partworks. London: Heron.

Higgs, R. 1994: Doctors in crisis: creating a strategy for mental health in health care work. *Journal of the Royal College of Physicians, London* 28(6), 538–40.

Matthews, K., Milne, S. and Ashcroft, G.W. 1994: Role of doctors in the prevention of suicide: the final consultation. *British Journal of General Practice* 44(385), 345–8.

Tylee, A., Freeling, P., Kerry, S. and Burns, T. 1995: How does the content of consultations affect recognition by general practitioners of major depression in women? *British Journal of General Practice* 45(400), 575–8.

FURTHER READING

PRIMARY CARE

Elder, A. and Holmes, J. 2002: *Mental health in primary care – a new approach.* Oxford: Oxford University Press.

This brings together a primary and secondary care approach, of the kind outlined in this chapter.

Kendrick, T., Tylee, A. and Freeling, P. 1996: *The prevention of mental illness in primary care.* Cambridge: Cambridge University Press.

This book provides an outline of the important issue of the prevention of mental illness.

WHAT IT'S LIKE TO BE MENTALLY ILL

Barker, P., Campbell, P. and Davidson, B. (eds). 1999: *From the ashes of experience: reflections on madness, survival and growth.* London: Whurr Publishers.

Dunn, S., Morrison, B. and Roberts, M. 1996: *Mind reading: writer's journey through mental states.* London: Minerva.

Read, J. and Reynolds, J. (eds). 1996: *Speaking our minds: an anthology of personal experiences of mental distress and its consequences.* London: Open University/Macmillan.

The new Open University course on mental health also has a good series of interviews, as does the book cited above in the reference to Brown (1996).

Rogers, A., Pilgrim, D. and Lacey, R. 1993: *Experiencing psychiatry.* Basingstoke: Macmillan/MIND.

A challenging study of the views of people who have been seriously ill.

DIFFERENT WAYS OF LOOKING AT MENTAL HEALTH

The Open University has produced books under the heading *Mental health and distress: perspectives and practice*:

Module 1: *The contested nature of mental health*, 1997.

Module 2: *The social and ethical context of mental health*, 1997.

PSYCHIATRY

Goldberg, D., Benjamin, S. and Creed, F. 1994: *Psychiatry in medical practice.* London: Routledge.

A good introduction, but to standard secondary care only.

Oxford University Press publish both a *Shorter* textbook and the longer *New Oxford textbook*.

American Psychiatric Association 1994: *Diagnostic and statistical manual of mental disorders*, 4th edn (DSM-IV). Washington DC: American Psychiatric Association.

COMMUNICATING

Corney, R. 1991: *Developing communication and counselling skills in medicine.* London: Routledge.

This gives a collection of good writing about communicating with distressed people.

NARRATIVE MEDICINE

Brody, H. 1987: *Stories of sickness.* New Haven: Yale University Press.

Greenberg, M., Shergill, S.S., Szmukler, G. and Tantam, D. 2003: *Narratives in psychiatry.* London: Jessica Kingsley Publishers.

Narrative in a secondary care case format.

Greenhalgh, T. and Hurwitz, B. (eds). 1998: *Narrative-based medicine: dialogue and discourse in clinical practice.* London: BMJ Books.

An interesting series of essays, but see particularly the contributions of Launer, Elwyn and Gwyn, and Holmes.

Launer, J. 2002: *Narrative-based primary care.* Abingdon: Radcliffe Medical Press.

A broad introduction.

Skills are essential to general practice. History taking and physical examination are the cornerstones of the consultation and require good communication and examination skills for the satisfactory management of patients. The general practitioner is expected to be competent in a range of skills, the most important of which are explained in this chapter.

LEARNING OBJECTIVES

By the end of this chapter, in relation to each of the skills listed in the training plan below, you should:

- know what the skill entails;
- understand the basic science that underlies the skill;
- know the clinical indications for using the skill;
- know the key steps in performing the skill, having previously rehearsed the procedure on a model, a volunteer, or in your mind;
- be aware of the pitfalls or hazards of performing the skill, and know how these can be avoided;
- know your level of competence at performing each skill by asking your tutor or other professionally competent person to assess you;
- feel competent to practise the skill in a variety of clinical settings;
- know that you treat patients with courtesy and respect when performing a skill.

SKILLS AND PROFESSIONAL RESPONSIBILITIES

Examining ears, measuring blood pressure, giving injections, taking blood and syringing ears are all in a day's work for a general practitioner (GP). Some GPs extend their service to patients by acquiring more specialized skills, for example minor surgery, doing electrocardiograms (ECGs) or undertaking proctoscopy for examination of the rectum – procedures for which other patients would be referred to hospital. With busy work schedules in general practice, the management of patients is often shared with other members of the primary health care team such as the practice and community nurses. Although their training demands high standards in skills performance, GPs are responsible for ensuring competence in staff to whom work is delegated.

Training in clinical skills involves not only the acquisition of specific technical competencies but also the development of an appropriate professional approach. It is an opportunity to practise both the art and the science of medicine. Patients should feel reassured and confident in your ability before you use your skills: giving information about the procedure and why it needs to be undertaken, giving your patient an opportunity to ask questions and discuss anxieties and, finally, obtaining your patient's *informed consent*. The basis of practice is that patients should be actively involved in their care. You have a responsibility to patients to allow them the right to refuse examination and treatment. You also have a professional responsibility to ensure that you are competent in all procedures performed on patients, and that these competencies are maintained and updated throughout your professional career.

ACQUIRING NEW SKILLS

When you acquire a new skill you will be working through a set of learning objectives, practising until you feel confident, and then performing the skill in a clinical setting. Skills training is an opportunity for task-based learning. By revising and applying relevant basic science to the process, you will gain a deeper understanding of both the principles and the components of that skill. Being 'let loose' on a patient is a real incentive for some preparatory anatomy reading!

Begin by practising on a model, then transfer to the consulting room. The adage of 'see one, do one, teach one' has been superseded by 'prepare, practise, perform and perfect'. This cycle should be repeated until you are ready for your tutor to assess your competence at performing the skill. If you fail to achieve a satisfactory standard, you will be required to repeat the assessment. However disheartening this may be,

minimum standards of competence are important for the safe practice of medicine. Doctors are now required to have a satisfactory annual appraisal of their professional practice and performance in order to revalidate registration on the Medical List.

HOW TO USE THIS CHAPTER

The skills described in this chapter are grouped into three sections. The level of undergraduate training at which you would be expected to start performing the skill is indicated in brackets. However the timing will vary according to the medical training programme.

- Basic professional skills.
    How to behave professionally *(all years)*.
    How to ensure patient confidentiality *(all years)*.
    How to obtain informed consent *(all years)*.
    How to follow a code of conduct for patient examination *(all years)*.
- Skills used in clinical examination and diagnosis.
    How to take a pulse and blood pressure *(year 1)*.
    How to measure height and weight *(years 3, 4, 5)*.
    How to take a temperature *(year 1)*.
    How to examine an ear *(years 3, 4)*.
    How to use dipsticks *(years 2, 3)*.
    How to use a mini-peak flow meter *(years 2, 3)*.
- Skills used in clinical management and treatment.
    How to give an injection *(years 3, 4, 5)*.
    How to syringe an ear *(PRHO, GP registrar)*.
    How to take a blood sample *(year 3)*.
    How to write a prescription *(year 5, PRHO)*.
- Special communication skills.
    How to write a referral letter *(year 5, PRHO)*.
    How to consult with special age groups:
    – children *(year 4)*
    – elderly people *(years 3, 4)*
    – patients with limited or no English *(all years)*.
    How to do a home visit *(year 2)*.
    How to sign a death certificate *(year 5 [observe], PRHO, GP registrar)*.

For each skill, you are invited to work through an exercise. The instructions take you sequentially through the steps involved in performing the skill. Each exercise is designed for use as a self-directed learning tool away from your tutor. If you have the chance to observe a competent practitioner demonstrate a specific skill, take the opportunity. On completion of each exercise, it is essential for your tutor to check your technique and approach.

Each exercise has the following format:
1. clinical indications for using the skill,
2. background information on relevant basic science,
3. a list of equipment required,
4. an outline of the procedure, described step by step,
5. points of practice in which commonly encountered problems are highlighted,
6. a practical exercise or thinking and discussion point to help reinforce your learning.

At the beginning of the chapter there is a training plan that includes a list of procedures and space for recording dates when each skill has been attempted and assessed. It may be advantageous for your tutor to sign-up your competence here as a record of achievement.

QUESTIONS TO ASK BEFORE YOU START EACH SKILLS EXERCISE

■ *What background knowledge do you need?* What do you need to know in order to understand the procedure? Think of your basic science knowledge – the anatomy involved in examining an ear, the biochemistry underlying the measurement of blood sugar.

Have you any previous experience? Are you already confident enough or do you need to improve? If so, how? Whom should you ask for guidance?

■ *What are your learning objectives?* What are you aiming to do? How should you do it? What standard of practice is expected for minimum competence? When should you ask to be assessed?

■ *What equipment do you need?* Check out exactly what you need before you start. Get the equipment ready.

■ *How do you get started?* Arrange for a 'dummy-run', preferably on a model, or practise first on a volunteer member of the staff or a fellow student. When you feel sufficiently confident, ask your tutor to observe you demonstrate your skill before transferring to a patient.

■ *How do you persuade patients to let you practise on them?* Your tutor, or supervising member of the primary care team, will introduce you to a patient. Some simple non-invasive skills such as blood pressure measurement may be practised in the surgery without tutor supervision if you have the patient's permission. Common courtesies are implicit to professional practice. Always introduce yourself. Always explain what you intend to do before and during the procedure. Always offer to help patients who need help positioning themselves on the examination couch. Always thank your patients afterwards for their co-operation.

Tutor quote

There are many students who surprise me with their knowledge. It is also good to see when a student is actually caring about patients and I have had lots of students who show little caring touches like helping an old lady to get dressed or helping somebody with a backache off the couch rather than leaving them until they fall off. This somehow always helps me to spot those doctors I believe to be the caring doctors who won't leave the nurses to go behind them to tidy up the patient.

■ *How do you handle difficult questions?* Some patients will confront you with statements or questions that challenge your experience. For example, if you are asked 'Have you done this before? If not, I don't want to be your guinea-pig', you should be honest. Over-confidently telling a patient you have undertaken a procedure numerous times when you are a novice is a travesty of experience and is not to be recommended. If the circumstances feel uncomfortable, consult your tutor.

■ *How can you improve?* After performing a skill, ask for feedback from your patient and

Tutor quote

tutor. If you are out of your depth, do not feel too shy to ask for help. Try to keep calm throughout, even if you are having technical difficulties.

Tutor quote

I remember a student who was terribly anxious about examining patients, to the extent that she was worse than I was when I took my first blood test. She was getting trembly and sweaty and I only realized when I watched her taking a blood pressure that she couldn't really do it. We went through it and in the end we simplified things right down to the point where she just sat with me and checked patients' pulses until she felt calm about holding people's hands and touching people, and that always struck me as being such a small bit of learning in terms of learning but so important as a hurdle to get over.

- *How do you know when you are competent?* When you have been assessed as performing satisfactorily by your tutor. Your tutor can help you to develop and improve your skills by:
- arranging equipment, suitable patients, and space to practise,
- supervising you,
- advising about correct techniques,
- monitoring your progress,
- checking your competence,
- signing your personal training plan/skills record (see later in this chapter),
- giving you feedback from the patient.

Tutor quote

Students with confidence ... they can do everything ... no problem ... 'Taking blood ... leave it to me ... I'll take the blood on this patient'. After a few minutes, I pop back to see how the student is getting on and I am horrified to see that there is blood all over the place. They have done the whole thing wrong: they have kept the tourniquet on with the needle out ... blood everywhere ... student not wearing gloves ... a good example of how tutors should make sure to supervise ... somebody should be watching the student.

BASIC PROFESSIONAL SKILLS

Throughout your medical career both as a student and a qualified doctor, you should aim to have good relationships with your patients and colleagues. This is essential for professional practice. You should:

- always treat patients with politeness and consideration,
- involve patients in decisions about their care,
- show respect for patients and colleagues without prejudice for background, language, culture and way of life,
- recognize the rights of patients, particularly with regard to *confidentiality* and *informed consent*.

HOW TO MAINTAIN PATIENT CONFIDENTIALITY AND OBTAIN INFORMED CONSENT

Background

Throughout your medical studies and career, you will have access to private and sensitive information about patients. Personal details will be shared with you in total confidence on the understanding that information will not be divulged to others except for the purposes of teaching and to other members of the health team who are involved in your patient's care. Patients have a right to expect that you will not pass on confidential information without their consent (General Medical Council, 2003a).

- Confidentiality is central to the trust between patients and doctors.
- Confidential information includes all personal details and data disclosed verbally, in writing or on computer.
- Confidential information may be used for teaching but must be *anonymized*. This means that all personal details have been removed from clinical notes, written and oral presentations and project work.
- Confidentiality should be maintained for all time, even after a patient's death.

Practical advice

When you wish to gain access to patient notes in the surgery, you must work directly from the clinical notes and not photocopy sections.

- Information removed from the surgery for study purposes must be anonymized and secured in a case or folder.
- If you photograph patients for projects, you must obtain their consent, and cover the eyes if used for presentation or publication.
- You must not discuss any patient's personal or clinical details in a public place where confidential information can be overheard. Remember:
- every patient has a right to confidentiality,
- every student has an obligation to respect that right,
- breaching confidentiality is a disciplinary offence.

Informed consent

Background

Before you examine, treat or care for competent adult patients, you must obtain their consent. Adults include all persons aged over 16 years. Consent must be given voluntarily and not under pressure from others. Consent may be written, oral or non-verbal. Children who fully understand what is involved in the proposed procedure can also give consent, although ideally their parents should be involved (General Medical Council, 2003b).

How to obtain informed consent from a patient

- Before you take a history or examine a patient, you should first obtain permission to do so from your tutor or supervisor.
- Introduce yourself to your patient by your full name, explaining that you are a student, stating your course and where you are studying. Explain your intentions – whether you wish to take a history, make an examination or carry out a procedure. Explain what is involved and the reason for doing it. Check that your patient understands. Offer an opportunity for questions and discussion. Assure your patient of confidentiality and anonymity. Ask your patient if he or she agrees that you may proceed. You should explain that a patient has the right to decline examination, and that this will not affect their management.

Consent for student undertaking an intimate examination of patient

- If examination involves an intimate area of the body, for example the breasts, genitalia, vagina or rectum, in addition to obtaining verbal consent as described above, you should make a record in the patient's notes of your examination and findings, and sign it and date it, recording that consent was given.
- You must examine in the presence of your supervisor and have a chaperone if advised.

Consent for student undertaking a surgical procedure or an invasive examination on a patient

- It may be the policy at your medical school that students obtain a patient's written consent before making an invasive examination of the body such as rectal or vaginal examination. If this is the case, ask your patient to sign and date a statement outlining the procedure to be undertaken or use an official consent form. This should be countersigned by your tutor, and filed in the patient's clinical notes.

HOW TO EXAMINE PATIENTS: FOLLOWING A CODE OF PRACTICE

Patient consultations in general practice tend to take place in more relaxed surroundings than in hospitals. Most GPs and practice nurses do not wear white coats or uniforms. Patients appreciate the informality of general practice. It encourages good rapport between patients and staff and facilitates patient-centred consultations. However, it is important that the patient–doctor relationship is maintained within professional boundaries. The informality of general practice places staff at risk of over-familiarity with patients and, exceptionally, this leads to misinterpretation of the professional doctor–patient relationship. Both students and staff should be cautious about creating ambiguous situations in which allegations of improper behaviour might arise. To avoid this, it is essential that all healthcare staff follow a code of conduct in clinical settings to ensure sound professional practice.

Being a student in general practice

- You should wear an identity badge prominently displayed at all times. You should check the accepted dress code with your GP tutor or trainer before starting the placement.
- You should be a member of a medical defence union. At most medical schools this is compulsory. Once qualified, you cannot be employed without membership of a medical defence union.

Consulting with patients in the surgery

- Dress appropriately for meeting and/or being seen by patients. Your tutor will help you.
- As a student, you should always obtain permission from a doctor or nurse before taking a history or examining a patient.
- Privacy is essential. When taking a history from a patient, conversations should not be overheard.
- The seating arrangement in the consulting room is important. It is preferable for the patient to be seated to the side of or at an angle to the doctor's chair rather than directly opposite and separated by the desk in a confrontational way (Fig. 6.1).
- Using computers: patients prefer to see the screen so that they can observe data entry, even if this means turning with your back to the patient while you use the computer. Introduce yourself to the patient by name and status. Explain that you are a medical student and where you are studying. A student should never pose as a doctor. A PRHO or registrar should explain that they are training in the practice.
- Non-verbal behaviour reveals much about you. Maintain eye-to eye contact throughout the consultation. Looking away momentarily is acceptable, but always refocus on the patient's face, even if not reciprocated. Encourage your patient to talk in response to questions. Listen attentively, indicating that you are hearing, such as a nod of the head, by murmuring or by facial expression. Smiling or showing surprise in response to appropriate conversation is interactive. Ensure your body is relaxed, particularly your arms, which

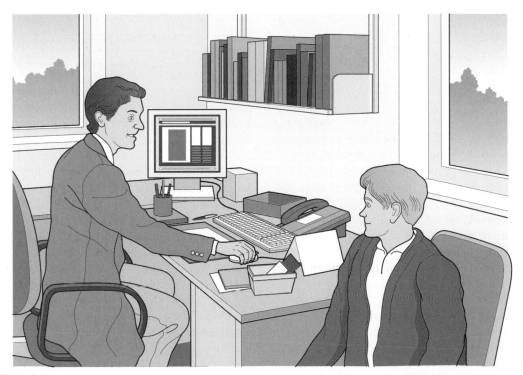

Figure 6.1 Recommended seating in a GP consulting room showing doctor and patient. Reprinted from MacLeod, 1983.

are best held open on your lap. Sitting forward, learning on your desk or folding your arms across your chest suggests aggression and is not conducive to open conversation.

- Avoid interrupting the patient's history until there is a natural pause. If patients talk incessantly or ramble, you may need to interrupt and summarize the salient points in the history to refocus the consultation.
- Keep discussion relevant. Avoid making personal or humorous comments about your patient and using terms of endearment. It is unprofessional to refer to your own personal circumstances for illustrative purposes, however tempting. Rather, phrase any personal experience in the context of a third person.
- Avoid writing notes or inputting data on the computer while your patient is talking.

Examining patients and professional etiquette

- Your patient should be allowed privacy to undress and dress. You should explain which garments should be removed and where they should be placed. You should draw the curtains around the patient and not observe the patient undressing.
- The examination couch must be covered by clean paper.
- Ask your patient to let you know when he or she is ready for examination. Minimize patient exposure by providing a cover for exposed parts of the body when not being examined. You should avoid examining patients underneath their garments.
- Keep discussion relevant to the examination.
- If your patient is uncomfortable, distressed or aroused, withdraws consent, makes inappropriate remarks or you feel ill at ease, discontinue the examination.
- After the examination is completed, assist the patient off the couch and ask them to dress.
- Explain your examination findings to your patient, and thank them for their co-operation.
- Ensure that the examination couch has a clean cover for the next patient.

When should you use a chaperone?

If you make an examination of a patient that involves an intimate body area such as the genitalia, rectum or female breasts, the patient should be offered a chaperone. This is essential if the examiner is of the opposite sex to the patient. In general practice, it may be difficult to find someone who can act as chaperone. In this case, one possibility is to offer an examination at a later time when the patient can return with a friend or relative as chaperone, or to offer the patient the option of being examined by a doctor of the same sex. Surveys have shown that adults of both sexes would prefer a nurse as chaperone and teenagers would prefer a parent. As a medical student, your chaperone could be your tutor or other member of staff, or another student, preferably of the same sex as the patient.

- Do not examine an intimate body area of a patient unnecessarily. This may be misinterpreted.
- If you are a chaperone, you should stand unobtrusively to one side of the couch. If you have concerns, you should tactfully discuss them with the examining student or doctor.
- If the patient asks for a chaperone and no one is available, it is preferable to postpone the examination rather than to place yourself at risk.

SKILLS USED IN CLINICAL EXAMINATION AND DIAGNOSIS

HOW TO TAKE A RADIAL PULSE

Taking an arterial pulse is one of the most fundamental skills in medical practice and is used in the baseline monitoring of a patient's clinical condition. You will be introduced to this skill in the first year of the undergraduate course. The arterial pulse can be measured at any anatomical site where a main artery runs close to the body surface and is accessible to palpation. These points include the carotid, brachial, radial, femoral, popliteal, posterior tibial and dorsalis pedis arteries. The pulse most routinely taken is the radial pulse because of its accessibility.

Background knowledge: the physiology of pulse measurement

When the left ventricle of the heart contracts, a column of arterial blood is ejected into the aorta and a pulse wave is transmitted into the arterial system. This pulse wave takes between 0.2 and 0.5 seconds to reach the feet, although the speed of the column of blood is about ten times slower. The form of the pulse wave is determined by the quantity of blood ejected into the aorta, the speed of ejection and the elasticity of the arterial wall.

The arterial pulse has four characteristics: rate, rhythm, volume and form. These are most accurately assessed in the main pulses that are closest to the heart i.e. the carotid, the brachial and the femoral pulses. The normal pulse rate in an adult is around 60–85 beats per minute. A rapid pulse, or tachycardia, is a pulse rate of 100 beats or more per minute. A slow pulse, or bradycardia, is one of less than 60 beats per minute. The pulse rhythm is the degree of regularity of the pulse. The pulse should be regular, although there may be a noticeable variation with respiration, known as sinus arrhythmia, in which the rate increases with inspiration and slows with expiration. A pulse is reported as regular or irregular. An irregular pulse is described as regularly irregular, for example when there are extra or ectopic beats, or irregularly irregular, as in atrial fibrillation when some ventricular contractions are too weak to be transmitted to the radial pulse. Pulse volume is difficult to assess at the radial pulse. However, a low-volume pulse can be described as 'weak', while a high-volume pulse can be described as 'bounding'. Peripheral pulse characteristics are modified by the properties of the arteries, as in arterial narrowing. Pulse form is a description of the character of the pulse wave, i.e. whether the wave is slow to rise, as in stenosis (narrowing) of the aorta, or falls rapidly, when it is known as a collapsing pulse, as in regurgitation of blood in the aorta.

Procedure for taking a radial pulse

■ A radial pulse is measured with the second, third and fourth fingers. The thumb should not used because pulsation in the thumb may be confused for the patient's radial pulse and lead to an inaccurate reading. This is less of a problem for stronger pulses such as the femoral and carotid.

■ Ask your patient to rest his or her forearm on a surface with the palm of the hand uppermost. The arm may be supported with your own hand.

■ Feel the patient's radial pulse along the outer border of the wrist by placing the three middle fingers along the length of the forearm.

■ The rate is measured with the second hand of a watch by counting the pulse beats in a defined period – usually 15 seconds – and multiplying (in this case by 4) to give the pulse rate per minute. If the patient has an irregular pulse, you should count the rate over 1 minute for greater accuracy, although measurement by auscultation will be more precise.

Practical points

■ Use a watch with a second hand for clinical teaching and examinations, otherwise you cannot take an accurate pulse measurement and risk failing a clinical examination.

■ Take the radial pulses on both sides of the body (Fig. 6.2). It is good practice to compare the two simultaneously, as weakness or delay in one will give a clue about arterial disease such as artery narrowing or blockage.

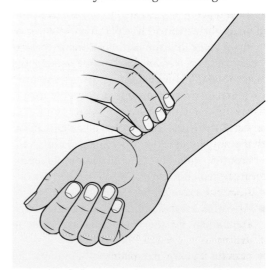

Figure 6.2 Method for palpating the radial pulse. Reprinted from John MacLeod, *Clinical examination: a textbook for students and doctors by teachers of the Edinburgh Medical School,* © 1983 Elsevier Ltd, with permission from Elsevier.

Tutor quote

A tutor was examining third-year students in an OSCE (Objective Structured Clinical Examination). The candidate was fashionably dressed in designer gear. The first question required the student to take the patient's pulse. The student looked at the watch and then at the examiner and exclaimed, 'I can't; my watch has no second hand!' The student scored no marks and failed. Fortunately for the student, the OSCE was an end-of-term formative assessment and not the final qualifying examination. Students cannot undertake full examination of patients in clinical practice without a practically designed watch.

HOW TO MEASURE BLOOD PRESSURE

This is one of the most commonly performed procedures. You may start blood pressure measurement in the early years of the medical course in physiology class or in the clinical setting. By the third year, you will be expected to measure blood pressure routinely on patients. Several methods are in use for blood pressure measurement, each with advantages and disadvantages, and levels of accuracy. The most familiar are the mercury column and the aneroid sphygmomanometers that require auscultation. The newer automatic devices use oscillatory methods. The mercury devices may be withdrawn because of fears of environmental mercury toxicity, and so you should prepare for this by becoming familiar with the different methods. Equipment varies from practice to practice and from country to country. In the UK, equipment should satisfy the stringent standards set by the British Hypertension Society (1999).

Common indications for blood pressure measurement include:

- screening at well-person checks,
- assessing fitness for employment or insurance acceptance,
- diagnosing hypertension,
- monitoring treated hypertension,
- monitoring high/normal or high readings in untreated patients.

Because a diagnosis of hypertension has life-long implications, it is important to measure it as accurately as possible. The instrument should have its accuracy validated and be correctly maintained and calibrated. It is recommended practice to measure and report blood pressure after a patient has been resting for 10–15 minutes. Your patient should have been sitting in the waiting room for about 10 minutes rather than rushing in off the street before the blood pressure is measured. If the blood pressure is raised at the start of the consultation, the reading should be repeated after several minutes.

A minimum of two measurements should be taken at each visit. Initially it seems complex in terms of co-ordination, but becomes straightforward with practice.

Background knowledge: anatomy and physiology of blood pressure measurement

All methods are based on the blood pressure changes that arise from compression of the brachial or radial artery to that above the systolic pressure and from decompression to that below the diastolic pressure (Figs 6.3–6.6). The pressure is applied using a cuff that encircles the arm and causes compression of the brachial artery. Digital wrist models compress the radial artery.

Systolic blood pressure is indicated by a tapping sound that originates in the artery distal to (away from the centre of the body) the cuff as

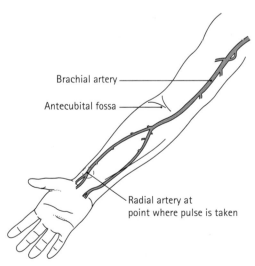

Brachial artery

Antecubital fossa

Radial artery at point where pulse is taken

Figure 6.3 Positions of the brachial and radial arteries in relation to surface markings (anterior view).

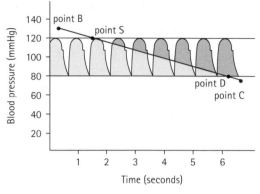

point S = systolic pressure
point D = diastolic pressure
⟍ = blood pressure in the cuff

Figure 6.4 The effect of falling pressure in the sphygmomanometer on the arterial blood pressure. Consider that the arterial blood pressure is being measured in a patient whose blood pressure is 120/80 mmHg. The pressure (represented by the oblique line) in a cuff around the patient's arm is allowed to fall from greater than 120 mmHg (point B) to below 80 mmHg (point C) in about 6 seconds.

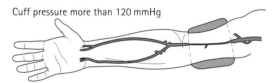

Figure 6.5 The effect of increasing the pressure in the sphygmomanometer above that in the brachial artery. When the cuff pressure exceeds the systolic arterial pressure (120 mmHg), no blood progresses through the arterial segment under the cuff, and no sounds can be detected by a stethoscope bell placed on the arm distal to the cuff.

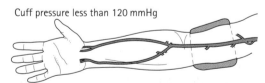

Figure 6.6 The effect of reducing the pressure in the sphygmomanometer below the diastolic artery pressure. When the cuff pressure falls below the diastolic arterial pressure, blood flow is restored to the brachial artery, arterial flow past the region of the cuff is continuous, and no sounds are audible. When the cuff pressure is between 120 and 80 mmHg, spurts of blood traverse the artery segment under the cuff with each heartbeat, and the Korotkoff sounds are heard through the stethoscope.

the cuff pressure falls below the peak arterial pressure. This allows blood to spurt into the compressed artery. **Diastolic blood pressure** is defined as the point at which sounds disappear as the cuff pressure falls below the minimum arterial pressure. This allows blood flow to become continuous.

Oscillatory methods

Oscillatory methods are used in automatic devices. They are based on the principle that blood flowing through an artery between systolic and diastolic pressures causes vibrations in the arterial wall that are transmitted to the air in the cuff. These are detected and transduced into electrical signals to produce a digital readout. Newer models use 'fuzzy logic' to decide how much the device should be inflated to start readings at about 20 mmHg above the patient's systolic pressure. Deflation of the cuff is automatic and occurs at a rate of about 4 mmHg per second. Oscillatory methods may seem slower than the auscultatory methods but are more accurate.

What you will need

- a sphygmomanometer of the standard mercury in glass type,
- an arm cuff with connecting tubing attached to a rubber bulb and to the sphygmomanometer,
- a stethoscope.

About the equipment

- A sphygmomanometer consists of a mercury manometer with a vertical scale, an inextensible cuff containing an inflatable bladder, rubber tubing, pump and control valve (Fig. 6.7).
- The manometer scale is indicated in millimetres of mercury (mmHg), from 0 to 260 in units of 10 mm. The manometer should be read from a distance within 1 metre, with your eye on a level with the meniscus (see Fig. 6.7). Conventionally, the reading is recorded to the nearest 2 or 5 mmHg. Recent guidelines recommend that it should be to the nearest 2 mmHg.
- Cuffs are of two types: one with a Velcro fastening, and another that is tapered and wraps

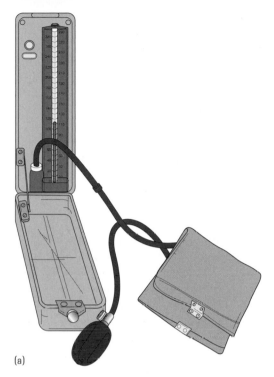

(a)

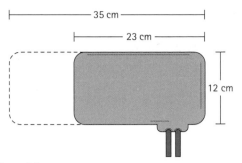

Figure 6.8 Diagram to show the dimensions of a sphygmomanometer cuff suitable for an arm circumference less than 33 cm.

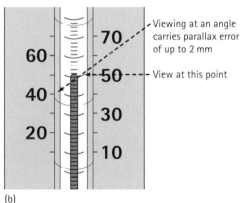

(b)

Figure 6.7 (a) A mercury sphygmomanometer. (b) Close-up of a manometer tube to show the scale.

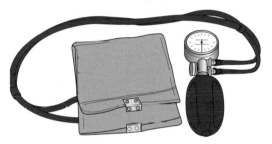

Figure 6.9 An aneroid sphygmomanometer.

around the arm, with the end of the cuff tucking under the encircling cuff. Cuffs are available in different sizes (Fig. 6.8). Each consists of a cloth and an enclosed inflatable bladder. The bladder should completely encircle the arm. If it does not, the cuff should be changed for a larger size. The recommended bladder width is 20 per cent greater than the diameter of the limb at the point where the cuff is applied. For an obese patient, you should use a larger cuff, and for a child, a smaller paediatric model. The cuff is changed by detaching the interconnector and replacing it with an appropriately sized cuff.

- Another type of sphygmomanometer is the aneroid model, which has a cuff and a pressure gauge. It is less accurate and less cumbersome than the upright model, and is easier to carry in an emergency on-call case (Fig. 6.9).

Procedure (Fig. 6.10)

- Allow your patient to rest for at least 10 minutes before taking the blood pressure.
- Explain the procedure and the reason for taking the blood pressure. If this is the first time your patient has had a blood pressure measurement, explain that inflating an arm cuff to a high pressure may feel slightly uncomfortable.
- Your patient should be seated with his or her arm at heart level. Select the arm closest to a supporting surface for measurement. Ideally,

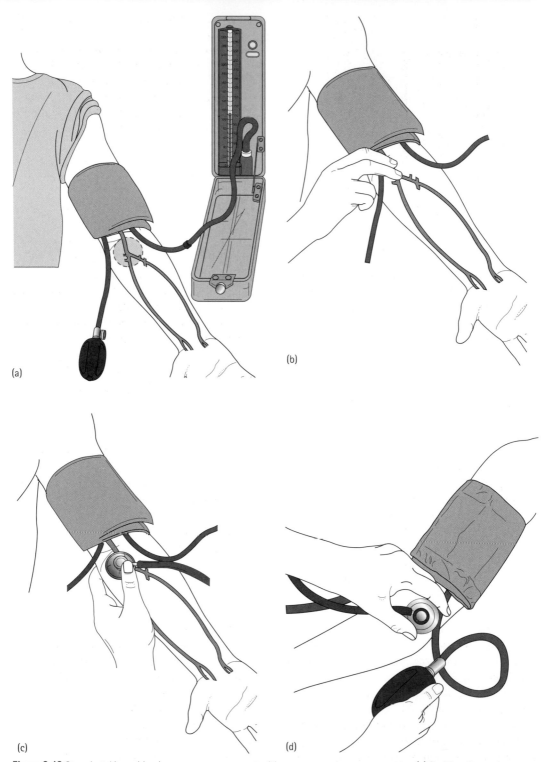

Figure 6.10 Steps in taking a blood pressure measurement with a mercury sphygmomanometer. (a) Position the equipment and cuff (anterior view). (b) Identify the brachial artery. (c) Place the stethoscope over the brachial artery. (d) Inflate the cuff to a level exceeding the pressure in the artery, as shown in (e).

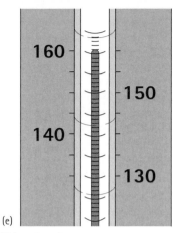

(e)

Figure 6.10 (*continued*).

all clothing should be removed from the arm. In reality, with the short consultation time in general practice, you will observe patients push (pull) the sleeve to just below the shoulder. You should check that the sleeve does not constrict the arm and that there is sufficient space distal to the encircling cuff for the stethoscope to be placed in the antecubital fossa without touching the cuff. For training purposes, the patient should remove the upper garment and rest the arm on a surface with the elbow slightly flexed and the palm of the hand uppermost.

- Wrap the cuff around the arm above the elbow, with the lettering on the cuff outermost. With an older model, the bladder is placed between the cuff and the skin over the brachial artery. This position is indicated by an arrow on the outside of modern cuffs. It is conventional to position the rubber tubes distal to the cuff, although if positioned proximal to the cuff (towards the centre of the body), it is easier to place the diaphragm of the stethoscope in the antecubital fossa.

- Open the manometer box with the mercury column vertically placed and facing you, with the middle of the scale, from 180 mm to 60 mm, at eye level. Check that the mercury meniscus reads zero. If not, report this and change your instrument.

- Locate the radial pulse over the lateral aspect (outermost) of the wrist using the index and middle fingers – not your thumb as this will

transmit your own pulse. To gain an approximate idea of the systolic pressure, close the valve where the bulb and tubing connect by turning the screw away from you. Inflate the cuff by repeatedly squeezing the rubber bulb. As you inflate, you will notice that the radial pulse disappears and that if you continue to inflate by about 20–30 mm above this pressure, then deflate, the radial pulse will reappear. This pressure indicates the approximate systolic pressure. Now deflate the cuff.

- Locate the brachial artery in the antecubital fossa by palpating around the medial (inner) part of the elbow crease (Fig. 6.10, a and b). Sitting opposite and slightly to the side of the patient, place your stethoscope in your ears and place the diaphragm over the brachial artery (Fig. 6.10c), steadying it with your thumb or a finger. While listening with your stethoscope, inflate the cuff to a level exceeding the pressure in the artery (Fig. 6.10, d and e). At this point you will not hear any sounds.

- Release the pressure in the bulb by turning the control valve slowly, aiming to achieve a fall in the mercury level at a constant rate of 2–3 mm for each heart beat. The column may fall jerkily until you have learnt to control the valve evenly. You will hear faint tapping sounds as the pressure falls. These are known as the **Korotkoff** sounds, named after the Russian surgeon from St Petersburg who first described them in 1905 (Fig. 6.11). Note the mercury reading at the point at which the sounds appear. This is the **systolic** blood pressure (**phase 1**).

- As the cuff pressure falls, you may notice a softening of the sounds (**phase 2**), which then become sharper again as the pressure continues to fall (**phase 3**), then more muffled (**phase 4**) and, finally, disappear (**phase 5**). The phases are very variable, with sometimes only phases 1 and 5 being distinctive. The point of complete disappearance of the sounds (phase 5) is defined as the **diastolic** pressure. There is less inter-observer error with phase-5 recordings.

- Record both the systolic (phase 1) and the diastolic (phase 5) pressures, writing systolic over diastolic, e.g. 120/80, recording to the

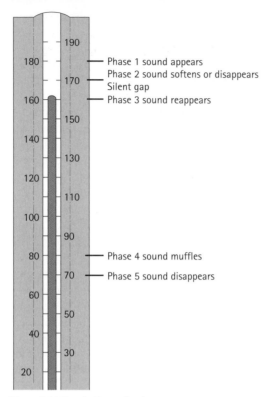

Figure 6.11 Korotkoff sounds, phases 1–5.

nearest 2 mm. For example, readings of 179 systolic over 143 diastolic would be written as 178/142. The blood pressure fluctuates around a mean that is individual for each patient. The mean varies with time and other factors such as the patient's position and degree of relaxation. Fastidiously recording to the nearest 1 mm suggests an accuracy that is misleading.

■ Recheck the readings at least twice. If the blood pressure exceeds 140/95 mmHg, repeat in the other arm and again after a further 5–10 minutes. Because the reading may have been taken at the maximum point in the patient's blood pressure range, the pressure should be checked on at least three separate occasions over a period of time of not less than 1 month before a firm diagnosis of hypertension is made.

You may find it helpful to watch a video or CD ROM recording of how to take a blood pressure (British Hypertension Society, 1999) or to do some further reading (e.g. Beevers et al., 2000).

Practical points

■ Use the correct cuff size. If the arm is too large for the cuff, use a larger size cuff.
■ The meniscus should be read at eye level.
■ Inflate the mercury column above the systolic by at least 30 mmHg to avoid taking the phase 3 sound as the systolic and thereby under-recording the blood pressure.
■ Readings should be taken with the mercury level *falling*, not rising, recording the systolic pressure first and then the diastolic pressure.
■ All bulbs leak slightly, but if the leakage prevents you from halting the mercury column as it falls, the pressure will be underestimated. Report the instrument as faulty and use another.

If the arm is unsupported, you will obtain a falsely high reading.

Oscillatory blood pressure devices

There are many different models (Fig. 6.12). They are battery driven, have automatic inflation and deflation with oscillometric precision measurement, and have display windows for blood pressure and pulse readings. Most have a memory recall facility for up to 14 readings.

Procedure

■ Wrap the cuff around your patient's upper arm, and secure the Velcro fastening.
■ Switch on the start button on the front of the machine and allow the cuff to inflate automatically until it reaches maximum pressure. The pressure will automatically deflate until the blood flows smoothly through the artery in the usual pulses without any vibration in the artery wall.
■ Take the reading from the digital display on the display panel that gives the systolic and the diastolic readings. The pulse rate may also be displayed.
■ Switch off the machine after completing the measurement to conserve the batteries.

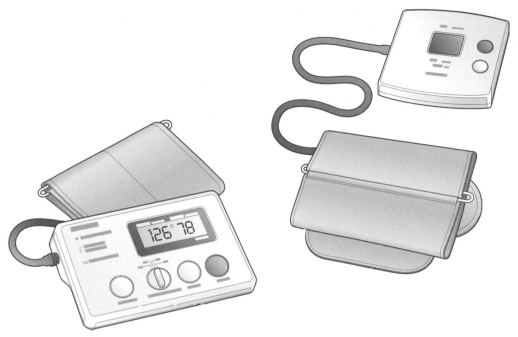

Figure 6.12 Oscillatory sphygmomanometers.

Practical Exercise

☐ Take blood pressure readings on a series of patients and record the Korotkoff phases for each of them. You may not hear them all. What effect will changing the cuff size have? Investigate the difference of the cuff size on the readings. Record the pressures using different cuff sizes.

☐ Take the blood pressures of patients of different ages, shapes and sizes. Do you notice any association of blood pressure with (a) age and (b) weight?

☐ Take blood pressure readings on the same patient, varying the position of the patient's arm, for example with the arm held horizontally unsupported, horizontally with support, in the overhead and dependent positions. Do you notice any differences?

☐ Take readings with the patient in the following positions: standing, sitting on a chair, lying supine (on the back), sitting on an examination couch with legs horizontal. Are there any differences?

☐ Investigate the effect of exercise and rest on blood pressure. Ask a patient to run up and down stairs several times and measure the pressure immediately after stopping, then every 2–3 minutes for 10 minutes. What do you notice happening to the readings, particularly the systolic? Now you can understand why you record pressure after a patient has been sitting still for at least 10 minutes!

☐ Find a patient with an irregular pulse, for example with atrial fibrillation. What effect does this have on serial recordings of blood pressure?

HOW TO WEIGH AND MEASURE A PATIENT

Background knowledge

Adult weight and height measurements are used for a number of reasons, including the long-term monitoring of weight in obesity, the recovery from illness when under-nutrition may be problem, and the assessment of growth in young adults. In general practice, weight measurements are most commonly used for monitoring obesity in adults. Babies and infants are weighed regularly by health visitors in order to monitor their growth and nutrition.

The relationship between weight and height is expressed as an index, the **body mass index (BMI)**. It is calculated by dividing the patient's weight in kilograms by the square of their height in metres:

$$BMI = \frac{weight\ (kg)}{height\ (m)^2}$$

The BMI is equally applicable to men and women. It is used with a set of charts and nomograms for adults (Fig. 6.13); there is a different

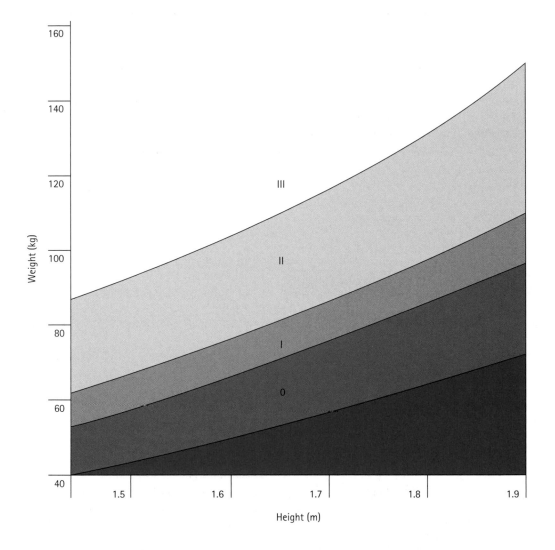

Grade	BMI	Classification
0	19–25	Normal range of weight
1	26–29	Overweight
11	30–39	Obesity
111	40 and over	Severe obesity

Figure 6.13 Use of the body mass index to show grades of obesity.

set for children. Apart from a few muscular individuals who may be wrongly classified as overweight, the BMI is a robust measurement index. Its categories are used to indicate whether weight is in the ideal range of 18.5–24.9 kg/m², is underweight, i.e. <18.5 kg/m², overweight or obese, i.e. >25 kg/m². The overweight category is further subdivided into: pre-obese class 1, 25–29.9 kg/m²; obese class I, 30.0–34.9 kg/m²; obese class II, 35–39.9 kg/m²; and obese class III, >40 kg/m².

Estimates suggest that most adults in England have a BMI above the 'normal' range and that a fifth are obese, with a BMI that exceeds 30 kg/m². As obesity is a risk factor for life-threatening medical conditions, weight is monitored as part of a weight management programme.

Procedure

Practical points

- A patient should be weighed and measured if possible on the same set of scales to allow comparisons over time. Readings on home or hospital scales cannot be compared with surgery or clinic readings because of differing sensitivities.
- A patient should be weighed each time wearing approximately similar garments, i.e. with or without coat or shoes. Although the most accurate comparisons would be made if weighed nude or in underclothes, this is not practicable in the surgery!
- Height should be measured with the patient in stockinged feet for greater accuracy, as shoe heels vary.
- Measurements should be read and recorded in the metric system. Despite the official change from avoirdupois to the metric system, patients continue to ask for a conversion to old units.
- If there is a choice of scales, a digital system is preferred because the facility of adjusting the reading to zero between readings leads to greater accuracy. Digital models also allow automatic conversion to the avoirdupois system that is quicker than referring to conversion charts. All machines should be checked annually for accuracy.

HOW TO TAKE A TEMPERATURE

The normal body temperature extends over a range of values that varies by the site of measurement, by individual and by time of day (Table 6.1). A temperature below the normal range is classified as **hypothermia**, i.e. below 35 °C. An abnormally raised temperature is defined as **pyrexia** and is above 37.5 °C. Although the body temperature can be estimated crudely by palpation, it is more accurately measured using a clinical thermometer.

The following methods are described.

1. *Palpation.* Body surface temperature can be measured with the back of the hand or fingers to give a crude estimation of local temperature as long as your hand is not cold. This method will detect a local rise in temperature and may offer a clue to underlying pathology that indicates increased blood flow to the area. This occurs with local inflammation, as with a skin infection, or increased blood flow in tumours. It will also detect local body cooling in comparison with the opposite side of the body. In a limb this may suggest arterial occlusion.

   In everyday practice, you may notice a clinician estimating body temperature by placing a hand on a patient's forehead and pronouncing a fever to be present. Such a crude method is unreliable. Body temperature is measured more accurately with a thermometer, several models of which are available, as described below:

2. *The mercury thermometer* (Fig. 6.14a). Mercury thermometers are commonly used, but, because of concerns about breakage and mercury toxicity, they may eventually become obsolete. They have a simple design, with a glass storage bulb for mercury and a connecting column along which expanding mercury flows when the temperature rises. Most have

Table 6.1 Normal temperature ranges by site

Axillary	34.7–37.3 °C	94.5–99.1 °F
Oral	35.5–37.5 °C	95.9–99.5 °F
Rectal	36.6–38.0 °C	97.4–100.4 °F
Ear	35.8–38.0 °C	96.4–100.4 °F

a graduated scale in degrees centigrade, extending from 35 to 42 °C. Some have a dual scale in Fahrenheit and centigrade. A special sub-normal reading thermometer that reads from 30 to 35 °C or lower is used for the diagnosis of hypothermia.

3. *The digital oral thermometer* (Fig. 6.14b). The digital thermometer is used for oral temperatures and is quicker to use than the mercury type. It is placed under the tongue, is made of plastic, is waterproof and battery driven. It has a tapered end, a metal sensor at the tip for measuring temperature, a body that displays the temperature in an easy-to-read window, and an on/off button. The temperature range is usually 32–43.9 °C. The body temperature is recorded within 10–15 seconds and a bleeper sounds when the

temperature has stabilized. Because neither mercury nor glass is used in the construction, digital thermometers are safer for use with children than the mercury types. Digital thermometers can also be used to measure body temperature under the arm or rectally (Fig. 6.14c).

4. *The ear thermometer* (Fig. 6.14d). The ear thermometer measures body temperature in the ear. It consists of a hand-held body with display window and control buttons for on/off and memory recall, and a cone for insertion into the ear, and is covered by a lens filter. When skin contact is made in the external canal, it will record the temperature within 1 second. This is the recommended method for use in children, when time and safety are important.

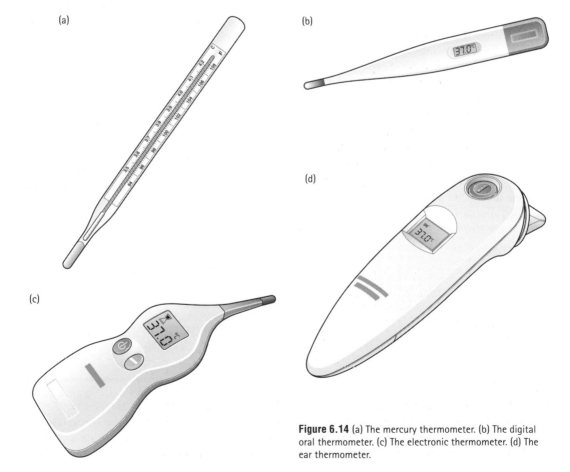

Figure 6.14 (a) The mercury thermometer. (b) The digital oral thermometer. (c) The electronic thermometer. (d) The ear thermometer.

How to take an oral temperature using a mercury or digital thermometer

Procedure

- The thermometer should be sterile. The tip should be sterilized in an antiseptic solution such as chlorhexidine, or a protective plastic cover should be used over the tip and stem of the thermometer.
- Place the tip of the thermometer under your patient's tongue, and ask the patient to close his or her mouth over the thermometer without clamping the teeth onto the glass or sensor tip.
- Mercury thermometers should be left in place for at least 1 minute to allow the reading to stabilize before removal, and digital thermometers for about 30 seconds or until a beeping sound indicates that the temperature has peaked.
- Remove the thermometer from the patient's mouth. To read a mercury thermometer, rotate the stem around its longitudinal axis until the mercury column is seen. The reading is taken from the graduated scale where the mercury column ends. For digital thermometers, take the reading from the display window.

Taking an axillary temperature

When taking an axillary temperature, the thermometer tip is placed in the pit of the axilla and the patient is asked to hold the arm against the chest wall.

Taking a rectal temperature

A rectal temperature is taken with the patient lying on the side. You should gently insert the thermometer into the rectum in a backwards direction for a distance of 3–4 cm. The end of the thermometer will protrude.

Practical points for all methods of temperature recording

- The thermometer reading should be returned to zero before use by shaking vigorously. For mercury thermometers, you should check that the mercury column has returned to about 35 °C. Failure to do this is a common cause of inaccuracy, particularly with mercury thermometers. For digital thermometers, the display window should be cleared using the on/off switch.
- The time to temperature equilibration varies according to the model. A mercury thermometer should be left in contact with the body for at least 60 seconds before reading; failure to do so causes under-recording of the temperature. The digital and electronic models are much quicker.
- Hot drinks taken immediately before the body temperature is recorded will cause a local rise in body temperature. You should check that the patient has not recently had a hot drink, otherwise you may erroneously diagnose fever when none is present and subject the patient to unnecessary investigations. Likewise, an iced lollipop may cause under-recording of a fever. However, it is not unknown for an occasional patient to use this trick to feign illness!

How to take an ear temperature

- Ensure that a clean probe cover is used with the ear thermometer for hygienic practice.
- Press the memory button on the handle to turn on the instrument.
- Tug on your patient's ear to straighten the external canal. This gives the thermometer clear access to the eardrum. For infants, the ear canal is straightened by pulling the ear lobe downwards and backwards. For adults, the ear canal is straightened by pulling the earlobe upwards and backwards.
- While tugging the ear, fit the probe snugly into the ear canal and press the activation button. This automatically measures the temperature.
- Release the button when you hear the 'temp beep' and note the reading.

HOW TO EXAMINE AN EAR

Examining an ear includes inspection of both the external ear and the tympanic membrane of the middle ear. The instrument used is known as an auriscope (otoscope).

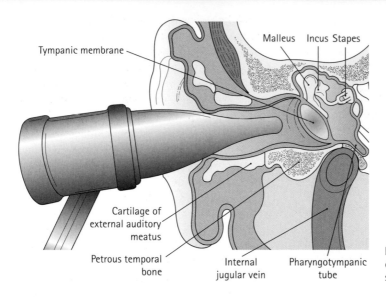

Tympanic membrane

Malleus Incus Stapes

Cartilage of
external auditory
meatus

Petrous temporal
bone

Internal
jugular vein

Pharyngotympanic
tube

Figure 6.15 The anatomy of the external and middle ear, coronal section.

Indications for examining the ear

- For diagnosis in patients with complaints specifically relating to the ear, for example pain (otalgia), itching (pruritus), difficulty hearing, blocked ear, discharge, or noises in the ear (tinnitus). The most common ear presentations in general practice are children with earache, ear discharge or suspected earache because of pulling at the ear.
- For diagnosis in infants with non-specific illness in whom the differential diagnosis includes middle ear infection (otitis media). Unexplained symptoms in an infant may be associated with an ear infection. Parents may have noticed that their child is 'grizzly' or irritable, cries more than usual, is not feeding or has an unexplained temperature. This is known as pyrexia of unknown origin (PUO).
- To check for wax before ear syringing.
- In the assessment of speech disorders to check whether the cause is impaired hearing, for example infants with delayed or poorly developed speech or adults with abnormal speech (dysphasia).
- In routine examination for insurance purposes, pre-employment medical for occupations such as telephonist, or for obtaining a licence to participate in certain sports, for example scuba diving, flying, gliding or parachuting.

Background knowledge

The ear comprises three parts: the outer, the middle and the inner.

The **outer** or **external ear** (Fig. 6.15) comprises the auricle, which projects from the side of the head, and the external acoustic meatus or canal, which leads to the tympanic membrane of the middle ear. In babies and infants, the auricle and canal are composed of cartilage. As adulthood approaches, only the outer third remains cartilaginous, and the inner two-thirds come to lie in the temporal bone. The canal is lined by skin and in the subcutaneous tissue are hair follicles, sebaceous glands and ceruminous glands that produce wax. In the adult, the canal is approximately 2.5 cm long and forms an S-shaped curve that is first directed medially (towards the centre), forward and slightly upward, and then passes medially, backwards and upward. To allow insertion of the auriscope, the canal needs to be straightened. This is done by applying traction to the auricle: in adults by pulling in a backwards and upwards direction, and in infants by pulling in a backwards and downwards direction. This is necessary because of changes in skull shape with growth.

The middle ear (Figs 6.15 and 6.16) consists of the tympanic cavity in the petrous part of the tympanic bone and three auditory ossicles: the malleus, incus and stapes.

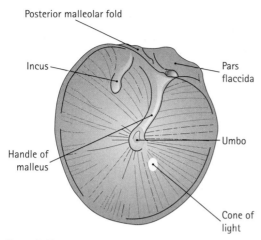

Posterior malleolar fold

Incus

Pars flaccida

Handle of malleus

Umbo

Cone of light

Figure 6.16 The tympanic membrane of the right ear as seen through the auriscope.

What you will see when looking through a auriscope into the ear

The part you will be examining is the tympanic membrane. This separates the outer ear from the ossicles of the middle ear. Although the membrane is round and faces downwards and forwards, it appears oval when looked at through the auriscope due to a parallax effect. In a patient with a normal ear, you will see the tympanic membrane as a glistening, semi-opaque sheet with a cone of light reflected from the lower anterior (towards the front) part. You will also see an oblique line passing in an anterior–posterior (forwards–backwards) direction. This is the handle of the malleus, which is attached to the tympanic membrane. Superiorly (towards the top of the head), the malleus forms a lax membrane, the pars flaccida. The remaining membrane is taut and concave where it is pulled inwards by the handle of the malleus.

What you will need

- An auriscope with efficient batteries. Check that there is a strong beam of light.
- Set of aural speculae (attachable plastic or metal cones of several sizes).

Procedure

Although most ears examined in general practice are those of children, it is more considerate first to gain experience by examining the ears of adults who are free of ear complaints. Children are more easily upset, tend to fidget and need a special approach (see below).

- Explain the procedure to your patient, demonstrating the auriscope and reassuring that the examination may be uncomfortable but not painful.
- Inspect the pinna and auricle for skin changes, signs of infection or discharge.
- Position your patient and yourself. With an adult, either ask the patient to turn the head to one side or, as the examiner, get up and move to the side of your patient. If you are right handed, it is more comfortable to examine the right ear holding your auriscope in your right hand, leaving your left hand free to pull on the auricle (Fig. 6.17). Examine the left ear holding the auriscope in your left hand and pull on the auricle with your right hand. If you are left handed, examine the patient's right ear holding the auriscope in your right hand, and examine the left ear with the auriscope in your left hand. Hand usage is not a hard or fast rule. You may prefer to hold the auriscope in your dominant hand for both sides, but note that when examining the contralateral ear, your arms will cross as you pull on the auricle. Which feels comfortable for you?
- Select a suitably sized speculum. This should be the largest that can be inserted into the canal without causing pain. A plastic speculum will be comfortably warm, but a metal type may be cold and before use should be warmed in warm water and dried.
- Turn on the auriscope light. Hold the auriscope between your thumb and index finger, either with the palm of your hand placed vertically or with your palm uppermost as if holding a soupspoon. This position difference is a matter of preference. Try both.
- With your free hand, draw the auricle upwards and backwards to straighten the canal. Insert the speculum gently into the external canal, advancing by a short distance at first. View through the lens in front of the speculum. Use the fourth and fifth fingers to steady the auriscope against the head. What do you see? The skin of the auditory canal should come

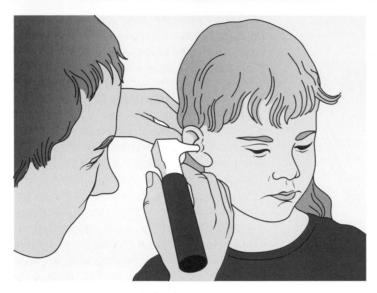

Figure 6.17 An auriscope held in the correct position.

into view. Sometimes you see deposits of yellow or brown wax. Beyond this you should see a small part of the tympanic membrane. Advance the auriscope along the canal by changing its angle and take another look. The whole of the tympanic membrane should come into view. It will look grey and opaque and you should see a shiny area known as the light reflex. If not, you may bring this into view by a slight change in direction of either the auriscope or the auricle. There may be abnormal appearances of the tympanic membrane. If red, it usually indicates inflammation. A fluid level or opaque circumscribed area suggests the presence of exudates; a hole in the tympanic membrane suggests a perforation. If you see only wax, the ear canal is probably blocked.

Examining a child's ear (without tears!)

■ This can be a frightening procedure for a young child. Because children move unpredictably, may be frightened or unco-operative, they have to be restrained during the examination. The child's head must be steadied to allow an adequate view of the ear and to minimize the risk of damage to the tympanic membrane by the auriscope. As preparation, explain the procedure to the parent and child.

■ Select a smaller (paediatric) speculum for the auriscope.

■ Befriend your young patient. Your aim is to avoid frightening the child and to examine without tears or before they appear. Chat to and reassure the child about your intentions, perhaps by demonstrating your auriscope light on clothing, a teddy, doll or the child's parent. Try turning the encounter into a game.

■ With the parent sitting facing you, ask the parent to sit the child across his or her lap with the child's head and inner arm against the parent's chest, and the parent's arm or hand held firmly across the child's head. The parent's other arm should be placed around the child's chest and outer arm. This is similar to a child's 'cuddling' position (Fig. 6.18).

■ You are now ready to examine. Use the same procedure as for the adult, except that to straighten the external meatus, pull the pinna downwards and backwards.

Practical points

■ If the ear is partly or wholly blocked with wax, try to remove this gently with a cotton bud. If not, the patient should be asked to introduce a few drops of oil into the canal daily over at least 3 days to allow the wax to soften, before returning for further examination or ear syringing.

■ If you are unable to view the whole tympanic membrane, this may be due to faulty equipment. Although the position of the auriscope

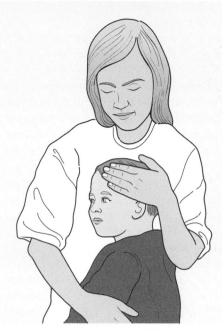

Figure 6.18 The correct positioning of the parent and child for examination of the child's ear.

in the auditory canal is correct, the main beam of light may not be directed out of the end of the speculum because the bulb carrier is bent. Try a different auriscope.

■ If a child screams throughout the consultation, how should you handle the situation? The kindest approach is to spend time comforting the child or allow a cooling-off period by sending the parent and child back to the waiting room to recover. In reality, you are working to a tight schedule, both in the surgery and on home visits. In this case, and regrettably, you may have no alternative but to do a 'go-for-it' examination with the crying child held firmly by an adult. But warning – avoid ensuing kicks!

Practical Exercise

Examine as many patients as possible. Select a wide range of shapes, sizes and ages.

Ask your tutor or other doctors to show you any patients with abnormal ears.

HOW TO USE DIPSTICKS

Dipstick analysis is an example of 'near-patient' or 'point-of-care' testing performed on urine or blood samples using commercially available disposable reagent strips or kits. You will notice these being used often in the surgery. Testing is convenient because it can be done during a consultation in the surgery, at a patient's home, or using 'away-from-patient testing' on samples taken beforehand but tested in the surgery. The dipstick method has the advantage of allowing results to be used in immediate management decisions. Tests are cheap, simple to use, and save time for both the doctor and the patient compared with sending a patient or sample for hospital testing. However, dipsticks using blood samples are not as accurate as laboratory analysis methods.

Advances in technology have led to the development of a wide range of laboratory tests. Some are available for use in the surgery and include equipment for blood analysis, for example undertaking full blood counts and blood chemistry. The equipment requires regular servicing for reliability and calibration to maintain quality control.

Clinical indications for dipstick analysis

1. Urine.
   ■ Screening for urinary proteinuria as found in nephrotic syndrome and nephritis, or for glycosuria as in diabetes (Multistix, Diastix).
   ■ Diagnosis of urinary tract infection, using dipstick urine analysis to detect nitrites and blood (Uristix, Multistix).
   ■ Checking diabetic control through the detection of glycosuria, ketonuria (Multistix, Ketostix, Keto-Diastix).
2. Blood.
   ■ Testing for random or fasting blood sugar (BM-Stix, Glucotide).

How do dipsticks work?

■ Test strips are made of disposable plastic with attached reagent areas that change colour when the substance to be tested is present in the sample. There may be one or several tests combined on each strip.

- In the diagnosis of a lower urinary tract infection, bacteria in the urine that reduce nitrate to nitrite can be detected by the nitrate reductase test. Pus cells in the urine are detected by the leucocyte esterase test.
- In screening for and managing diabetes, the glucose test is based on a double sequential enzyme reaction involving the oxygenation of glucose to gluconic acid and hydrogen peroxide by a catalyst, glucose oxidase. A second enzyme, peroxidase, catalyses the reaction of hydrogen peroxide with a potassium iodide chromogen to produce colours ranging from green to brown.
- Ketone testing is based on the reaction between acetoacetic acid with nitroprusside to produce colours changing from buff pink, indicating a negative result, to maroon, if positive.
- BM-Test 1–44 is based on the glucose reaction described above.

What you will need

- Reagent stick with the associated reagent bottle and colour-coding strip.
- Patient sample container, e.g. for urine.
- A lancet for obtaining a blood sample from the patient.
- A watch or timer that measures in seconds.

Procedure for testing urine

Each test includes simple instructions. An outline of the procedure is as follows.

- Obtain the sample to be tested from your patient. A urine sample may be passed into any clean receptacle. However, if in addition to dipstick testing a midstream urine specimen is to be sent to the bacteriology laboratory, the sample must be passed into a sterilized laboratory bottle and a small volume of this used separately for the dipstick test.
- Select the appropriate reagent. Check the expiry date on the unopened bottle; if it has expired, discard it. Sticks should be used within 6 months of first opening the bottle.
- Collect a fresh sample as described above.
- Open the reagent bottle and remove one strip. Immediately replace the cap on the bottle. Hold the plastic end of the strip. Note the

time interval required for the dipstick reading on the instructions.
- Now you are ready to start the test. If the sample is to be sent for bacteriological culture, the urine should be dripped onto the test stick over a sluice or tray, otherwise you will contaminate the urine by dipping the stick into the sample. Note the time with a second hand immediately after testing the sample.
- After the stated time interval, read the strip by visually matching the colour on the stick to the colour on the bottle to give you a reading.
- Record the results in the patient's notes.
- Dispose of the sample in the lavatory or sluice, not the washbasin used for hand washing, as this would compromise hygiene.
- Wash your hands after completing the test.

Procedure for testing blood

A blood sample is obtained by puncturing a finger or the ear lobe with a lancet, and applying pressure to obtain a drop a blood that is then allowed to drip onto the surface of the analysis strip.

Each test kit has instructions written on the side and an enclosed instruction sheet. It is important to follow all instructions carefully to avoid faulty results (Fig. 6.19).

Practical points

- Always check the date on the reagent bottle to ensure that it has not expired, as this will give an unreliable reading. When first opening a bottle, write the date on the side and do not use from 6 months beyond this date.
- Because the tests are not as reliable as laboratory analyses, they should not be used alone for diagnosis. They are useful for supplementing a high diagnostic index of suspicion from the history and examination.
- If the colour on the stick falls between two colour strips on the bottle, take an estimate between the two colour ranges. Always read in good lighting.
- False-positive and false-negative readings occur, but because the enzymatic methods are chemically specific and quite sensitive,

Getting the best from BM-test 1–44

Good technique is essential in obtaining accurate results. It is important to follow **all** the instructions below, **carefully**

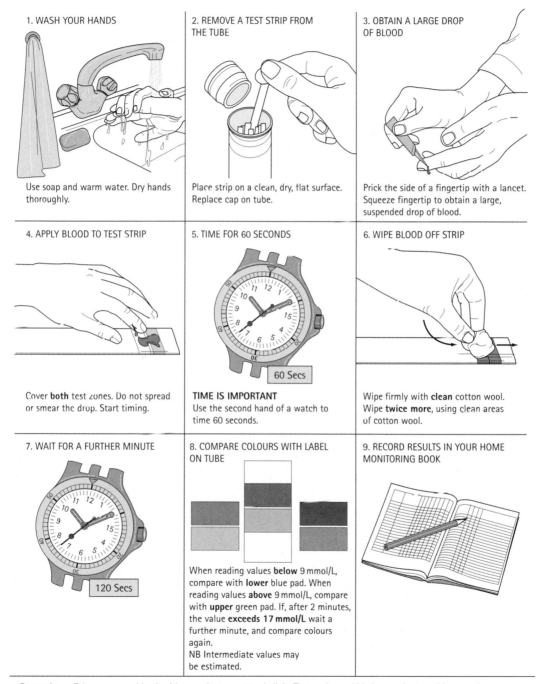

1. WASH YOUR HANDS

Use soap and warm water. Dry hands thoroughly.

2. REMOVE A TEST STRIP FROM THE TUBE

Place strip on a clean, dry, flat surface. Replace cap on tube.

3. OBTAIN A LARGE DROP OF BLOOD

Prick the side of a fingertip with a lancet. Squeeze fingertip to obtain a large, suspended drop of blood.

4. APPLY BLOOD TO TEST STRIP

Cover **both** test zones. Do not spread or smear the drop. Start timing.

5. TIME FOR 60 SECONDS

60 Secs

TIME IS IMPORTANT
Use the second hand of a watch to time 60 seconds.

6. WIPE BLOOD OFF STRIP

Wipe firmly with **clean** cotton wool. Wipe **twice more**, using clean areas of cotton wool.

7. WAIT FOR A FURTHER MINUTE

120 Secs

8. COMPARE COLOURS WITH LABEL ON TUBE

When reading values **below** 9 mmol/L, compare with **lower** blue pad. When reading values **above** 9 mmol/L, compare with **upper** green pad. If, after 2 minutes, the value **exceeds 17 mmol/L** wait a further minute, and compare colours again.
NB Intermediate values may be estimated.

9. RECORD RESULTS IN YOUR HOME MONITORING BOOK

Remember... Take your record book with you when you attend clinic. The results could help your doctor achieve good control of your diabetes.

Figure 6.19 Patient instruction sheet on how to use a glucose test strip on blood samples.

these are unusual. However, high levels of vitamin C may cause false negatives in the Clinistix and Diastix methods, whereas reducing sugars, such as lactose, fructose and galactose, drugs such as aspirin, tetracycline, cephalosporins and nalidixic acid, and detergents may cause false positives.

■ If you are colour blind, is the accuracy of the reading affected? Impaired colour vision affects the interpretation of these strips, especially if you have a red/green or mixed colour vision deficiency. In these circumstances, the interpretation of a glucose test strip is unreliable. Blue/yellow defects have little effect on interpretation of the strips. If in doubt, check your colour vision with the Ishihara test. Colour blindness also has implications for self-testing for patients, especially diabetics.

Practical Exercise

❑ Sit in the diabetic clinic and offer to test blood and urine samples with available test strips. You will note a wide range of positive readings. For blood sugar, how do the stick readings compare with results from the glucose meter?

❑ Sit in a screening clinic, well-person clinic or a general surgery and test all urine samples offered by patients for routine dipstick testing.

HOW TO USE A MINI-PEAK FLOW METER

Portable mini-peak flow meters are used to diagnose and monitor obstructive airways disease, for example asthma, chronic bronchitis and emphysema. Several models are available, but the most commonly used is the portable mini-Wright peak flow meter. They are a reliable and cheap method of measuring airway obstruction, and are as essential to the monitoring of chronic respiratory problems as the sphygmomanometer is to blood pressure. Available on prescription, the meters allow patients to participate in monitoring their condition at home. Meters are calibrated in low ranges for use with children.

Background knowledge

Expiratory flow can be measured using the maximum peak expiratory flow rate (PEFR) or the forced expiratory volume in 1 second (FEV_1) The peak flow meter measures the maximum flow of exhaled air in a forced expiration. This is known as the peak expiratory flow rate (PEFR). Changes in chronic bronchitis and asthma increase airways resistance and produce a fall in PEFR. This can be monitored satisfactorily in the surgery with the mini-peak flow meter, although very sensitive changes will only be detected by more sophisticated spirometry. The PEFR and FEV_1 are similar but not identical physiological measures. FEV_1 is measured on a maximally forced expiration using a spirometer and is a more accurate measure of lung function than that taken with a peak flow meter. The FEV_1 is disproportionately reduced in patients with airway obstruction. Fixed large airway obstruction is seen most easily in a display of flow against volume (Fig. 6.20). The diagnosis of asthma is made by establishing reversibility of airways obstruction in response to a bronchodilator.

What you will need

■ Mini-peak flow meter (Fig. 6.21).
■ A disposable cardboard mouthpiece or plastic mouthpiece that has been disinfected.
■ A chart to show normal peak flow readings in adults and children (Fig. 6.22).

Using a peak flow meter involves two steps: using or demonstrating the use of the meter yourself, and teaching your patient how to use the meter (Fig. 6.23). The second skill is an

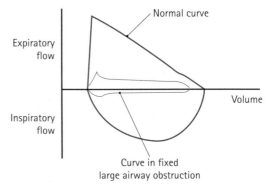

Figure 6.20 Flow–volume curve in a normal patient and in one with fixed large airway obstruction.

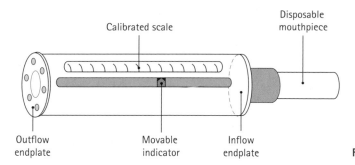

Figure 6.21 A peak flow meter.

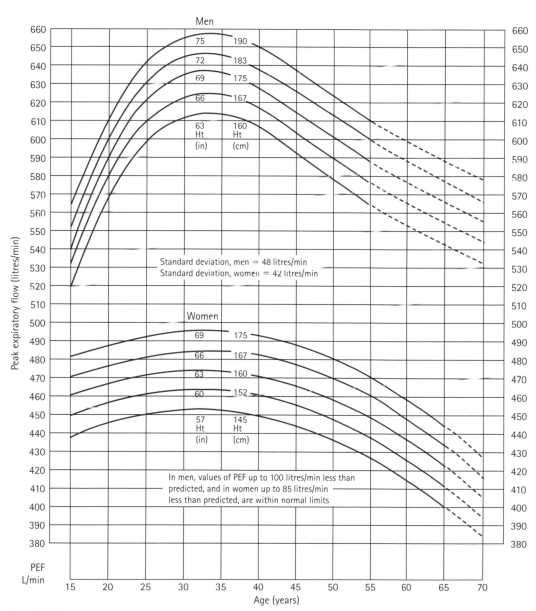

Figure 6.22 A graph used for comparing actual and predicted peak expiratory flow rates.

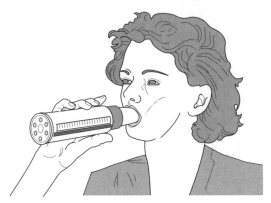

Figure 6.23 A patient using a mini-peak flow meter.

extension of the first and is not quite as straightforward as you might think.

Tutor quote

A third-year medical student was asked by his tutor if he knew how to use the peak flow meter. 'Certainly', he replied. 'I've had asthma since I was 7 years of age and often use one.' His demonstration involved three separate steps. 'Stand up, take a deep breath and blow as fast as you can down the tube, like this.' He was then asked to explain to a patient with asthma how to use the meter in preparation for home monitoring. He was surprised that the patient was unable to reproduce his three-stage skill in a way that was reliable. Teaching the same technique and checking the patient's understanding took 12 steps (as described below).

Procedure

- Explain to your patient the importance of measuring the breathing capacity of the lungs, showing the mini-peak flow meter.
- Select two separate disposable, or sterilized plastic, mouthparts and insert one into the meter. This will be your demonstration model. The other will be for your patient.
- Stand up and demonstrate in slow motion how to use the mini-peak flow meter.
- With one hand, hold the meter in the horizontal position, ensuring the indicator is free to move. Explain the requirement to take as deep a breath as possible and to hold it.

Place your lips over the outside edge of the mouthpiece as if pouting, making a seal between the tube and the lips.

- Breathe out down the mouthpiece as fast and as forcefully as possible, allowing the indicator to move as far as possible. It is not necessary to continue exhaling until the residual volume is reached, since the peak flow occurs at the start of the process. Repeat this procedure twice more and take the best of three readings as the PEFR.
- Return the needle to zero.
- Remove your mouthpiece and replace with your patient's. Hand the meter to your patient.
- Ask your patient to stand and repeat the demonstration three times, checking technique and returning the indicator to zero after each attempt.
- Take the maximum recording in litres/ minute.
- Use the peak expiratory flow chart (see Fig. 6.22) to plot this value on the ordinate against your patient's age on the abscissa. Determine your patient's predicted PEFR for age and gender on the height curve. You may now compare the actual with the predicted PEFR. Express this as a percentage.
- Record readings in the patient's notes or computer record. There is usually a separate asthma file for monitoring long-term treatment.

Practical points

- Hygiene: disposable mouthpieces are preferable, but if plastic models are used, they should be disinfected for each patient.
- Under-recording will occur if air leaks around the mouthpiece. It is therefore important to check that the lips are well sealed on the outside of the tube. Lips may be wrongly positioned inside the mouthpiece.
- Air escapes down the nose, causing under-recording. You can use a nose clip if this is problem.
- The handgrip impedes the movement of the indicator. Reposition the grip on the meter.
- Poor respiratory effort or low-force blowing causes under-recording. This is more likely in

patients who are older or who have a painful chest wall, for example broken or bruised ribs.

■ Use of a spitting action down the mouthpiece will move the indicator further than if the flow meter is used correctly. This gives an artificially high reading.

Practical Exercise

Investigate the effects of exercise on PEFR of yourself or a colleague.

❏ Take a baseline reading with the mini-peak flow meter.

❏ Exercise vigorously for at least 6 minutes, for example by running up and down stairs or, if there is a nearby park, take a run. When you feel out of breath, take another reading. Is there any difference? If the post-exercise reading is reduced, is this significant? What criteria would you use for the diagnosis of asthma?

For further reading, see Rees and Kanabar (1999).

SKILLS USED IN CLINICAL MANAGEMENT AND TREATMENT OF PATIENTS

Injections given in general practice are most commonly by the intramuscular or deep subcutaneous route, although occasionally intradermal or intra-articular routes are used. Most vaccines are given by intramuscular or deep subcutaneous injection. Local anaesthetic for minor surgery is given subcutaneously. Injections are sometimes required on emergency home visits for the control of distressing symptoms, for example a patient with intractable vomiting may be managed with an intramuscular injection of an anti-emetic drug such as prochlorperazine.

Background knowledge

A knowledge of surface landmarks, skin structure and the anatomy of muscles is essential if injections are to be given safely. Be aware of the positions of important structures, which, if traumatized with the injecting needle, could be

irreparably damaged or result in serious complications such as haemorrhage.

Intramuscular sites

■ *Thigh* (Fig. 6.24). Lateral and antero-lateral aspects are formed by the vastus lateralis or rectus femoris muscles, two of the four components of the quadriceps femoris muscle (the others are the vastus medialis and vastus intermedius), the main extensor muscle of the leg. Inject into the antero-lateral aspect of the thigh into the vastus lateralis or rectus femoris.

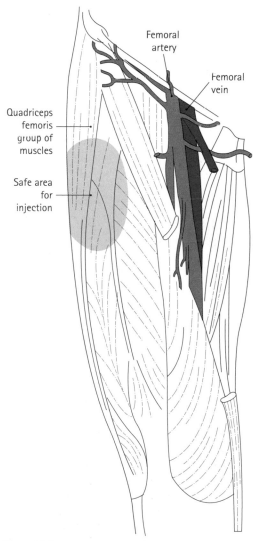

Figure 6.24 Site for intramuscular injection into right thigh (anterior view).

Dangers: avoid the femoral artery and vein (which lie immediately medial to the rectus femoris), and the branch nerve to the vastus medialis.

■ *Buttock* (Fig. 6.25). The contour is formed by the gluteus muscles (maximus, medius, minimus, arising from the posterior gluteal line of the ilium and iliac crest), the natal line and the lateral surface of the greater trochanter.

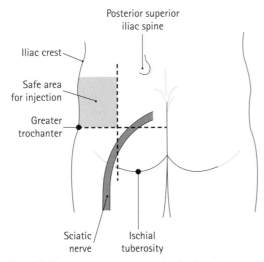

Figure 6.25 Site for intramuscular injection into left buttock (posterior view).

The landmarks are: the iliac crest superiorly, posterior superior iliac spine supero-medially, ischial tuberosity infero-medially and greater trochanter of femur laterally.

Dangers: sciatic nerve, located inferiorly to two imaginary lines: (i) from posterior superior iliac spine to greater trochanter, (ii) from iliac crest to ischial tuberosity. The 'safe' area for injection is in the upper, outer quadrant of the buttock.

■ *Upper arm* (Fig. 6.26). The contour of the upper arm is formed by the deltoid muscle, which originates from the anterior aspect of lateral third of clavicle, the acromion and the spine of scapula and is inserted into the deltoid tuberosity on the lateral side of the shaft of the humerus.

Dangers: anterior branch of axillary nerve (supplies deltoid muscle), which winds posteriorly around the surgical neck of the humerus, below the capsule of the joint, approximately 6–8 cm below the bony prominence of the acromion.

Intradermal, subcutaneous and intramuscular injections (Figs 6.27–6.29)

What you will need

■ Syringe of suitable size: 1 mL, 2.5 mL or 5 mL, depending on the volume to be injected.

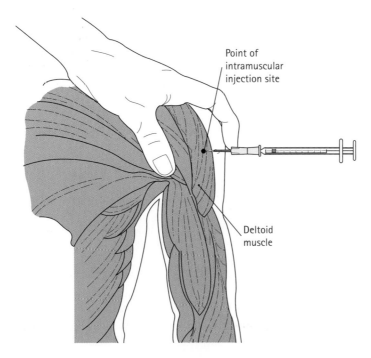

Figure 6.26 Site for intramuscular injection into the upper arm (anterior view).

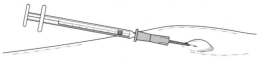

Figure 6.27 The intradermal route.

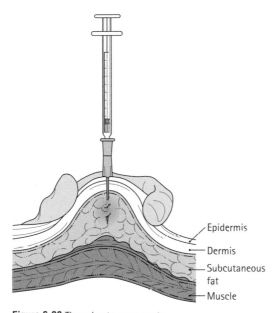

Epidermis

Dermis

Subcutaneous fat

Muscle

Figure 6.28 The subcutaneous route.

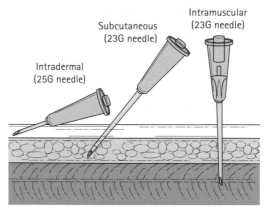

Intradermal (25G needle)

Subcutaneous (23G needle)

Intramuscular (23G needle)

Figure 6.29 Needle orientation for intradermal, subcutaneous and intramuscular injections (refer to Fig. 6.28).

■ Needle of suitable size: 21G (green) or 23G (blue) for intramuscular or subcutaneous injections. For intradermal injections, a 25G needle should be used.
■ Cotton-wool swab.
■ Ampoule of drug to be given.
■ Elastoplast.
■ Sharps box: this is a plastic box, usually yellow, for the safe disposal of needles and syringes.

Choosing the site for an intramuscular injection

Choice of an intramuscular site is a personal matter for the administrator when injecting adults, but in infants the antero-lateral aspect of the thigh or the upper arm is recommended. Injection into the fatty tissue of the buttock has been shown to reduce the efficacy of hepatitis B vaccine.

Needle orientation

The needle orientation for intradermal, subcutaneous and intramuscular injections is shown in Figure 6.29.

Procedure for an intramuscular injection

Practise first on models. An old orange or grapefruit is suitable, as the consistency of the peel approximates that of human skin. Take care to dispose of this after your session to avoid poisoning your colleagues!

Before you start:

■ Wash your hands: consider using protective gloves as a precaution against contamination with blood or other body fluids.
■ Check your equipment.
■ Check the name and dose of the drug on the ampoule. Double-check and, if possible, treble-check by asking a third-party professional such as a nurse to confirm the drug and dose. Time spent checking may save much anguish for the patient, relatives and doctor and minimize the risk of litigation.
■ Draw up the drug into the syringe in the following way. Tap the top of the ampoule, or flick your finger against the side, causing the contents to run into the base. Break off the top of the ampoule by snapping the glass at the neck. Sometimes a black dot is present at the neck of the ampoule, indicating the weakest point at which the glass will fracture most easily. With the needle tip positioned below the surface of the solution, draw up the contents into the syringe by pulling back the plunger. Tilt the ampoule initially to avoid withdrawing air, returning to a vertical position towards the end of the withdrawal process. Upturn the syringe and tap the side

to allow air bubbles to coalesce. Advance the plunger to expel air bubbles. The solution should be correctly drawn up and ready for injection.

Select the injection site and proceed as follows.

- Prepare your patient: explain the procedure, stressing that pain will be minimal.
- Position your patient according to the chosen injection site. For the buttock: lay your patient in the prone position (face down). For the arm: have your patient sitting with the arm relaxed at the side. This can be done in the standing position, but could be traumatic if the patient faints. For the thigh: have your patient lying on one side or standing, leaning over a couch.
- Assess the distance between skin and muscle by pinching the skin at the point of planned entry and assessing the depth of subcutaneous fat.
- You are now ready to give the injection. Hold the syringe between the fingers of your dominant hand. Steady the skin at the planned injection site by making it taut.
- Using a single puncture entry point, advance the needle with the bevel uppermost through the skin at an angle of 90 degrees (see Fig. 6.29). The needle will pass through the underlying structures of the superficial fascia, deep fascia and into the muscle. Each tissue has a characteristic tension or 'feel' about it. The depth will depend on the size of the patient and the site. Withdraw the plunger of the syringe to check that blood is not aspirated. If it is, the needle may be positioned in a blood vessel, in which case the needle should be withdrawn until no further blood is obtained on withdrawing the plunger.
- Advance the plunger, emptying the contents into the muscle. Withdraw the needle rapidly. Dispose of the syringe and attached, uncapped needle into the sharps bin. You should not try to re-cap the needle because if you miss, you may have a needlestick injury. If the needle has to be re-capped, for example during a home visit, do so with the cap lying on a surface in the horizontal position, and insert the needle into the cap.

- Record details of the injection in the patient's notes, to include name of drug, dose, method and site of injection, manufacturer's number from the side of the ampoule and date of expiry.

Procedure for a subcutaneous or intradermal injection

For a subcutaneous injection, follow the above procedure, except that the entry approach of the needle should be at an acute angle of approximately 45 degrees, with the bevel uppermost. The needle is advanced through the epidermis and dermis into the subcutaneous tissue, where the injection is given. For an intradermal injection, the needle approach is an acute angle of about 10 degrees to the skin, with the bevel uppermost. When the needle is positioned in the dermis, the solution is injected, and will cause the overlying skin to form a raised area. This disappears as the injected solution is absorbed.

Practical points

- Contrary to expectation, it is less painful to use a wider-bore needle than the finest available. Can you think of an explanation? The pressure exerted through a fine-bore needle is higher than that through a larger-bore needle in order to deliver the same volume of injectable material. This higher pressure is more painful.
- Should you use an alcohol swab to clean the skin at the injection site? Nowadays, alcohol swabs are considered unnecessary, although you may wish to use a dry cotton-wool swab to apply pressure to the entry point if bleeding occurs.
- How should you remove air trapped in the syringe? Do so by upturning the syringe with the neck uppermost and tapping on the syringe side. Bubbles of air will coalesce, move to the top and escape.
- If you are unable to break the neck of the ampoule, use a small metal blade to etch a scratch at the neck. The glass will usually break at this point.
- If you have a blood spillage, follow the procedure described in the section 'How to take a blood sample'. If you have a needlestick injury,

you should report this to your tutor or trainer and take their advice in following the standard work-place procedure.

■ After some injections, commonly immunizations, a small hard nodule persists at the injection site for 2–3 weeks. This is harmless and will resolve.

■ Could your patient faint?

Student quote

The first time I gave an injection I was quite nervous, but not, it seemed, as nervous as my patient! First, my tutor made me practise on a grapefruit. Quite simple! Then, the nurse introduced me to Mr W. She ran through the procedure and, as a routine precaution, showed me the resuscitation tray, pointing out the adrenaline syringe to use in the event of anaphylaxis from a severe allergic reaction. She told me this was so rare that she had never seen a case. I reassured my patient that the injection would not hurt, although he did tell me he occasionally felt queasy at the sight of needles. Everything went well until I withdrew the needle. My patient collapsed across the couch. He turned ghostly pale. It occurred to me he might have 'dropped dead', although having never witnessed that, I wouldn't have known. My next thought was that he was in anaphylactic shock but the nurse made no move to grab the resuscitation tray. I somehow felt everything would be all right because she was there. She turned my patient on to his back, placed his legs on the couch, and as he opened his eyes she said, 'Just a little faint, Mr W. Take some deep breaths. Can I get you a cup of tea?'. What a relief!

HOW TO SYRINGE AN EAR

The purpose of syringing an ear is to remove wax or cerumen that is blocking the external auditory meatus, causing pain or hearing impairment. Cerumen is produced by the ceruminous glands of the outer third of the meatus as a waxy protective substance. Wax production is variable and the wax is normally expelled by chewing movements. However, sometimes this process does not occur and the accumulating wax blocks the meatus. It is easier to remove wax that has been softened with oil for 3 or more consecutive days prior to syringing. Olive or almond oil is recommended, although some patients prefer to obtain an over-the-counter proprietary preparation.

Background knowledge

The anatomy of the ear has been described (see Fig. 6.15).

Syringing should be performed with water at or slightly above body temperature (37–38 °C). Water warmed or cooled to 7 °C above or below body temperature will stimulate the labyrinthine system by creating a convection current in the endolymph. This will stimulate the sensorineural epithelium within the ampulla of the horizontal semicircular canal and cause nystagmus (repetitively jerking eye movements), associated with a sensation of imbalance, vertigo and nausea. Patients find these symptoms extremely unpleasant. They are, however, put to good effect when assessing labyrinthine function in a procedure known as the 'caloric test' used in ear, nose and throat departments.

What you will need

■ Auriscope and specula.
■ Ear syringe with set of nozzles (hand-driven or electric model).
■ Collecting dish or receptacle.
■ Towel or waterproof cape to place around the patient's neck.
■ Water source.
■ Water container (reservoir box with electric model; jug with manual model).

About the equipment

Ears can be syringed using an electric pump or a manually operated model. The manual syringe is more cumbersome to use than the electric model and causes soreness and fatigue of the fingers from repeated movements of the plunger. There is also an increased risk of perforating the tympanic membrane through inadvertently dislodging the metal nozzle of the syringe. For these reasons, the electric pump has become the preferred method for ear syringing in most practices, with the manual syringe being increasingly obsolete. However, in the event of equipment or power failure, and in preparation for different styles of practice, both methods are described.

Procedure

- Take a history of any previous ear problems. Has your patient had a chronic ear discharge, a perforated eardrum or any ear operations, particularly a mastoidectomy for disease within the mastoid cavity?

  If there is any possibility of a perforated tympanic membrane, do not syringe, because of the risk of introducing infection into the middle ear or damaging the ossicles.

- Examine your patient's ear to confirm the presence of wax.
- Explain the procedure to your patient, emphasizing that you should be informed if dizziness occurs.
- Position your patient on a chair with the ear to be syringed facing you and the head tilted slightly away from you (Fig. 6.30). Place a towel or waterproof cape around your patient's neck and shoulders. Decorative earrings should be removed.
- Ask your patient to hold the receptacle below the ear to be syringed, pushing it against the skin to prevent water dripping down the neck.

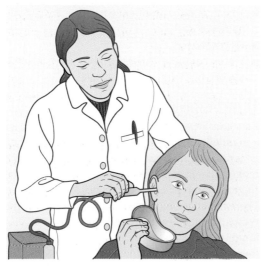

Figure 6.30 The correct position in which to use an ear syringe.

Using the electrical ear syringe

- Plug in the electrical pump and turn on the power (Fig. 6.31). Fill the reservoir of the syringe pump with tap water at body temperature or slightly higher – 38 °C is ideal. (Normal saline or sodium bicarbonate can be used instead of water.)
- Select a nozzle of a size suitable for your patient's ear. Attach the nozzle to the syringe handle.
- Turn on the water supply through the nozzle by switching the control dial on the pump to the 'on' position and adjusting the pressure control dial. Test the flow of water through the nozzle with the stream directed into a sink or receptacle. The flow should be moderately gentle and not too ferocious. Practise controlling the water flow by depressing and releasing the button on the handle of the syringe.
- Position the spout of the nozzle in the auditory canal with the tip facing upwards and backwards, while simultaneously applying traction on the auricle in an upwards and backwards direction (Fig. 6.32).
- With the water stream turned on, direct the flow gently towards the roof of the auditory canal. At first, water will be deflected by the wax and run back out of the ear into the receptacle, but as the wax is displaced, water should flow along the roof of the auditory canal and track around the wax deposit (Fig. 6.33).
- As you continue syringing, flecks of yellow-brown wax will appear in the water. These will become larger, until a single or several larger chunks of wax appear, an indication that you may have successfully removed all the wax. When you stop syringing, the patient may express delight that hearing has returned. Use the auriscope to check whether the meatus is clear. If you can see the tympanic membrane, stop syringing; if not, continue, refilling the reservoir with water as necessary. Examine the ear periodically until the wax has been cleared.
- Dry the meatus by mopping excess water with gauze or cotton wool. A wet meatal lining predisposes to infection of the external

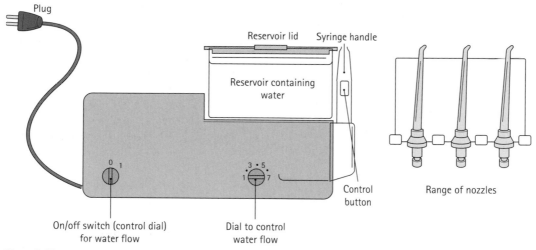

Figure 6.31 An electric pump and syringe.

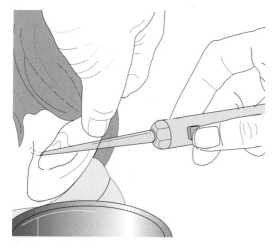

Figure 6.32 The pinna being pulled up and back to straighten the external auditory meatus.

canal and may cause otitis externa (infection of the outer ear).

■ Finally, clean the instruments. Wipe the nozzle with gauze or tissue paper, and detach and place in a sterilizing solution of chlorhexidine. Clean wax out of the auriscope speculum and place it in the same solution for 20–30 minutes. Allow it to dry thoroughly before re-using. This minimizes bacterial contamination from patients' ears.

Using the manual ear syringe

The same principles apply if using the manual ear syringe (Fig. 6.34). The models are made of stainless steel and each is supplied with a set of metal nozzles that, unlike the plastic nozzles, are not angled. A jug is used as a water reservoir for filling the syringe; tap water is satisfactory.

■ Select a suitably sized metal nozzle. Attach it to the neck of the syringe.

■ Screw the base with fixed grip rings to the barrel end. By placing your index and middle fingers in the base rings and your thumb in the plunger ring, you will be able to move the plunger relative to the barrel. Check that the syringe plunger moves freely inside the barrel. Wetting the plunger with tap water or smearing Vaseline on the plunger head will facilitate this movement. Leave in the closed (pushed-in) position.

■ Fill the reservoir jug with tap water at body temperature. Gauging the temperature with your own hand is sufficient, although testing with a thermometer will check your accuracy.

■ Position the tip of the nozzle below the surface of the water in the reservoir. Using your dominant hand, place the index finger in the plunger ring. Using your non-dominant hand to grasp the barrel, withdraw the plunger. This will draw up water into the barrel of the syringe. Avoid air entering the barrel. When full, hold the syringe horizontally to minimize leakage.

■ Change your handgrip on the syringe, placing your thumb in the plunger ring and

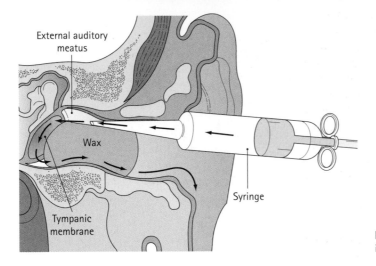

Figure 6.33 The direction of water flow in the external canal.

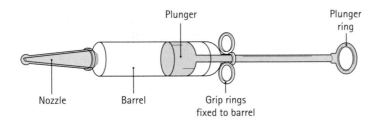

Figure 6.34 A manually operated ear syringe.

your index and middle fingers in the barrel rings. This frees the non-dominant hand.

■ Advance the nozzle into your patient's external auditory meatus while simultaneously, with your non-dominant hand, applying traction to the auricle in an upwards and backwards direction to straighten the auditory canal.

■ Advance the plunger into the barrel by moving the handle towards the barrel base, approximating the thumb, index and middle fingers. This movement empties the barrel of water. Direct the flow into the auditory meatus towards the roof of the canal.

■ When you have emptied the syringe, withdraw it. Examine the canal with the auriscope to check for the persistence of wax.

■ Continue this process of filling the barrel with warm water and syringing the ear until the wax has cleared. This may take as many as 8–12 syringes.

■ Dry the canal by mopping with gauze or cotton wool.

■ Clean the syringe with alcohol, particularly the nozzle. Allow it to dry thoroughly before using it on the next patient.

Practical points

■ It is essential to use water at body temperature to avoid an attack of caloric-induced vertigo.

■ Keep an eye on the water level in the patient-held receptacle. You may be so engrossed in the syringing that you fail to notice that the receptacle has overflowed, with the consequent soaking of yourself and the patient!

■ With the electric model, remember to turn off the water flow in the nozzle when inspecting the ear. If you do not, a jet of water will shoot across the room, targeting anyone in its path, including your tutor or the practice nurse!

■ When you have successfully unblocked the ear, your patient may remark about the sudden loudness of extraneous noise, especially high-frequency sounds. This abnormal sensitivity to sounds is known as hyperacusis, and will settle after several minutes.

Patients or their companions will warn you when syringing their ears that water is almost certain to shoot out of the opposite ear! This intimation of lack of cerebral content is a joke enjoyed throughout the world. Such hyperbole should not be dismissed without considering the care needed to avoid perforating the tympanic membrane during the syringing process. How could this happen? It is less likely with electric syringes because the angulation of the nozzle tip diverts water away from the tympanic membrane. With the hand syringe, however, unless the stream is directed posteriorly along the roof of the auditory meatus, it is possible for the water to impinge on the tympanic membrane with sufficient force that it causes a perforation.

HOW TO TAKE A BLOOD SAMPLE (VENEPUNCTURE)

Venous blood is used for most pathology testing; arterial blood is used for the measurement of blood gases; capillary blood from superficial sites such as the ear lobe for blood sugar; and heel prick samples in neonates for screening of phenylketones. Blood samples are taken from the plexus of veins in the antecubital fossa.

The process of taking blood from veins is called venepuncture or **phlebotomy** and the technician trained to undertake this procedure is a **phlebotomist**. It is common practice in the UK, whether in hospital or general practice, to use a vacuum system (Vacutainer) in which blood flows directly from a vein into a closed tube. This minimizes the risk of contamination from patients' blood.

The use of protective gloves

It is important to take precautions to minimize the risk of contamination of yourself and the immediate environment such as work surfaces, particularly for hepatitis B and C viruses and human immunodeficiency virus (HIV). For this reason, it is recommended that you wear protective disposable gloves during venepuncture. Even if you consider a patient to be in a low-risk category for transmissible disease, you can never be sure, as described in the following incident.

> **Tutor quote**
>
> *A doctor had a needlestick injury after injecting the shoulder of an 84-year-old patient. She thought this would be of little consequence as the patient was of 'low-risk' status. However, the patient had been transfused 8 pints of blood during a hip replacement operation some years ago. As this was immediately prior to the appearance of acquired immunodeficiency syndrome (AIDS), the laboratory had followed her up as a high-risk patient, testing her several times for HIV. Fortunately, all tests were negative and the doctor concerned was hepatitis B immune, having been previously immunized.*

'High-risk' patients include those who are:

- known or strongly suspected of being hepatitis B surface antigen (HBsAg)-positive,
- intravenous drug abusers,
- exhibiting high-risk behaviour for HIV,
- on haemodialysis,
- suffering from acute and/or chronic liver disease,
- institutionalized or have Down's syndrome.

The necessity for protective gloves is contentious; you will see some doctors and phlebotomists taking blood without wearing gloves. It is an individual decision and an individual risk, but it is better to be safe than sorry. If you decide to take the risk, you should always wash your hands both before and after taking blood.

All medical students, medical staff and medical personnel who have direct contact with patients or who handle blood products should be immunized against hepatitis B, and their hepatitis B immune levels should be checked 1 month after completing the primary immunization course. Current guidelines recommend a single booster dose of vaccine every 5 years after the primary course. Medical staff on units where invasive procedures are undertaken (e.g. obstetrics, surgery) may be required to have hepatitis C and HIV testing.

Anatomy

Figure 6.35 shows the superficial veins of the upper limb.

What you will need

- A pair of protective disposable gloves.
- A tourniquet: usually an elasticated strip with fastening buckle, or a length of rubber tubing.

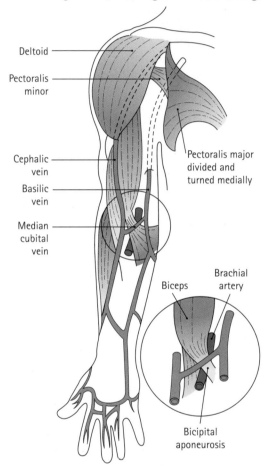

Figure 6.35 The superficial veins of the upper limb (anterior view).

- Vacutainer system: needle 21G (green), needle holder, blood collection tubes.
- Pathology request forms.
- Sealable plastic specimen bag for transport.
- Soft ball or other object for patient to grip (optional).
- A sharps bin: this is a yellow plastic bin with a white swing-top opening into which are disposed needles or other equipment such as syringes that have been in contact with blood or body secretions. These bins are collected by the Clinical Waste Collections Service in Britain and are incinerated according to the recommendations of the Committee on Substances Hazardous to Health.
- For the traditional method: disposable sterile propylene syringe and metal needle.

Taking blood with the Vacutainer system

The Vacutainer system is shown in Figure 6.36.

Procedure (Fig. 6.37)

- Explain the procedure to your patient.
- Select the blood sample bottles for the tests, checking that the labels are blank. Note from the label diagram the volume of blood required for each bottle.
- Check that the request form has been completed.
- With your patient sitting, select the arm for taking blood. This should preferably be the patient's non-dominant side or the arm closest to a supporting surface. You may

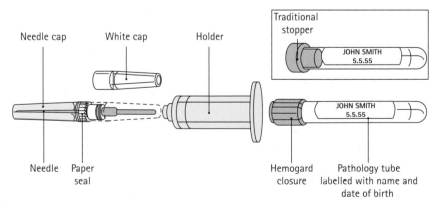

Figure 6.36 The Vacutainer system.

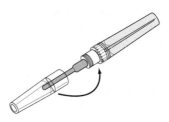

1. **Check paper seal is intact as proof of sterility. If seal is broken, DO NOT USE.** Holding the coloured section of the needle shield in one hand, twist and remove the white section with the other hand **AND DISCARD.**

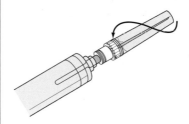

2. Screw needle into holder. Leave coloured shield on needle.

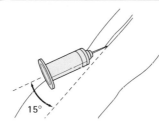

3. Prepare venepuncture site. Remove the coloured section of needle shield. Perform venepuncture in the usual manner with the arm in the downward position.

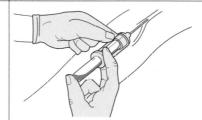

4. Introduce the tube into the holder. Placing your forefinger and middle finger on the flange of the holder and the thumb on the bottom of the tube, push the tube to the end of the holder, puncturing the diaphragm of the stopper. Remove the tourniquet as soon as blood begins to flow into the tube.

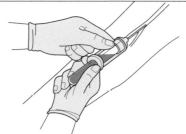

5. When the vacuum is exhausted and blood flow ceases, apply a soft pressure with the thumb against the flange of the holder to disengage stopper from the needle and remove the tube from holder. If more samples are required repeat from step 4.

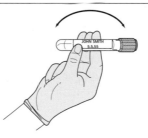

6. While blood is flowing into succeeding tubes, gently invert previously filled tubes containing additives 8 to 10 times to mix additives with blood. Do not shake. Vigorous mixing may cause haemolysis. Remove last tube from the holder before withdrawing needle from vein.

> Dispose of needles in accordance with local
> Control of Infection Protocols.
> Used needles are dangerous; be safe not sorry.

Figure 6.37 How to take blood with the Vacutainer system.

support the arm on a small supporting pillow. Apply the tourniquet to the patient's upper arm, about 10 cm above (proximal to) the elbow. The tourniquet should compress the veins but not be so tight distally that the arterial circulation is obstructed. The pulse should be palpable distally. With the arm extended and supported, ask the patient to clench the fist or grip a soft object. This helps to make the veins more prominent. Select a vein for venepuncture in the antecubital fossa. If the veins are compressed for longer than 3 minutes, the results of blood tests may be invalid. If this is the case, release the tourniquet for a few minutes and reapply prior to taking the blood samples.

- Put on a pair of suitably sized disposable gloves.
- Select a 21G needle, checking that the paper seal is intact as a sign of sterility. **If the seal is broken, do not use it**; discard the needle into the sharps bin. Holding the coloured section of the needle in one hand and the white section in the other hand, twist and remove the white cap and discard it.
- Screw the needle into the holder, leaving the coloured shield on the needle. Remove the cap from the needle. Approach the patient's arm with the needle bevel facing upwards. With the needle and Vacutainer at an angle of approximately 15 degrees from the surface, puncture the skin and advance the needle about 1 cm through the skin to ensure that it is completely inside the vein. Pushing the needle too far may perforate the opposite wall of the vein.
- Introduce the sample tube into the holder. With your forefinger and middle finger astride the base of the holder, place your thumb at the end of the tube and exert steady pressure, pushing the tube towards the end of the holder until you have punctured the stopper at the end of the tube. As soon as blood flows into the tube, remove the tourniquet.
- Allow the tube to fill to the required level. Apply gentle pressure with your thumb against the base of the holder, and remove the tube and stopper from the needle. When

the vacuum is exhausted, the blood flow stops.

- For further samples, successively substitute the remaining tubes using the same technique: first tubes without additives, next coagulation tubes, and finally tubes with additives. The latter should be gently inverted about eight to ten times to allow mixing with the blood. Do not shake, as this may cause haemolysis of the blood.
- When the last tube has been removed from the holder, withdraw the needle from the patient's vein. Apply a steady pressure, or ask the patient to apply pressure over a cottonwool swab at the puncture site with the elbow extended for 1–2 minutes. Discard the swab into a clinical waste container. If the puncture site is oozing blood, apply a small plaster. Flexing the arm as a method of applying pressure may lead to bruising at the venepuncture site.
- Dispose of the needle directly into the sharps bin (Fig. 6.38) without re-capping. It is also recommend that needle holders be discarded,

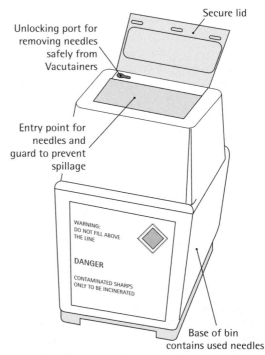

Secure lid

Unlocking port for removing needles safely from Vacutainers

Entry point for needles and guard to prevent spillage

WARNING: DO NOT FILL ABOVE THE LINE

DANGER

CONTAMINATED SHARPS ONLY TO BE INCINERATED

Base of bin contains used needles

Figure 6.38 A sharps bin for the safe disposal of contaminated needles.

although they may be washed in warm soapy water and dried before re-using. If there is no sharps bin available, for example when taking blood at a patient's home, you will need to re-cap the needle, which is best attempted by placing the cap on a flat surface and directing the needle into the cap in the same plane. In this situation, an empty soft drinks can makes a good temporary container, and this can be disposed of later with clinical waste at the surgery.

- Label the sample tubes with a ballpoint pen, completing the patient's details. Include full name, date of birth, hospital number and other information requested. Ask the patient to confirm his or her full name and date of birth, and check the details against the request form. Place the samples in a plastic, self-sealing transport bag. These usually have a pouch separate from the sample compartment for request forms. Blood from a high-risk patient should be labelled 'high-risk', and this should also be indicated on the request form.

Practical points

- *What if I do not obtain sufficient blood?* An under-filled tube may invalidate the test result. Tubes should always be correctly filled according to the diagram on the label.
- *How do I know if the needle is in a vein?* As soon as you push the pathology tube onto the holder, if the needle is in the vein, blood will flow immediately. If nothing happens, draw the needle back slightly and, if you subsequently enter the vein, blood will appear.
- *How do I know whether the vacuum in the sample tube has been lost?* As long as the needle remains under the skin, the vacuum is maintained. If the needle slips outside the skin, use a new tube.
- *What should I do if the vein collapses?* Remove the tube, leaving the needle in place in the vein. When the pressure returns in the vein, re-insert the tube.
- *What if the veins are too difficult to enter?* This happens with obese patients or patients with sclerosed veins from repeated phlebotomies or intravenous treatments such as

chemotherapy. After two or three unsuccessful attempts to collect blood, it is advisable to send a patient to the hospital phlebotomy service. Winged blood collection sets with thinner-gauge needles and multiple sample adapters for connection to a Vacutainer holder are available in hospitals.

- *What if I puncture the opposite wall of the vein?* A bruise (haematoma) may form at the site. You may have already obtained your sample; if not, it may be possible to continue the phlebotomy. After withdrawal of the needle, the patient should raise the arm above shoulder height, which will cause the veins to collapse and prevent further bleeding into the tissues.
- *What if I spill blood on myself or the immediate environment?* Wash the blood off your person with plenty of soapy water and an alcohol solution (70 per cent) if available. Use sodium hypochlorite solution 10 000 ppm (bleach, Milton) to wipe down contaminated surfaces and leave in contact for 30 minutes. Report any spillage or accidents involving blood or other body fluids to the practice nurse, sister in charge or occupational health officer.

Note. A video recording of phlebotomy will give you a better overview. A copy may be obtainable from your local hospital phlebotomy department.

Taking blood using the traditional needle and syringe

Taking blood with the traditional needle and syringe is done less often nowadays because use of the Vacutainer system reduces the risk of contamination. However, it is sometimes necessary to use the traditional method, for example when a blood sample is required at a home visit or the Vacutainer is not available. The patient is prepared as described above.

- Protective gloves should be worn. This is more important because of the increased risk of contamination.
- Select a pre-packed, sterile, disposable needle (size 21G) and propylene syringe of sufficient volume for the blood tests (10 or 20 mL). Remove from the packaging.

- Attach the needle to the syringe. Check that the plunger of the syringe can be withdrawn.
- With the plunger in the closed (pushed-in) position, remove the cap from the needle.
- Steady the selected vein by applying pressure with your non-dominant hand to the antecubital fossa. With the needle bevel uppermost, puncture the skin over the vein and advance the tip into the vein along its longitudinal axis for about 1 or 2 cm and stop.
- Steady the syringe against the patient's arm with your non-dominant hand and slowly withdraw the syringe plunger with your dominant hand. Blood should enter the barrel of the syringe. Withdraw the required volume.
- Release the tourniquet. Withdraw the needle and attached syringe as an entire unit from the patient's arm using a quick motion. Apply pressure with a cotton-wool swab to the puncture point, with the patient's arm extended as described above.

Practical points

- If there is insufficient blood for the test, you may need to take a second sample. It is preferable to re-puncture the patient than to attempt to disconnect the needle from the syringe in situ and replace it with another syringe. Only in extreme circumstances should this be considered, for example in emergencies or when vein availability is very poor. This procedure will always result in contamination with blood. **Protective gloves are essential in these circumstances.**
- Surfaces contaminated with blood should be cleaned with sodium hypochlorite.

SPECIAL COMMUNICATION SKILLS

HOW TO WRITE A REFERRAL LETTER

Communicating information about patients to health professionals is integral to clinical practice. Increasingly in general practice, patients with continuing problems may be managed by several healthcare professionals working in primary or secondary care. When a GP involves another professional in patient care – whether for an opinion, transferring clinical responsibility, for investigation, reassurance or management – it is essential to transfer information to the professional involved in a way that is helpful and effective. Conversely, the same applies when a specialist communicates with a GP.

Although informal referral can be made by telephone or face-to-face contact, for operational reasons and for record-keeping purposes, referral should be made by letter or, if available, by electronic booking. In this system, patient referrals from general practice to hospital specialists use tick-box protocols in web-based hospital links. On receipt of data, a central appointments system returns appointment details for the patient, and forwards the electronic referral to the specialist clinic. This provides a faster referral service for patients.

Until electronic referral replaces written referrals, the art of letter writing will continue to be an important skill. Writing good referral letters is difficult and needs practice. Written information should be clear, concise and presented in a logical way. The process involves abstracting information from personal knowledge of the patient and their health record, and presenting this as a summary. The letter should have maximum impact in as short a space and time as possible. Time constraints are equally relevant for both the specialist and the GP. If the letter is too long, the specialist may not have time to read it.

Although everyone has a personal writing style, there are a few rules that should be observed.

- Write in clear, coherent sentences, expressing the problems as accurately as possible.
- Use short words and phrases, rather than long words and rambling sentences.
- Use simple language, avoiding colloquialisms. It is acceptable to use the patient's expressions when describing the presentation.
- Avoid medical jargon, for example use 'breathing' not 'pulmonary ventilation'.
- Avoid abbreviations: not everyone understands them.
- Make it legible: type if possible.

Practical Exercise

Part 1. Think of a patient you have seen with your tutor who needs referral to a specialist. Imagine you are the specialist and have just received the letter. What information would you need from your tutor to allow you to respond appropriately to the request for help? Jot down the information points before continuing with this section. Write a model referral letter for your tutor. Stop here, and attempt to write your letter before reading on. Your outline should have included the following.

❏ *Patient details*: name, age, sex, National Health Service (NHS) number, ethnic background, hospital number.

❏ *Details of GP*: name, address, telephone number.

❏ *Reason for referral*: what help is the GP requesting? What question is being asked of the specialist?

❏ *Degree of urgency for appointment*: state if an urgent appointment is indicated.

❏ *Clinical problem.*

❏ *Important clinical and previous history.*

❏ *Findings on physical examination*: include key points and significant positive and negative findings that support your diagnosis or reason for referral.

❏ *Findings on investigation*: photocopies of results should be included.

❏ *Medication and drug sensitivities.*

❏ *Psychosocial history*: include this if it is likely to help the specialist's management; for example if an elderly patient lives alone, include details of the living circumstances and key carer.

❏ *Explanation given to the patient about the condition and the reason for referral*: this is helpful if the diagnosis may involve breaking bad news, for example if a diagnosis of cancer is likely.

❏ *Expected outcome of the referral.*

❏ *Desirable follow-up*: indicate whether you are expecting the patient to be returned to your care as soon as possible, or prefer the specialist to provide on-going management.

Part 2. Now check your referral letter using the above outline. If you have omitted vital information, amend your letter. Check its suitability and format with your tutor. If your tutor agrees, you could have the letter typed, ready to send to the specialist, remembering that your tutor will need to sign it. When your tutor receives a reply, ask if you may see the letter. Did the specialist interpret the letter correctly? Were all the questions answered? Have you learnt anything from the reply?

Part 3. Recent guidelines for good clinical practice have recommended that patient referral letters from GPs to specialists and replies from specialists to referring GPs should be copied to patients. This has been introduced in some areas.

❏ Can you list at least five benefits to patients of receiving copies of letters?

❏ What factors would a doctor need to take into account in the style and content of the letter?

❏ Are there issues of confidentiality to be addressed in introducing this practice?

HOW TO SIGN A MEDICAL CERTIFICATE OF CAUSE OF DEATH (DEATH CERTIFICATE)

Background knowledge

When a patient dies, there is a procedure for registering the death and for arranging the burial. It is a time of personal distress for the deceased's family, and the role of the family doctor is to provide support and guidance to the family (for whom a helpful booklet is available: Benefits Agency, 2000) and to follow the legal procedures for the registration of the death. Before a death can be reported in England and Wales, there must be either a Medical Certificate of Cause of Death, commonly referred to as a death certificate, or, if the death was unexpected, a certificate from a coroner after appropriate investigations into the cause of death have been made. A coroner is a lawyer or doctor responsible for investigating deaths.

It is the statutory duty of a registered medical practitioner to complete a death certificate stating to the best of his or her knowledge and belief the cause of death. The certificate is a legal document. If a doctor gives a cause of death that he or she knows to be untrue, charges of perjury and making a false declaration may follow.

If the death was *expected* and the patient died of *natural causes*, the procedure is as follows.

■ *Confirmation of death* of the patient by an examining doctor, who may be the patient's medical practitioner or an on-call doctor.

■ Arrangements for *removal of the body* by a funeral director (undertaker) to a funeral parlour. The deceased's family or representative is responsible for deciding on a funeral director.

■ The provision of a *Medical Certificate of Cause of Death* that states the cause of death. This is signed by the attending doctor and is provided free of charge. It must be delivered to the Registrar of Births and Deaths in the sub-district where the deceased lived. It is the responsibility of the doctor who signs the death certificate to deliver it in person or by post to the local Registrar of Births and Deaths. In most instances, however, the doctor arranges for this to be done by an informant of the deceased. A list of eligible persons who can act as informants is given on the reverse of the formal notice of death on the medical certificate. They are usually a relative, a person present at the death or the person who is arranging disposal of the body.

■ The provision of a formal notice of death entitled *Notice to Informant*. This is attached to the Medical Certificate of Cause of Death as a 'tear-off' section, and is completed by the doctor who signs the death certificate. It is provided free of charge.

■ If cremation is to take place, the provision of a *Cremation Certificate*, signed in two parts by two doctors who practise independently of each other, one of whom will have signed the death certificate. There is a fee for this certificate that is paid to the signatories by the funeral director and is included in the funeral costs.

If the death was *unexpected*, or the patient died of *unnatural* or *suspicious causes* (see below), the procedure is as follows:

■ *Confirmation of death* by an attending or on-call doctor.

■ Reporting of the death to the local *Coroner's Office* by the attending or emergency doctor. If there are suspicious circumstances, the doctor must *inform the police*. Where there are doubts, the doctor should discuss details with the coroner, who has the discretion to decide whether it is permissible to provide a death certificate or to proceed with a post mortem.

■ *Removal of the body to a mortuary*: the Coroner's Office will make arrangements for this.

■ Investigation into the *cause of death* by the coroner, who will provide the necessary certification. An *inquest* may be necessary to determine the cause of death. Doctors must co-operate fully with any formal inquiry into the treatment of the patient, and not withhold any relevant information.

Unnatural or suspicious causes of death must be referred to the coroner and include a death:

■ which was violent, unnatural or occurred under suspicious circumstances,

■ for which the cause is unknown or uncertain,

■ which occurred while the patient was undergoing an operation or before full recovery from an anaesthetic, was related to anaesthesia, or followed a fracture or fall,

■ caused by an industrial disease or industrial poisoning,

■ which occurred as a result of a medical procedure or treatment, or from a termination of pregnancy,

■ which may have been due to lack of medical care or where there were allegations of medical mismanagement,

■ where the deceased was not attended by a doctor during the terminal illness or was not seen during the last 14 days of life,

■ which occurred as a result of self-neglect or neglect by others,

■ which occurred in prison or in police custody.

The Medical Certificate of Cause of Death

This may be the first time as a student that you are observing your tutor sign a death certificate. As a PRHO or registrar, it may be the first time you are signing a death certificate in general practice. A book of Medical Certificates of Cause of Death (Form 66) is normally kept in the practice and is supplied by the Registrar General through the local Registrar of Births and Deaths. The same form is used in hospitals and the community and for all deaths occurring after the first 28 days of life. A different form is used for the deaths of live-born children occurring before 28 days. The Births and Deaths Registration Act of 1953 requires the form to be completed and signed by the medical practitioner who attended the patient during his last illness and saw the patient in the last 14 days of life. The certificate has to be accepted by the registrar. If the certificate has not been completed accurately or is unsatisfactory, it cannot be accepted.

Procedure

- Are you eligible to sign the death certificate? If so, you will be registered with the General Medical Council (GMC) either provisionally as a PRHO or with full registration as a GP registrar. You will have attended the deceased in his or her final illness and have seen the patient in the last 14 days of life. It is not a requirement for you to have seen the body after death. This is necessary only if you sign the cremation certificate.
- Start with the Medical Certificate of Cause of Death (Fig. 6.39). Do you know the cause of death? Do you feel confident that death was due to natural causes? If 'yes', you may sign the death certificate. Hand write in ink the following where requested: the full name of the deceased, the date of death as stated to you, the age of the deceased, the place of death, and the date when the deceased was last seen *alive* by you.
- *If you do not know the cause of death*, or did not attend the patient in the last 14 days of life, or you consider that the death was due to violence or unnatural causes, or was a sudden death of unknown cause, you must notify the Coroner's Office immediately. This includes the deaths of patients who sustained a fracture, had an accident or an operation, or had not recovered sufficiently from an anaesthetic. In these circumstances, you should not complete the death certificate.
- You are next asked to circle an appropriate digit or letter in two lists: *confirmation by post-mortem examination* and a *statement that the deceased person was seen or not seen after death*. For information about post mortem, you should indicate one of four

options: (1) whether the cause of death takes account of information obtained from post mortem, (2) whether information from post mortem may be available later, (3) a post mortem is not being held, or (4) you have reported the death to the coroner. Information about whether the deceased was seen after death offers three options: (a) that you as signatory saw the body, (b) that another medical practitioner saw the body, or (c) that the body was not seen after death by a medical practitioner. If you have reported the death to the coroner for further action, you should initial Statement A on the reverse of the form.

- The next section asks for details of the *cause of death*. It is completed in two parts: Part I deals with the actual or conditions leading to the cause of death, and Part II asks for information on other significant conditions contributing to the death but not related to the disease. Part I may confuse even the most experienced doctor. The form asks for the 'underlying cause of death' to be completed in I(c) and the disease or condition directly leading to death in I(a). You are asked to indicate at I(b) any other condition, if any, leading to I(a). The 'underlying cause of death' is the disease or injury that initiated the series of morbid events that led to the death. In I(a) you are asked for the disease, injury or complication causing death and not the mode of death, as in asphyxia. If two conditions have contributed to the death, both causes should be written on the certificate. An example is 'I(a) Chronic bronchitis, coronary atheroma'. If you are awaiting further information for confirmation of cause of death, such as a histology report, you should initial Statement B on the reverse of the form.
- On the right-hand side and opposite the section 'Cause of Death', you will notice a box in which you are asked to state the approximate interval between the onset of each condition listed and death. Below is an example.

I(a) Myocardial infarction	5 days
I(b) Coronary atheroma	5 years
I(c) Influenza	2 weeks
II Chronic bronchitis	18 years

BIRTHS AND DEATHS REGISTRATION ACT 1953

(Form prescribed by the Registration of Births, Deaths and Marriages (Amendment) Regulations 1985)

MEDICAL CERTIFICATE OF CAUSE OF DEATH

For use only by a Registered Medical Practitioner WHO HAS BEEN IN ATTENDANCE during the deceased's last illness, and to be delivered by him forthwith to the Registrar of Births and Deaths.

Register to enter
No. of Death Entry

Name of deceased ....

Date of death as stated to me .... day of .... 19..... Age as stated to me ....

Place of death ....

Last seen alive by me .... day of .... 19.....

1	The certified cause of death takes account of information obtained from post-mortem.	*Please ring appropriate digit(s) and letter.*
2	Information from post-mortem may be available later.	a	Seen after death by me.
3	Post-mortem not being held.	b	Seen after death by another medical practitioner but not by me.
4	I have reported this death to the Coroner for further action.	c	Not seen after death by a medical practitioner.

[See overleaf]

CAUSE OF DEATH

The condition thought to be the 'Underlying Cause of Death' should appear in the lowest completed line of Part I.

These particulars not to be entered in death register

Approximate interval between onset and death

I(a) Disease or condition directly leading to death† ....

(b) Other disease or condition, if any, leading to I(a) ....

(c) Other disease or condition, if any, leading to I(b) ....

II Other significant conditions CONTRIBUTING TO THE DEATH but not related to the disease or condition causing it. ....

The death might have been due to or contributed to by the employment followed at some time by the deceased.

Please tick where applicable

†*This does not mean the mode of dying, such as heart failure, asphyxia, asthenia, etc: it means the disease, injury, or complication which caused death.*

I hereby certify that I was in medical attendance during the above named deceased's last illness, and that the particulars and cause of death above written are true to the best of my knowledge and belief.

Signature .... Qualifications as registered by General Medical Council ....

Residence .... Date ....

For deaths in hospital: Please give the name of the consultant responsible for the above-named as a patient. ....

(Form prescribed by the Registration of Births, Deaths and Marriages Regulations 1968)

NOTICE TO INFORMANT

I hereby give notice that I have this day signed a medical certificate of cause of death of

....

Signature ....

Date ....

This notice is to be delivered by the informant to the registrar of births and deaths for the sub-district in which the death occurred.

The certifying medical practitioner must give this notice to the person who is qualified and liable to act as informant for the registration of death (see list overleaf).

DUTIES OF INFORMANT

Failure to deliver this notice to the registrar renders the informant liable to prosecution. The death cannot be registered until the medical certificate has reached the registrar.

When the death is registered the informant must be prepared to give to the registrar the following particulars relating to the deceased:

1. The date and place of death.

2. The full name and surname (and the maiden surname if the deceased was a woman who had married).

3. The date and place of birth.

4. The occupation (and if the deceased was a married woman or a widow the name and occupation of her husband).

5. The usual address.

6. Whether the deceased was in receipt of a pension or allowance from public funds.

7. If the deceased was married, the date of birth of the surviving widow or widower.

THE DECEASED'S MEDICAL CARD SHOULD BE DELIVERED TO THE REGISTRAR

COUNTERFOIL

For use of Medical Practitioner, who should complete in all cases.

Name of deceased} ....

Date of death ....

Age ....

Place of death ....

Last seen alive by me ....

Post-mortem}* 1 2 3 4
Coroner

Whether seen after death* a b c

Cause of death:—

I (a) ....

(b) ....

(c) ....

II ....

Please tick where applicable

Employment? ☐

B. Further information offered? ....

Signature ....

Date ....

Ring appropriate digit(s) and letter.

Complete where applicable

PERSONS QUALIFIED AND LIABLE TO ACT AS INFORMANTS

The following persons are designated by the Births and Deaths Registration Act 1953 as qualified to give information concerning a death:—

DEATHS IN HOUSES AND PUBLIC INSTITUTIONS

(1) A relative of the deceased, present at the death.

(2) A relative of the deceased, in attendance during the last illness.

(3) A relative of the deceased, residing or being in the sub-district where the death occurred.

(4) A person present at the death.

(5) The occupier* if he knew of the happening of the death.

(6) Any inmate if he knew of the happening of the death.

(7) The person causing the disposal of the body.

DEATHS NOT IN HOUSES OR DEAD BODIES FOUND

(1) Any relative of the deceased having knowledge of any of the particulars required to be registered.

(2) Any person present at the death.

(3) Any person who found the body.

(4) Any person in charge of the body.

(5) The person causing the disposal of the body.

*"Occupier" in relation to a public institution includes the governor, keeper, master, matron, superintendent, or other chief resident officer.

A

I have reported this death to the Coroner for further action.

Initials of certifying medical practitioner.

The Coroner needs to consider all cases where:

The death might have been due to or contributed to by a violent or unnatural cause (including an accident);

or the cause of death cannot be identified;

or the death might have been due to or contributed to by drugs, medicine, abortion or poison;

B

I may be in a position later to give, on application by the Registrar General, additional information as to the cause of death for the purpose of more precise statistical classification.

Initials of certifying medical practitioner.

or there is reason to believe that the death occurred during an operation or under or prior to complete recovery from an anaesthetic or arising subsequently out of an incident during an operation or an anaesthetic;

or the death might have been due to or contributed to by the employment followed at some time by the deceased.

LIST OF SOME OF THE CATEGORIES OF DEATH WHICH MAY BE OF INDUSTRIAL ORIGIN

MALIGNANT DISEASES	Causes include:
(a) Skin	– radiation and sunlight; – pitch or tar; – mineral oils
(b) Nasal	– wood or leather work; – nickel
(c) Lung	– asbestos; – nickel; – radiation
(d) Pleura	– asbestos
(e) Urinary Tract	– benzidine; – dyestuff; – chemicals in rubbers
(f) Liver	– PVC manufacture
(g) Bone	– radiation
(h) Lymphatics and haematopoietic	– radiation; – benzene

POISONING	
(a) Metals	e.g. arsenics, cadmium, lead
(b) Chemicals	e.g. chlorine, benzene
(c) Solvents	e.g. trichlorethylene

INFECTIOUS DISEASES	Causes include:
(a) Anthrax	– imported bone, bonemeal, hide or fur
(b) Brucellosis	– farming or veterinary
(c) Tuberculosis	– contact at work
(d) Leptospirosis	– farming, sewer or under-ground workers
(e) Tetanus	– farming or gardening
(f) Rabies	– animal handling
(g) Viral hepatitis	– contact at work

BRONCHIAL ASTHMA AND PNEUMONITIS	
(a) Occupational asthma	– sensitising agent at work
(b) Allergic Alveolitis	– farming

PNEUMOCONIOSIS	– mining and quarrying; – potteries; – asbestos

NOTE:—The Practitioner, on signing the certificate, should complete, sign and date the Notice to the Informant, which should be detached and handed to the Informant. The Practitioner should then, without delay, deliver the certificate itself to the Registrar of Births and Deaths for the sub-district in which the death occurred. Envelopes for enclosing the certificates are supplied by the Registrar.

Figure 6.39 Medical Certificate of Cause of Death.

■ Below the section 'Cause of Death' is a box in which you are asked whether the death may have been due to or contributed to by the employment followed at some time by the deceased. It does not ask you to provide details, only to tick the box, although you may have listed this under Part II. Details of some of the categories of death that may be of industrial origin are given on the reverse of the death certificate and in fuller detail at the back of the certificate book. However, you should have medical confirmation that this is the case because the coroner will ask you to submit a medical report. In the event of a suspected industrial disease, there will probably be an inquest.

■ Sign and date the form, certifying that you were in attendance during the deceased's last illness and that the details on the form are true to the best of your knowledge and belief. You are asked to give your qualifications as registered by the GMC, and to state your residence: this means the general practice address, not your home address.

■ You should complete the counterfoil attached to the book that asks for a copy of the details on the medical certificate.

■ Finally, you should check whether the *back of the certificate form* needs to be completed: Statement A that you have reported the death to the coroner; Statement B that you may be in a position later to provide the Registrar General with additional information as to the cause of death for statistical purposes.

Practical points

■ A symptom or a mode of dying such as heart failure is not acceptable as a cause of death. The underlying disease must be stated.

■ When recording a tumour, you should state the histology and whether benign or malignant.

■ Avoid the word 'accident', as in 'cerebrovascular accident', as this alarms relatives and implies violence. Instead you are advised to use 'stroke'.

■ Avoid ambiguous statements such as the cause of death was 'old age'. The registrar has a list of accepted causes of death and if your stated cause of death is not included on the list, the registrar is required to notify the coroner. This may cause distress to the relatives and it would have been more considerate to discuss the wording with the Coroner's Office first.

Communicating with relatives

It is good practice to see or telephone the deceased's next of kin to explain the details on the death certificate, and to enquire about who will be the informant. This contact provides an opportunity for relatives to ask questions about the cause of death and for you to clarify concerns. You should check that the informant knows what to do with the death certificate and the Notice to Informant. It is also an opportunity to enquire about the relatives' health and to offer support. Finally, thanking or commending the family if they have provided care will assist the bereavement process and will be appreciated.

HOW TO CONSULT WITH SPECIAL AGE GROUPS: CHILDREN AND ELDERLY PEOPLE

Consulting with patients at the extremes of age requires an adaptation of your approach with adults. Though separated by an age span of several decades, there are similarities in history taking when consulting with infants and elderly people who depend on others for part or all of their care. With both groups, communication involves a third party – babies with their parents or guardian, elderly dependent people with a relative or other key person with caring responsibilities. The sharing of information takes place as a trio of doctor, patient and informant. Even if your patient cannot talk, you can establish rapport non-verbally through eye contact, by touching, miming or writing if the patient can read. Use information gleaned from observing your patient, interaction with the carer and the home environment to supplement your history. The malodours of an incontinent patient, young or old, are distinctive. A healthy baby with normal muscle tone handles differently from the ill, floppy child. Nurses in close contact with immobile elderly patients describe how they intuitively 'feel' their patient's condition; for example patients with a stroke and disabling loss of speech (aphasia/dysphasia) may offer greater than normal resistance to being positioned if suffering pain.

Consulting with infants and elderly people requires special skills, which you will develop with experience.

Consulting with children

General approach

- Every child has the right to be treated as an individual with particular needs and potentialities.
- Every child has the right to have his or her wishes taken into account, and the right to speak and be listened to.
- It is the duty of professionals to take account of age, sex, health, personality, race, culture and life experiences when planning services for children (Children Act, United Kingdom 1989).

These principles underpin the approach to managing children. Whatever a child's age, each consultation is a partnership between the child, the child's parent(s) or guardian(s) and the doctor.

Children's personalities, behaviour and ability to communicate vary widely and are dependent on their stage of development, cultural background and intelligence. In addition, children and their parents may have unpredictable responses to illness. Parents often seem unduly upset and communicate a great deal of anxiety when their children are ill, to a degree which may appear disproportionate to the child's state of health. With the intense early bonding between parents and babies, it is emotionally disturbing to observe a previously responsive child deteriorate and, furthermore, frustrating when a child is unable to describe symptoms. Parents have an innate fear of losing a child – a fear that may be fuelled by sensationalist reporting in the media, particularly during epidemics. In addition, parents may be exhausted through disturbed sleep in caring for their child, leaving them emotionally vulnerable. These factors need to be considered when consulting with parents and children. Each consultation should be handled sensitively and with an individual approach tailored to the needs of each situation.

Children and babies are particularly fickle. They may appear ill one moment and bouncing with energy the next. They may be fractious in the consulting room and difficult to talk to, or they may be so excited when visiting the surgery that they show a dramatic improvement. Parents will often say that the child 'just wasn't like that when I left home. He's proving me a liar!' Remember, however, that parents are the experts in their child's health, and are the most qualified to give an accurate description of their child, even if not confirmed in the surgery. Communicating with children calls for patience and flexibility. Praising good behaviour throughout the consultation encourages co-operation.

As children grow older, communication patterns with parents and people in authority change in a complex way that reflects their move towards independence. While some teenagers appear to be forthcoming in the consultation, others may display a grudging resentment, play a manipulative 'game' with their parents or doctor, or be overwhelmed by anxiety and embarrassment, especially if asked about personal matters or required to undress. All this is a normal part of growing up and needs to be allowed for in the consultation by offering an explanation for the reasons for your questions or examination. The age at which teenagers prefer to consult alone varies according to the nature of the presenting symptom, the degree of maturity and the relationship with their parents and doctor. Over the age of 16, teenagers have legal responsibility for their personal medical care. Despite this, many prefer to be accompanied in the consultation. To respect confidentiality, teenagers should be given the opportunity to talk alone when accompanied. Older children are quick to identify adults as patronizing through what might be misinterpreted glances of disapproval or comments. For this reason, it is advisable to avoid personal comments or passing judgement.

Practical tips

- Greet your young patient by name in a friendly way, introduce yourself and explain where he or she should sit.

■ Observe the child's behaviour and interaction with his or her parents and with yourself as you bring the family into the consulting room. This will provide useful information before you begin the consultation. Is the child shy, avoiding eye-to-eye contact, hiding behind or clinging to the parent, or is the child friendly, confident and chatty from the start? Nowadays, children are drilled into not talking to strangers so that, if this is your first contact, the child will probably appear unfriendly while at the same time recognizing your tutor as a familiar. To understand how to respond to such a typical child, it will help to consider the impact of entering your consulting room.

Thinking and Discussion Point

❏ Spare a thought for the child. Imagine yourself as a small person in a grown-up world. Think of how the doctor and the consulting room would appear to you, looming at your small feet as you walk in through the door, holding the hand of a towering adult. Literature affords many illustrations of disproportionate sizing – *Alice in Wonderland*, *Gulliver's Travels* and *Mrs Pepperpot*!

❏ Show restraint. Children need time to adjust to 'strange' people seated in what appears to be a vast room dominated by intriguing instruments and computers. At first, avoid overwhelming the child with personal comments or by being over-friendly, as this approach may be rejected and the child may burst into tears rather than reciprocate. While initially greeting the child by eye contact and name it is preferable to initially focus attention on the parents and allow the child time to absorb the surroundings. Once you have passed the test of acceptability, your small patient may begin to relate, and you can then shift the consultation from a two-way to a three-way exchange.

❏ Physical contact. It is sometimes tempting to pick up babies, but they may sense unfamiliarity and not settle. Parents may also object if you treat their baby as a cuddly toy. Unless they ask you to help by holding their baby, or you wish to examine the baby, it is advisable to leave the infant undisturbed in the parent's arms. Likewise, with older children it is best to avoid physical contact unless they spontaneously climb onto your lap. Exceptionally, parents may misinterpret contact as manhandling of their child rather than an expression of your goodwill.

❏ Diversions. Toys help divert attention and encourage a child to settle into the consultation. Children usually prefer to discover toys alone rather than having them thrust into their hands. A nearby box containing a small number of toys appropriate for a range of ages or a toy temptingly placed on a stool may help. When examining a child, diversionary games such as 'peek a boo', demonstrating examination procedures on a doll or teddy or, if none is available, on a parent will reassure and encourage co-operation. Sometimes the whole consultation has to be turned into one big game in order to obtain the necessary information and enlist co-operation, but this is often hard work and time consuming.

History taking and examination of a child

Having settled the family group into the consulting room, you can proceed with history taking. The use of open questions helps identify the parent's expectation from the visit early on in the contact. The age when a child is sufficiently mature to give a reliable history varies, but may be around the age of 10, although even at this age the child may not share the parents' concern about his or her medical condition. With a younger child, questions should be directed towards the parent or escort, while allowing the child to contribute spontaneously. It is wise to check the child's information with the adult and, conversely, to check the adult's information with the child.

It is acceptable to examine children in an opportunistic way rather than follow a systems procedure, particularly when time is limited. You may be able to examine a child more thoroughly if the child is co-operatively sitting or lying on the parent's knee than if he or she is distressed, lying on an examination couch. If you need to examine the ears or chest, do so first, because once a child starts to cry these procedures will be difficult. Procedures that may be uncomfortable, for example inspecting the mouth or taking blood, should be left to the end of the examination.

A common difficulty is knowing how to express to a child the parent's concern without making the child feel ashamed or guilty. It is best to address the problem and the parent's anxiety directly, while involving the child in the decision-making process. For example with a 7-year-old child who is bed-wetting (nocturnal enuresis): 'Charlie, mum is worried about you wetting the bed at night. Many children do this at your age. They can't help it. One day they will grow out of it; it will stop and everything will be all right. Because it's a lot of work for mum to wash the sheets, shall we see if we can find someone to help you get dry?'

Practical Exercise

During your time in general practice, try to gain experience in taking histories from the following groups:
- ❑ a parent/parents and baby,
- ❑ a parent/parents and toddler,
- ❑ a parent/parents and primary school child,
- ❑ a parent/parents and pubertal child aged 12–15 years,
- ❑ an adolescent consulting alone.

Compare the contributions made by the child towards the consultation at each age.

Consulting with elderly patients

Most elderly people take care of themselves, plan their own lives and make their own decisions. However, a small proportion suffer from serious conditions such as stroke or Alzheimer's disease, which have such a devastating effect on their life that they need help to cope with everyday needs. For some, communication is made difficult by deafness, speech disorders or memory impairment.

Thinking and Discussion Point

Taking histories from this age group allows you to assess your attitude towards older people. How do you regard elderly patients?
- ❑ With affection as you would your grandparents or an aunt or uncle?
- ❑ With respect or fear because of their great age, wisdom and dignity?
- ❑ With curiosity as a source of history pre-dating your own existence?
- ❑ With frustration because speech and hearing loss prevent effective communication?
- ❑ With contempt because they have no role in life, may be unkempt, incontinent or grumpy?
- ❑ With disdain because they appear old-fashioned, speaking and dressing differently from you?

If 'ageism' is defined as prejudice or discrimination against people of a certain age, consider how the outcome of a consultation with an elderly patient may be influenced by the negative views of the interviewer.

At times you may experience some negative feelings when communicating with elderly people. Negative feelings must be addressed, even in the most adverse circumstances, for example when visiting a neglected patient in distressingly dirty conditions. It helps to understand why patients live in this state. What are the medical circumstances? What were this person's previous personality and lifestyle? How can their quality of life be improved despite having an irreversible medical condition? Whatever the patient's state, courtesy is essential. Elderly patients dislike being patronized, but they may be too courteous to tell you so.

The question of whether to address an elderly patient by first name or surname with title sometimes arises. Although you may feel rapport would be established more quickly by using first names, most older people believe the use of surnames is a mark of respect. If in doubt, the use of names should be discussed with your patient. What is important is that both you and your patient feel at ease.

Observation provides clues about communication difficulties. Spotting a hearing aid may prompt you to adjust your voice, but if you do this, check that the patient can hear before proceeding with the interview. A patient with a hemiplegia may have visual loss on one side (hemianopia), and you may need to change position if your patient is to see you.

A keen eye during home visits may supplement your history taking and provide valuable information about a patient's social circumstances. Is the house clean or cluttered? How do the relatives and patient interact? Are there signs that the patient is not coping with everyday activities?

COMMUNICATING WITH PATIENTS WITH LIMITED OR NO ENGLISH

The UK population has become increasingly cosmopolitan and multi-racial. Patients with limited or no English are more likely to present in metropolitan and tourist areas, although increasingly this may be the case throughout the UK. Patients with language difficulties represent a range of circumstances: people working on secondment from overseas, migrant workers from abroad seeking short-term employment, refugees or asylum seekers, holiday visitors, and relatives visiting families in the UK. All groups are entitled to registration with a GP. Holiday visitors register temporarily with the NHS if their country of origin has reciprocal arrangements with the UK, or privately if this is not the case. Refugees are entitled to the full range of NHS healthcare services free of charge and are encouraged to have permanent registration with a GP. The registration system in general practice encourages continuity of care and is helpful for managing patients with language difficulties.

Communicating with patients with limited English is fraught with difficulty and may cause misunderstanding and frustration for both the healthcare professional and the patient. These patients are additionally disadvantaged because of lack of information about the healthcare system. They may originate from a country where expectations and experience of medical care differ from the UK and may, for example, expect direct access to specialist care rather than accept GP care.

It is important for healthcare professionals who consult with patients with limited or no English to understand the cultural differences and the patient's expectations. Tolerance of cultural and racial diversity is essential for making effective contact. This is particularly so for refugees and asylum seekers, who may have difficulty accessing health care and communicating needs. Refugees represent diverse populations. They include people applying for refugee status, those allowed temporary admission to the country while immigration status is considered, and those with the right to stay indefinitely. Refugees are a vulnerable group because many have health problems that are complicated by personal and psychological distress arising from separation from their families, loss of status, poverty and the 'cultural bereavement' of leaving their country of origin.

Receptionists may identify patients with language difficulties on first contact. Special arrangements can be made by booking the patient to see a doctor who speaks the same language, if available; by asking that the patient be accompanied by a friend or relative as interpreter; or by offering a professional interpreter from the UK interpreting service Language Line. Many health authorities publish public directories of local GPs that include languages spoken. Additionally, patients may belong to an ethnic group that states a preference to consult with a doctor of the same gender. Muslim and Hindu women prefer a woman doctor when consulting with gynaecological problems, and this request should be respected.

For reasons of confidentiality, patients should be offered the choice of a professional, a relative, or a friend as interpreter. However, use of a close family member as an interpreter raises confidentiality issues and may not be in the patient's or relative's best interests. The use of children may pose particular problems, as patients may need to discuss sensitive topics of a sexual or personal nature or which, in the case of refugees, may involve brutality or torture in their persecuting country, which may be upsetting. Professional interpreters are prebooked through Language Line for the patient's appointment time, and are remunerated on a pro-rata hourly rate, usually by the NHS. Telephone interpreting is preferred because it is more time efficient than the interpreter visiting the surgery.

How is the interpreting service used?

Prior to the start of the consultation, telephone contact is made with the interpreter. With the patient in the consulting room, the doctor will begin the consultation and use the telephone for a three-way communication between the patient, doctor and interpreter.

Interpreting services vary from area to area, but most offer a wide range of languages from all continents, particularly in metropolitan areas. If no interpreter is available, or the patient is seen without forewarning of language difficulties, communication may need to be non-verbal, using facial expression, miming or drawing. Although this may establish rapport with the patient and addresses basic needs, it is an unsatisfactory and unreliable way to conduct a consultation.

Consulting through an interpreter is difficult, time consuming and stressful for the doctor within the constraints of short consulting times in general practice. The logistics of arranging an appointment with doctor, patient and telephone interpreter simultaneously are not easy. It is recommended that appointment times be extended up to 30 minutes for patients with language problems because of the increased time needed.

Your approach

Before the consultation begins, you will need to check that an interpreter has been pre-booked to coincide with the patient's appointment. Using a telephone interpreter, once the line has been accessed, the interpreter will introduce themselves by first name and give you their interpreter's reference number. Start by introducing yourself and checking the interpreter's language. Give the interpreter a brief summary of the patient's age, nationality and gender from the registration details, and any clues you have about the clinical problems.

You are now ready to start the consultation. Being open and sympathetic builds up trust with your patient and is important. Welcoming the patient by shaking hands and indicating where he or she should sit will help to break down barriers. If a personal interpreter accompanies the patient, indicate where they should sit. It is preferable to seat the patient closest to yourself with a full view of your face so that lip reading and facial expression can enhance communication. The interpreter should sit next to the patient, facing you. Check that the patient consents to the use of an interpreter. If a telephone interpreter is used, the consultation will involve a three-way process of communication, passing the telephone from the patient to you and allowing time to talk to and listen to the interpreter for a translation. Allow the patient plenty of opportunity to talk about presenting problems. Interpreters are familiar with the structure of the consultation and will initiate the process. A good start is to acknowledge the patient's problems.

Supplementing verbal exchange by observing body language will provide clues about symptoms such as pain, distress, anxiety, depression or the anatomical location of symptoms. Keep communication to a minimum and give instructions clearly via the interpreter, especially when you have made a diagnosis and need to explain your management. At this stage you should check the patient's understanding of the UK health service and, if necessary, explain how the system works, particularly in relation to general practice. It is helpful to write down the diagnosis and instructions in English so that the patient has the option of getting a translation later, and include drawings and diagrams. If you give the patient a prescription, you should explain the location of the pharmacy. Information leaflets in the patient's language are helpful, but if not available, a leaflet in English allows later translation. Information on health care is available for refugees through the National Information Forum and copies may be available in the practice. It is helpful to write down your name for the patient for follow-up. Before you say goodbye to the interpreter, offer your patient a last chance of asking questions. Finally, thank your interpreter and note their reference number in case you need to contact them again for further visits. Interpreters visiting the surgery will ask you to countersign their claim form, stating the duration of the interpreting time.

HOW TO DO A HOME VISIT

As a student, you may visit patients at home for a variety of reasons. You may make a pre-arranged visit alone or paired with a student colleague to gain experience in routine history taking from a housebound patient, to follow up a patient recently discharged from hospital, to undertake a project, to accompany your tutor or other member of the primary healthcare team to assess a chronically ill patient or to gain emergency 'on-call' experience.

Visiting a patient at home is a very special experience. Indeed, it is a privilege enjoyed by few. Although some members of the primary healthcare team (for example community nurses, midwives and health visitors) visit defined patient groups, what makes general practice unique is the access doctors have to the homes of registered patients. Patients are a microcosm of society, representing all backgrounds and ages. Doctors have the advantage of being invited and usually welcomed into the home. Many students feel nervous about home visiting, partly because of feelings of insecurity, lack of self-confidence about social and communication skills and, partly, with pre-arranged visits, a feeling of imposing on patients. However, most patients enjoy talking to students, there being mutual benefits.

Chapter 10 discusses home care in general practice.

Thinking and Discussion Point

Can you think of other occupations whose members have access to homes? Under what circumstances would visits be made?

Every home reflects individual and family values. Visiting a cross-section of society, you may be surprised at the wide range of lifestyles and living conditions. Some visits will fascinate, as they offer insight into cultures different from your own, but in other homes you may react adversely, particularly where a patient's personal cleanliness is compromised due to incontinence or cognitive impairment. Whatever your impression, you need to handle the situation sensitively, remembering that you are a guest and that you are there to help a patient made vulnerable by illness or disability. Whoever and whenever you visit, you need to be prepared for all eventualities.

Common questions from students about home visiting

■ *How safe will I be?* Because you are in an unprotected environment when visiting, you should be aware of personal safety, especially when travelling (Metropolitan Police, 2001). Observe the same ground rules as you would when socializing in the community generally. Avoid risks such as walking alone in alleyways, being confrontational with strangers or appearing lost. Obtain clear directions before you set out to visit. Look confident without appearing arrogant. Always inform someone of where you are going and when you expect to return. Take the surgery telephone number with you in case you need help, and a mobile phone if you have one.

■ *Should I carry identification?* Patients, especially elderly people, are naturally suspicious of strangers who knock at their door. They have a right to expect confirmation that you are the student sent by your tutor. A student identity or railcard with attached photograph is adequate. Additionally, a letter of introduction from the surgery is reassuring. Patients appreciate a quick telephone call before you set out. When the patient opens the door, announce clearly who you are, where you are from and why you are visiting. Greeting the patient by name is courteous and provides further reassurance. Check whether there is a relative in the house and, if so, that he or she is aware of your presence before starting your interview. If you are visiting a patient living in sheltered housing, a residential or nursing home, always introduce yourself to the warden or director as a security measure.

■ *What shall I wear?* This is a matter to discuss with your tutor beforehand, as dress codes may differ from practice to practice. Patients expect you to be clean and tidy; they may feel threatened if you appear in the latest outrageous fashions. For safety reasons, avoid appearing too conspicuous in the area you are visiting – not too smart in a depressed area, not too scruffy in a smart part of town.

■ *How shall I respond if a patient is abusive or I feel threatened?* Occasionally the interview may go wrong. Your patient may misunderstand or misinterpret your conversation through no fault of your own. If you sense that you are no longer welcome, or that the relationship with your patient or a relative feels uncomfortable or threatening, leave the house as soon as is courteously possible. There is a tendency to underestimate feelings of resentment, so it is better to leave rather than attempt to repair the situation. If possible, sit between the patient and the entry door of the room so that, in the event of a patient becoming physically aggressive, you can make a speedy exit.

■ *What happens if the conversation runs dry?* Many students worry about this more when taking a history in a patient's home than in hospital or the surgery. This is probably because the patient has greater control in the home situation. The use of open questions and summarizing techniques will maintain conversation. Pauses in the conversation are quite natural and may be helpful. They may seem embarrassingly long, but they are usually much shorter than you imagine.

■ *Should I examine the patient?* The current recommendation is that you should not examine a patient at home unsupervised by your tutor. There is no insurance cover for this in the event of an accident, for example if the patient falls or makes a false allegation.

■ *What shall I do if the patient becomes acutely ill during the visit?* Patients who become acutely ill may agree to continue with a student visit so as not to disappoint. If the patient feels unwell, it is best to stop the interview and offer help. You may need to call a relative in the house. If you are unsure, ask the patient's permission to use the telephone to call the surgery for advice.

Checklist for home visits

■ The patient's name, address and telephone number.
■ The carer's name, address and telephone number, if appropriate.
■ The practice telephone number.
■ A map of the area being visited; directions for finding the patient's address.
■ Personal identification; a letter of introduction.
■ Patient notes, if required.

After a pre-arranged visit, it is courteous to write and thank the patient.

SUMMARY POINTS

To conclude, the most important messages of this chapter are:

■ the patient is at the centre of your learning and must be treated with courtesy and respect;
■ general practice requires an understanding of the basic science underlying any skill;
■ be aware of the clinical indications for using a skill;
■ to learn a skill, you need close supervision and expert knowledge;
■ it is important to rehearse and repeatedly practise any skill.

REFERENCES

British Hypertension Society 1999: *Blood pressure measurement* CD-ROM. London: British Medical Journal Publishing Group.

Beevers, G., Lip, G.Y. and O'Brien, E. 2000: *ABC of hypertension*, 4th edn. London: British Medical Journal Publishing Group.

Benefits Agency, April 2000: *What to do after a death in England and Wales. A guide to what you must do and the help you can get.* A leaflet for relatives of the deceased.

General Medical Council 2003a. *Confidentiality: Protecting and providing information.* London: General Medical Council. www.gmc-uk.org

General Medical Council 2003b: *Seeking patients' consent: the ethical considerations.* London: General Medical Council: www.gmc-uk.org

MacLeod, J. 1983: *Clinical examination: a textbook for students and doctors by teachers of the Edinburgh Medical School.* Edinburgh: Elsevier.

Medical Certificates of Cause of Death (Form 66). Notes for Medical Practitioners. (Copies are available from the local Registrar of Births, Marriages and Deaths.)

Metropolitan Police 2001: *Stay safe. Your guide to personal safety.* London: COI Communications. (Also available from local police stations.)

Rees, P.J. and Kanabar, D. 1999: *ABC of asthma*, 4th edn. London: BMJ Books.

Summative Assessment 2003: *The structured trainer's report.* Winchester: National Office for Summative Assessment. www.nosa.org.uk

FURTHER READING

Levenson, R. and Coker, N. 1999: *The health of refugees. A guide for GPs.* London: Kings Fund Publishing.

National Health Service 2002: *Reference guide to consent for examination or treatment.* London: Department of Health. www.doh.gov.uk/consent

National Information Forum 2000: *Signposts. Information for asylum seekers and refugees.* London: National Information Forum. www.nif.org.uk

National Information Forum 2001: *How to make a new life in the UK. A self-help guide for young refugees and asylum seekers.* London: National Information Forum. www.nif.org.uk

APPENDIX: THE ASSESSMENT OF PRACTICAL SKILLS IN GENERAL PRACTICE

Medical schools implement their own methods of assessment for the core clinical skills and procedures that medical students are expected to have acquired on graduation. Some will be acquired predominantly in hospital and others in general practice. Small group or individual teaching in general practice makes this setting ideal for the learning and assessment of skills. Many schools have student logbooks in which core skills and procedures are listed. Some are records of satisfactory completion of skills training on demonstration of satisfactory performance of skills competencies to a tutor.

UNDERGRADUATE LEVEL

Practical skills are assessed by observation of a student's performance of the skill by an examining practitioner of that skill. Evaluation of skills competencies may be through 'in-course' assessment, as in the end of term sign-ups in a skills logbook, or 'end-of-course' assessment, as in an Objective Structured Clinical Examination (OSCE). You are required to demonstrate minimum competence in the skill being assessed. You are also required to demonstrate that you have achieved a standard required for safe clinical practice with patients.

What constitutes minimum competence? Assessment of a skill is undertaken against standards of performance that are shared by the community of practitioners of that skill. This process is known as criterion-referencing and involves an observer checking your performance against a set of listed criteria.

You may find it helpful to cross-check your skills against these OSCE questions.

Measurement of pulse and blood pressure

Instructions to candidate. Please examine this patient's pulse and blood pressure using the equipment provided and report your findings to the examiner.

Marking schedule: criteria for the measurement of blood pressure and pulse.

          Adequate/Inadequate/Not performed

- Introduces him/herself to patient.
- Establishes rapport with patient.
- Explains procedures and ensures consent.
- Ensures patient has rested for 10 minutes where appropriate.
- Positions patient and equipment appropriately.
- Applies cuff correctly.
- Locates brachial pulse.
- Puts stethoscope in antecubital fossa.
- Blows up cuff to appropriate level.
- Measures systolic and diastolic readings in mmHg.
- Removes cuff.
- Reports reading and interprets correctly.
- Encourages patient's questions and deals with them appropriately.
- Acknowledges patient's concern.
- Uses appropriate language.
- Documents blood pressure.

Peak flow measurement and instructions to patient on use of an inhaler

Instructions to candidate. Assess this patient's peak expiratory flow rate using the equipment provided and instruct him in the use of an inhaler.

Marking schedule: criteria for assessing measurement of peak flow and instructing patient on use of inhaler.

          Adequate/ Inadequate /Not performed

- Introduces him/herself to patient.
- Establishes rapport with patient.
- Explains importance of technique and ensures understanding.
- Checks patient's understanding of asthma.
- Prepares meter appropriately.
- Asks patient to take deep breath and seal lips around mouthpiece.
- Asks patient to blow as fast as possible into meter.

- Reads meter correctly.
- Checks peak flow against standard chart or patient's personal record.
- Indicates whether peak flow is a satisfactory technique and comments on its value.
- Suggests reasons for inhaler to be used.
- Shows patient how to shake inhaler.
- Asks patient to breathe out fully before using.
- Shows patient how to co-ordinate inhaler action while breathing in.
- Instructs patient to hold breath for 10 seconds after inhalation.
- Explains how to repeat after 1 minute.
- Indicates how often to use inhaler.
- Uses appropriate language.
- Checks patient has understood procedure.
- Encourages patient's questions and deals with them appropriately.
- Acknowledges patient's concerns.

Urine analysis

Instructions to candidate. Test this urine sample and report your findings to the examiner.

Marking schedule: criteria for assessing urine analysis.

          Adequate/Inadequate/Not performed

- Puts gloves on.
- Ensures urine sample is fresh.
- Checks container for correct stick and expiry date.
- Opens container and takes single stick out, closing bottle.
- Dipsticks urine for 1 second and taps off excess urine.
- After dipping, holds strip horizontal until test is complete.
- Reads stick after appropriate time.
- Records the result.
- Disposes of stick and gloves.
- Washes hands.
- Interprets results appropriately.
- Acknowledges need to send urine to laboratory or otherwise.

Measurement of blood glucose

Instructions to candidate. Measure the blood glucose and report your findings to the examiner.

Marking schedule: criteria for assessing measurement of blood glucose.

Adequate/Inadequate/Not performed
- Introduces him/herself to patient.
- Establishes rapport with patient.
- Explains procedure and ensures consent.
- Ensures patient is sitting or lying down.
- Assembles equipment.
- Inserts strip and calibrates machine as appropriate.
- Chooses an appropriate place for test and ensures warm and well perfused.
- Washes hands and puts on gloves.
- Takes lancet and inserts sharply into skin, drawing blood.
- Obtains a hanging drop of blood without undue squeezing of puncture site.
- Drops blood onto test strip.
- Waits until the machine records a reading.
- Disposes of sharp safely.
- Checks haemostasis.
- Disposes of strip and gloves.
- Reads appropriately and records.
- Appropriate interpretation of value.

Ear examination

Instructions to candidate. Examine this patient's ear including the use of the auriscope.

Marking schedule: for assessing ear examination.

Adequate/Inadequate/Not performed
- Introduces him/herself to patient.
- Establishes rapport with patient.
- Explains examination to patient and ensures consent.
- Enquires about hearing loss, characteristics and impact on life.
- Enquires about associated features, tinnitus and vertigo.
- Enquires about possible causes.
- Tests hearing with speech.
- Tests with tuning fork.
- Holds auriscope and patient's ear correctly.
- Identifies normal anatomy.
- Appropriate use of questions, open, closed and clarifying.
- Acknowledges patient's concerns.
- Encourages questions from patient and deals with them appropriately.
- Appropriate summary and analysis of findings.

POSTGRADUATE LEVEL

At postgraduate level, the national requirement for the demonstration of competence in the range of skills required for completion of postgraduate training in general practice is outlined in the Summative Assessment document known as *The structured trainer's report* (Summative Assessment, 2003). This has to be completed satisfactorily by the registrar's trainer before the end of the training year to provide evidence that a registrar has reached the standards for independent general practice in the UK. The Summative Assessment has two parts: a Formative Assessment record for use during the year and a Final Assessment sheet that should be completed in month 11.

There are 35 skills in Summative Assessment, grouped in seven parts:
- Part 1: Specific clinical skills
  - Mental state
  - Using an auriscope
  - Using the ophthalmoscope
  - Using the sphygmomanometer
  - Using the stethoscope
  - Using the peak flow meter
  - The vaginal examination
  - Using the vaginal speculum
  - The cervical smear
  - The rectal examination
  - Venous access
  - Intramuscular and subcutaneous injection.
- Part 2: Making a diagnosis
- Part 3: Patient management
- Part 4: Clinical judgement
- Part 5: Organization skills
- Part 6: Professional values
- Part 7: Personal and professional growth.

Only specific clinical skills are included in this chapter. It is recommended that these skills are completed in the early part of the training year. As a registrar, you should practise the skills throughout training and ask your trainer to assess you at intervals during the year as a formative assessment. You should check that your trainer has a copy of the Summative Assessment at the start of your training year so that regular assessment can take place. Your trainer will need to collect sufficient information to allow him or her to make a judgement as to whether you have achieved the necessary standard for the skill and can interpret the findings. Your trainer should sign you up, stating the method of observation and date of assessment, and should include comments on potential improvements. The Summative Assessment also lists sources of assessment other than your trainer, e.g. practice nurse, family planning trainer or consultant. Included under each skill is a list of criteria for failure to reach the required standard. Your trainer is unable to sign the Final Assessment if any of the fail criteria are outstanding. When your trainer has signed the Final Assessment, the evidence collected for proficiency is complete.

CHAPTER

7

DIAGNOSIS AND ACUTE MANAGEMENT IN GENERAL PRACTICE

Although there are many facets of general practice, sound diagnostic reasoning and effective and informed decision making are cornerstones of good medical care. This chapter shows how your clinical skills are the starting point for developing your management plan with the patient. It explores the ways in which investigations, referral and therapy contribute to the process of management. Understanding ways of using research evidence and linking this to good clinical judgement will inform your decision making and help you to provide high-quality care for each of your patients.

LEARNING OBJECTIVES

By the end of this chapter, you will be able to:

- understand the nature of diagnosis;
- use elementary clinical skills to diagnose many of your patients' problems;
- learn the nature of investigations and how to ensure you use them effectively;
- plan a programme of management for your patients;
- understand the place of referral in patient management;
- understand the role of evidence-based medicine and guidelines in supporting patient care in general practice.

THE PATIENT WALKS INTO THE ROOM ... WHAT NEXT?

In general practice, the reason that the patient has walked into your consulting room is that he or she has taken the decision to consult a doctor.

This is very different from hospitals, where a patient can only be seen by referral from another doctor (with the exception of accident and emergency/casualty and certain other self-referral clinics). In general practice, the patient makes the decision to see the doctor and the reasons vary widely, as discussed in the chapter on common illnesses in general practice (Chapter 4). In this chapter, we consider the processes of making diagnoses and managing patients with acute problems. The principles of patient diagnosis and management are common to many clinical situations; here, we focus on those that are of special significance or different in the primary care setting.

Reasons for seeing the doctor include:

■ a new medical problem or issue;
■ an acute episode in a chronic problem;
■ follow-up of a previous acute consultation;
■ reassurance about a symptom;
■ discussion of a visit to another doctor;
■ discussion of investigation results;
■ repeat medication;
■ a medical examination (e.g. for life insurance);
■ a form or letter.

Practical Exercise

Make a record of each consecutive patient you see during a surgery. What was the main reason for consulting? Was this a valid reason for coming to the doctor? Compare with your tutor each of your perceptions of the reason for consultation and whether it was an appropriate use of general practitioner (GP) time. Later, you will use this list again to consider which of these consultations would have been better undertaken by other members of the primary healthcare team.

WHAT IS A DIAGNOSIS?

I stood at the end of the bed and said, 'This is Obstreosis of the Ductal Tract! It's a tertiary case and Coreopsis has set in'. They were all amazed of course but it was a barn door case ... '.

(After James Thurber, 1965.)

It is not unusual to hear this sort of claim, usually from a registrar trying to impress someone. Sooner or later, they find they are talking to their beer and starting to believe their own stories.

Perhaps surprisingly, it is unusual to make an absolute diagnosis. Most diagnoses are actually a balance of probabilities, based on evidence drawn from a number of sources. This is part of the evanescent entity called clinical judgement. When patients are better, the fact that they were treated with medication appropriate to the working diagnosis lends confirmation to the diagnosis. If the patient has either recovered or died, there is less pressure to make a definitive diagnosis. If the patient fails to improve, the problem is explored further and further explanations are proposed until a diagnosis is made or events render it unnecessary.

WHY MAKE A DIAGNOSIS?

Whilst it is academically satisfying to make a precise diagnosis, the overriding reason for our work as doctors is that of helping our patients. In this light, a firm diagnosis is helpful but not the sole or even necessarily the most important consideration. For instance, we are taught to differentiate between direct and indirect inguinal hernias; in practice, clinical differentiation is of little practical importance, as it does not alter the management. Or consider the problem of an elderly smoker with an acute exacerbation of chronic obstructive pulmonary disease (COPD). He is treated with antibiotics, bronchodilators and steroids, and recovers. Was this bronchitis or bronchopneumonia? Since the presentation and management are more or less identical in each case, the precise diagnosis is immaterial. If the diagnosis lies between acute bronchitis (often with a lot of bronchospasm) and asthma, it is of much more significance, as longer term management will be different. In other situations, it may be important to act before making a diagnosis. For instance, temporal arteritis presents with a severe headache, but the symptoms are not pathognomonic. Definitive histological diagnosis by temporal artery biopsy will take several days. Treatment is by high doses of steroids with potentially serious side effects, but the risk of delaying is of sudden and irreversible blindness. Treatment is therefore commenced on clinical suspicion.

In each of these cases, the safe management of the patient is the critical issue, as part of which making a formal diagnosis has varying levels of priority.

LEVELS OF DIAGNOSIS

We can think of diagnoses as being made at various levels, as in Table 7.1. As a student, you should be able to get progressively to higher levels as your learning proceeds, but for all doctors there are situations in which they are only able to make an elementary diagnosis, and in those situations it is more important to have a strategy for handling that situation based on a sensible working hypothesis, rather than being 'stuck' on making a diagnosis.

You should only make the inferences that the diagnostic information you have collected allows you to make. If you assume that you have to make a firm diagnosis when the information is simply not strong enough, you will help neither the patient nor yourself. Rather, you need to use the information that you have obtained as a summary of your thinking so far. Unless you are clear of what you do and don't understand about your patients' problems at each point, you will be unable to ask the right questions to take you to the next stage.

WHAT ABOUT DIAGNOSES IN GENERAL PRACTICE?

Because of the nature of general practice, diagnoses are more frequently of the 'working hypothesis' kind. This is sometimes crudely interpreted as hospital doctors making 'proper' diagnoses and GPs failing to do so. However, the nature of general practice is such that diagnoses will rarely be as clear when a patient first presents to the surgery as they will be when the patient goes to a hospital clinic. There are a number of reasons for this.

- The patient presents at an earlier stage of the illness at the surgery than at the hospital when symptoms and signs are less developed.
- The patient is less clear in his or her mind at presentation as to the nature of the problem. As this is discussed with the patient's primary care physician, the nature of the problem is clarified.
- The GP is considering the whole patient, the psychological, the social and the physical;

Table 7.1 Levels of diagnosis

Diagnostic level	Features	Examples
Pathological diagnosis	Pathological material has been examined which is pathognomonic of the condition	Dermatophyte infection from culture of affected skin Crohn's disease from surgical specimen of diseased bowel
Clinical diagnosis	Symptoms and signs of condition are so suggestive that treatment can be confidently undertaken	Acute asthma attack

Differential diagnosis	Several possibilities exist which are listed in order of likelihood	An acute abdomen:
		    peritonitis
		    acute pancreatitis
		    perforated peptic ulcer
		A chronic running nose:
		    allergic rhinitis
		    vasomotor rhinitis
		    chronic sinusitis

Problem list	The various problems cannot be made to fit into a diagnosis or diagnoses by the doctor or student	An unhappy child:
		    headache
		    tummy ache
		    just changed schools
		    awake at night with cough

specialists, by their very nature, focus on one aspect of the patient's problems.

Tutor quote

Somebody came in with a cough who was a grandmother of 54. I asked if she smoked and, yes, she did. She smoked excessively, and she said she had to smoke because of the stress. I made some enquiries about the stress and she said she was stressed out because her son drank excessive amounts of alcohol and he was beating his wife. They had two children, a baby of 4 months and one of 7 years. The outcome of the consultation was that she needed a place of safety for those two children. So the consultation went from the presentation of a productive cough to, within 10 minutes, the need to alert the social workers and get a Place of Safety Order for the children.

HOW ARE DIAGNOSES MADE IN GENERAL PRACTICE?

Doctors in any situation have three essential tools to help them understand their patients' problems:

- they listen to the patient's story and views of their illness: the history;
- they physically examine the patient: the examination;
- they perform various kinds of tests: the investigations.

Different disciplines use these approaches in varying amounts. Some doctors, such as haematologists, rely heavily on investigations to make diagnoses (how else can you work out the cause of an anaemia?); others, such as surgeons, place considerable reliance on the examination (how else do you diagnose a lump in the groin?); but the most important basic information, even in these disciplines, is obtained from the history, and every clinician relies on this as the major diagnostic tool. It has been estimated that 80 per cent of all diagnoses are based on the history, 15 per cent on the examination and 5 per cent on investigations.

THE HISTORY IN GENERAL PRACTICE

Practical Exercise

Listen to your tutor take a history from some patients. To which part of the history does your tutor give greatest weight:
- ❏ the presenting complaint?
- ❏ the systems review?
- ❏ the past history?
- ❏ the family history?
- ❏ the therapeutic history?
- ❏ the social history?
- ❏ the patients' knowledge and beliefs about their conditions and their attitudes to them?

Often, a GP does not need to take past, family or therapeutic histories, as these are well known to them. This is one of the features of the *continuing care* relationship found in general practice. In well-organized GP records, these details are recorded on a summary sheet, usually fastened to the front of the notes and increasingly automatically produced by the software that maintains computer-held records.

As a medical student, you will probably have been taught to carry out a systems review on each patient you clerk. This is the endless shopping list of potential symptoms in different systems that students reel off like a priest trying to get through Mass quickly. It rarely offers additional diagnostic information and its only major area of importance is as a screening exercise for patients who are being prepared for surgery. The advice of a former president of the Royal College of Physicians is to abandon it (Hoffbrand, 1989): 'The greatest argument against the systems review is that experienced clinicians do not use it'. You will rarely hear of it being used in general practice.

Tutor quote

So what I am thinking about is a student who was just unable to get out of the way of asking leading questions, technical questions. So, after a battle, we agreed that he would say nothing, that he would introduce himself and say hello to the patient and that he would say nothing, and he was completely flabbergasted by what happened then. He was shocked by how much patients told him. We then had this sort of game using just gestures to encourage people to say things. He also had a list of phrases that he could use, like 'Tell me more about that' and 'Is there anything else you want to tell me?' And so we went through this list of questions and we agreed it and he really thought this was cracked and he went along with it because I used my authority to force him. But he was just completely flabbergasted by this and shocked. It was very exciting for me, too, as it seemed to me that the questions that were left out of the clinical examination are 'Tell me all about it', 'Is there anything else you want to tell me?', 'What did it feel like?', 'What did it look like?' and so on. And the second part of the agreement that I made with this particular student was that before he could ask any technical questions he had to summarize back to the patient what the patient said, and so he would summarize by saying, 'Now, if I have heard you right, what has happened to you is this and I would like to ask you some questions, but before I do is there anything else you want to tell me?' So that was a revelation for both of us really.

Where does this leave the GP? There are two key areas.

The history of the presenting complaint is the information around which your understanding of the patient's problems is built. Each symptom presented is analysed until you are clear you know exactly what the patient means. The time course of the condition is carefully mapped. Nothing is accepted at face value; you must be sure you know what the patient means at every stage. For instance, the patient who tells you of his 'duodenal ulcer playing up' may, indeed, have a duodenal ulcer. Alternatively, he may have a gastric ulcer, oesophagitis, irritable bowel syndrome, diarrhoea or almost anything else. The patient may be using 'duodenal ulcer' to impress the doctor with its seriousness. (How many of us have called a head cold 'flu' to add *gravitas* to our suffering?) The patient may think that describing the symptoms as a 'duodenal

ulcer' is putting the problem in a language the doctor can understand. He may have once had a duodenal ulcer and it may seem the same this time. The critical thing is to arrive at a shared understanding with the patient as to the precise meaning of the symptoms.

The patient's knowledge, beliefs and attitudes about the condition is a key part of any history and one of the parts most frequently omitted. It is perhaps of greatest importance in general practice, in that patients have chosen to see you for reasons of their own. It is crucial to be clear about what those reasons actually are. When you are clear, you are in a position to help your patient, even if you and your patient may sometimes differ about what are the most important things. Sometimes patients won't be clear about what has made them come to see you. Finding out what those reasons are may be the first step in helping them. Too many doctors make the mistake of assuming they know why the patient is there; they may come up with brilliant diagnoses, but if they have not dealt with the patient's concerns, the job is only half done.

CASE STUDY 7.1

A 73-year-old woman was admitted to hospital about every month for investigations of sudden acute chest pain. It didn't sound cardiac and the electrocardiogram and cardiac enzymes were always normal. Her husband had died of a heart attack some years previously. She was reassured by everyone that 'your heart's fine' and sent back to her flat. If reassurance was all it took, she had overdosed on it. But back she came again month after month. One day, the house-man sat down with her and naively asked, 'What do you think the problem is?' After a prolonged silence, she said, 'It's cancer, doctor'. 'Why do you say that?' 'My brother had lung cancer.' The houseman (wising up): 'Did he have pain with it?' 'Terrible pain.' 'Was it like yours?' 'It was *exactly* the same!'

Everyone was absolutely right to diagnose that there was no organic pathology, but wrong in assuming that it was her heart and the memory of her husband's death that had precipitated her symptoms.

Thinking and Discussion Point

Why does telling a patient there is 'nothing wrong' often not result in the reassurance that the doctor was intending?

THE EXAMINATION IN GENERAL PRACTICE

'He never examined me' is a frequent complaint of patients who found a consultation unsatisfactory. There is little time for each consultation in general practice; the average consultation length is still little more than 8 minutes per patient (Wilson, 1991). GPs respond by honing their clinical technique to include only those things that are of significant diagnostic value. As we saw above, the examination only contributes 15 per cent to the diagnosis, as opposed to 80 per cent from the history.

Practical Exercise

As your tutor talks to successive patients, decide what examination (if any) you would make. Compare this with what your tutor does and discuss the differences with him or her. You should not assume that the tutor's decision is necessarily the only one. Often, a number of approaches could be made, and understanding the differing merits and objectives of each is useful.

❑ Discuss with your tutor how useful it is to: take the blood pressure of a patient complaining of headache; listen to the chest of a child with a cough; palpate the abdomen of a young man with acute diarrhoea.

❑ Why else might you want to examine the patient apart from to make a diagnosis?

❑ What is the value of carrying out a 'full physical' as a screening exercise?

You should think of an examination in the same way as an investigation: how will carrying out this examination improve my understanding of the patient's problems? Does the patient need the examination for reassurance?

INVESTIGATIONS IN GENERAL PRACTICE

Thinking and Discussion Point

'General practitioners under-investigate and hospital doctors over-investigate'. Discuss the truth (or otherwise) of this assertion with your tutor and with a hospital doctor. How will you ensure you investigate appropriately?

Investigations can be used in two main ways: for diagnosis and for management. For instance, a single random blood sugar test is useful for the *diagnosis* of diabetes. It will detect the bulk of cases (although a blood sugar taken 2 hours after eating is better still). However, in the *management* of diabetes, the blood sugar changes so quickly that a single test is of little value, especially since the result may not be available for some days. In managing diabetes, a rapid assessment of blood sugar is required and must be repeated frequently if it is to inform management. Indicator strips used for the self-measurement of blood sugar are much more useful, even though they are considerably less accurate. Where precision is required for diagnosis, an immediate result is more important for management.

Interpreting results: normal or abnormal

Few investigations give an absolute result or are pathognomonic. For the most part, they will help you build up your evidence for a diagnosis, but only when interpreted in the light of the whole of the patient's story. For instance, an electrocardiogram (ECG) is a useful test in suspected myocardial infarction, but it does not always show characteristic changes in a confirmed myocardial infarction, and it sometimes shows changes when no infarction has taken place. This under-diagnosis or over-diagnosis by the test are known respectively as the **sensitivity** and **specificity** of the test. Whilst one does not need to know the exact values, it is important to have an approximate idea of the limitations of any test. An awareness of sensitivity and specificity is helpful in judging these limitations. (There are definitions of sensitivity and specificity in the glossary section of this book.)

Often, sensitivity and specificity are inversely related. For instance, the erythrocyte sedimentation rate (ESR) is a *sensitive* test but a very poorly *specific* one. It is reliably elevated to high levels in a condition such as polymyalgia rheumatica (it is *sensitive*), but is frequently elevated for a host of unrelated reasons (poorly *specific*). A Paul–Bunnell test is very *specific*: when positive, it is highly indicative of glandular fever, but many people with established glandular fever have a negative test (it is *insensitive*). Other assays (such as assays of thyroid-stimulating hormone) are both specific and sensitive and, as such, approach the ideal. Any test you order should be done in the light of your knowledge of its limitations of specificity and sensitivity.

When presented with an individual who has a positive result in a screening test, what may be of more interest to a clinician are the **positive** and **negative predictive values** (see the glossary for definitions).

Who's for screening?

With increasing access to private health care, there has been a considerable increase in the vogue for 'screening' tests. With modern laboratory technology, a large number of tests can be done quickly and relatively inexpensively on a single sample of blood. American medicine (see any relevant soap opera) gets through acres of such tests. As well as American medics, there are British house officers ordering every test under the sun in case the consultant should ask for it. There are problems with this approach. Every test has a probability of producing a false-positive result. The more tests carried out, the more false-positive results you will obtain. You then have to deal with these, sometimes by ordering more elaborate, expensive or invasive tests. To minimize spurious results, only carry out a test when there is a clear clinical indication. An example of the failure of screening tests comes from the early days of human immunodeficiency virus (HIV) infection. With the disease then relatively rare and tests relatively unsophisticated, there was considerable political pressure from some quarters to screen

people for HIV *en masse*. The number of undiagnosed true positive cases in the community was below the rate of false positives for the test. At the same time, there were significant numbers of false negatives, both because of the technical limitations of the test and because it was unable to detect early infections. Thus the test caused distress to people who would turn out to be uninfected, whilst failing in its aim as a screening test.

Effects of tests on awareness of health

Another reason to avoid unnecessary tests is that they can increase anxiety and concern about health. Stoate (1989) showed that screening for blood pressure increased anxiety about health reflected in an increased frequency of consultations in those screened. In the case of blood pressure, such screening arguably justifies the health anxiety caused; for many tests done 'just to see', it certainly does not.

Deciding whether to request a test

As a student or doctor, the most important question you can ask about any investigation is, 'Will it change my management?' If the answer is 'yes', you then need to ask, 'Could I get the same information cheaper, quicker or less invasively another way?' If the answer is 'yes', you should think again.

In the same way as guidelines for treatment have been devised to aid clinicians' rational decision making, there are a number of guidelines available on when to use investigations, for instance those produced by the Royal College of Radiologists (2003).

Who is the investigation for: patient or doctor?

We have stated that investigations have the two prime functions of diagnosis and management. In addition, you may have seen investigations used to 'reassure the patient'. It is important to consider whether or not the patient will be reassured by your action. In the same way as doctors sometimes assume rather than ask what their patients' real worries are, they equally may assume that a patient will be reassured by a negative test (such as a cranial X-ray to reassure the patient that there is no brain tumour). The same message applies: find out what the issues are that actually concern the patient and deal with those. As a *British Medical Journal* editorial put it, 'Unless their true fears are addressed, diagnostic tests may leave them more anxious than before' (Fitzpatrick, 1996).

The range of investigations available in general practice

An increasing range of investigations is available to GPs. These may be carried out in the following ways.

- By the patients themselves: for example blood sugar monitoring using indicator strips, peak expiratory flow rate monitoring via mini peak flow meters (both available on prescription).
- In the doctor's surgery: for example indicator strips for urine testing for a wide variety of substances, immunological detection kits for pregnancy testing, ECGs and audiograms; there are mini auto-analysers available allowing 'near patient testing' for basic biochemical and haematological indices such as cholesterol, haemoglobin and creatinine.
- In a clinical laboratory (usually based at a hospital, but sometimes contracted out to an independent laboratory): some complex or unusual assays, such as certain endocrine or genetic tests, are only carried out at specialist centres. The availabilities of laboratory-based tests to GPs vary from laboratory to laboratory.
- In specialist departments: most kinds of X-rays are available directly to the GP; other sophisticated tests, such as endoscopy and echocardiography, are examples of an increasing range of tests often available directly to GPs without consultant referral. The exact availability varies from area to area, depending on factors ranging from the availability of the investigation locally to the prejudices of the person in charge of the investigating unit. The reasons why certain tests are not available may be highly idiosyncratic. The hospital may believe that to allow GPs to use certain tests would be to waste money (this assumes the GPs are using them excessively or inappropriately). It may be 'protectionism', as a specialty tries to protect its interests from others treating those conditions. In the better-regulated establishments, a dialogue will be established between the laboratory or department offering the test and the GPs and others who wish to use it to ensure it is correctly used and appropriately available.

Do 'good' doctors use more or fewer investigations?

There can be a kind of machismo in ordering every investigation under the sun or, conversely, refusing to have anything at all to do with them. There is a certain feeling, prevalent amongst house officers starting their first job, that more is always better. If you are used to using an investigation, you can get blasé and use it more frequently than justified by the clinical situation. Huge numbers of routine urea and electrolyte samples taken during inpatient stays have little clinical value. Conversely, examinations may be under-used by those who are not aware of the potential they offer. Thus, you cannot judge a doctor by the quantity of investigations he or she uses, but by the quality of use. So aim to know the potential and the drawbacks of each investigation and, armed with that knowledge, *investigate appropriately.*

WHAT ARE YOUR OBJECTIVES IN PLANNING YOUR PATIENTS' CARE?

Two first-year medical students gave the following opinions after a visit to a hospice.

Student quotes

It was depressing, all those people dying and nothing the doctors could do.
It seemed incredibly peaceful; although people knew they were dying, they seemed really peaceful and content.

The two views above show completely different opinions on what was going on. Too often, our views of what constitutes management are from one direction only. Let us look at the different goals that a doctor might be trying to achieve in managing a patient.

1. *To cure the patient's disease.* This is the most usual view of the doctor's role. Television soaps, society in general, patients, relatives and sometimes the doctors themselves believe this is their role. Sometimes it is: if you have bacterial meningitis, you want the doctor to move fast and eradicate the organisms before they do you permanent harm.

2. *To prevent disease.* If one can prevent a disease developing, it is far better than curing it once it is there. This is a prime role for the GP, who has access to a population in both sickness and health, as described in Chapter 11 ('Health promotion in general practice'). There is an opportunity to intervene with screening, education and lifestyle advice before disease starts. Cervical screening, education about safe sex and advice on smoking have all had an important impact on the lives of individuals. However, this role is unglamorous. There is a much less tangible reward for the GP preventing coronary artery disease than for the surgeon with a large team and high-tech facilities.

3. *To prevent complications.* It may be impossible with existing medical knowledge to prevent or cure a disease. Chapter 9 deals with the care of those with chronic illness. As important as preventing or curing a disease may be the prevention of its complications. Diabetes is a good example. Insulin-dependent diabetes can neither be prevented nor cured at present, but the important aims of management remain to prevent the serious complications of blindness and gangrene and fatal ones of renal disease and myocardial infarction.

4. *To alleviate symptoms.* Some illnesses are brief and self-limiting; they do no long-term harm, but are unpleasant whilst they are there. An example is sore throat. Approximately 65 per cent of cases are viral (Ross et al., 1971) and no antiviral treatment is available. Thirty-five per cent are bacterial, but studies of antibiotics show that they only reduce the duration of symptoms by 1 day. Thus curative treatments are either non-existent or limited in their efficacy. Prevention is not a practical possibility. To enable patients to function as well as possible whilst they have the infection is the objective. Thus treatment is with analgesics, antipyretics and anti-inflammatories, most conveniently provided by aspirin, which has all three effects (although this is not used in children under 16 years of age because of the association with Reye's syndrome). Paracetamol is a safe alternative, being an analgesic and antipyretic, and despite the absence of anti-inflammatory properties, it is probably of comparable efficacy. Locally acting agents such as soothing or local anaesthetic throat pastilles or sprays may be helpful. It will usually also be one of the doctor's management objectives to educate the patient as to the nature of the condition and how the patient can manage his or her own condition without the need to see the doctor in the future.

Alleviating symptoms has an equally important role to play in major illnesses. The management of pain resulting from a terminal illness or surgery is of tremendous importance to the patient. The doctor may have other priorities, especially if a patient is having difficult or dangerous postoperative problems. Historically, doctors have not always managed pain very well, whether disregarding it in favour of what they consider to be more pressing issues, or being poorly informed about its management. An important goal of the hospice movement has been to develop ways of alleviating symptoms for which there is no ultimate cure.

5. *To educate and inform.* The doctor has an important role in educating patients and thus helping them to manage their own illness. In the example of a sore throat, patients need to learn to manage their problem, but this is equally important in major illnesses.

Diabetes management crucially relies on the patient's understanding of his or her and its management. The aim is for the patient to understand how to manage the illness from day to day by the use of an appropriate diet and exercise, by monitoring blood sugar values and by manipulating the insulin regime. To do so, the patient needs to understand something of the nature of the illness, but doctors who interpret this as a lecture on the pathophysiology of the condition have missed the point.

In many conditions, patients are encouraged to take a more active role in their own management, and there is a vocal lobby from patient groups demanding such changes. Whilst this appears laudable, it is not always clear how effective it is. For instance, numerous studies attempting to educate patients about asthma have shown little effect in preventing hospital admissions or symptoms.

Thus, in managing any patient, there are a variety of objectives that may be pursued, and often more than one. Being clear about which objective you are pursuing will help to ensure that each aspect of the patient's problem is appropriately dealt with.

MANAGEMENT IN GENERAL PRACTICE

ASSESSING THE PATIENT

The first step in managing your patient is your assessment of the patient's situation. Taking the history, making the examination and arranging diagnostic investigations are the major part of this process, as discussed above. Your further assessment will depend upon the objectives you have established for your patient's management.

If, for example, your objective is patient education, you will need to assess what the patient understands about his or her condition. You will have some knowledge of this from the history, especially your exploration of the patient's ideas, concerns and expectations about the condition. But you may need to go into more detail at this stage, and begin a dialogue with the patient comparing your understanding of the condition to the patient's.

If your objective is the alleviation of symptoms, you will need to have measures of their severity against which the effects of your therapeutic manipulations can be compared. For instance, for the patient with intermittent claudication, you need measures of exercise tolerance (such as how many stairs can be climbed before the pain starts). Attempt to quantify your patient's symptoms in terms that have a meaning for both you and your patient. (For a patient living in a bungalow, the above may be unhelpful, and the number of stops on the way to the shop may be better.) This allows you and your patient to have a way of comparing progress. Laboratory investigations may define this more precisely, such as Doppler imaging and angiography in the case of the patient with intermittent claudication, but they should augment clinical understanding rather than attempt to replace it.

CASE STUDY 7.2

A 19-year-old man, Mr G, complains of breathlessness and a night-time cough. You have assessed the patient by taking a history that has revealed an episodic pattern of breathlessness, worse early in the morning and when playing football. It is worse in the spring when the pollen count is high and much worse when he visits his aunt and her cats!

On examination, there are no physical signs in the chest, but he has a peak flow of only 300 L/min. He believes he has asthma, but is alarmed by the reports he has read in the paper of the rise in asthma deaths. You lend him a peak flow meter, which later shows consistently lower morning than evening values, and arrange skin tests, which confirm his allergies to cats, pollen and additionally to house dust mite.

PLANNING TREATMENT

Having assessed your patient's condition, you are now in a position to initiate treatment. Consideration of any treatment's effectiveness is vital. Much treatment offered to patients is of no proven efficacy. Later in this chapter we consider how evidence-based medicine and clinical guidelines ensure your patient receives treatment that is likely to be of benefit.

WHAT ARE THE RISKS AND BENEFITS OF TREATMENT?

What are the possible adverse consequences of the treatment you are proposing? Will your treatment be worse than the disease it is intending to cure? If the treatment is important but side effects inevitable, how will you ensure your patient is compliant with that treatment? You and your patient need to take a view of the risks and benefits of the treatment you are considering. For a rapidly fatal disease like meningitis, the antibiotic chloramphenicol with its associated risk of aplastic anaemia may be a justifiable risk. (Chloramphenicol is now virtually never used in the UK. However, in the developing world it remains an affordable and effective antibiotic choice.)

So far, we have assumed your patient requires drug treatments, but other treatments are possible and often desirable. A change in lifestyle may be of considerably greater importance for the insomniac patient than the prescription of any drugs. Relaxation techniques, such as yoga, can produce significant and sustained falls in blood pressure that may be more acceptable to the hypertensive patient than a lifetime of tablets. A spectrum of treatments from the orthodox, such as surgery and physiotherapy, through osteopathy and chiropractic to acupuncture and homeopathy are all offered with more or less scientific justification. (These options are discussed further in Chapter 8, 'Prescribing in general practice'.)

Your job as a doctor is to help patients find a treatment that:

■ they find acceptable,
■ has good evidence for its efficacy, and
■ has acceptable adverse risks.

NEGOTIATING WITH THE PATIENT

If your plan for the management of the patient is to go ahead, the patient is the person most responsible for implementing it. Following through your management plan requires not just telling your patient about it, nor even listening to their concerns, but is an active process of negotiating with the patient around the various options that are available and the benefits and shortcomings of each.

Tutor quote

I was running a seminar with some students. We were talking about compliance and the word 'bargaining' came in. Some students went for it; some students said that they would bargain. One student said that we should be ashamed of our view. He said, 'We should say "This is what you need, these are the tablets, this is the dose you take", and the patient will take it if you tell them'. So the discussion went on, and I said, 'But aren't patients different? Different patients make decisions in a different way'. What he said then was, 'If you give all patients exactly the same information then their decisions will be identical'. Now we were coming to the crunch, so I said, 'What do you mean? If you took a 40-year-old man who has recently lost his wife because she took penicillin and died of anaphylactic shock and somebody who had recently had a child who recovered from pneumonia because of penicillin and if you gave them the same information, would they make the same decision?' and he said, 'Yes, if you give them the statistics, they will still make the same decision'. So he was still not prepared to accept that patients make decisions differently. So then he said that he believed that they would make the same decision as him. So one of the other students then said, 'You want your patients to be like you?' and that is what stopped him – 'Do I want the patients to be like me? Does everybody have to be like me for me to accept them?' I could see that there was this expression change. I said to him that, as a doctor, you respect the patient, that they are different, they have autonomy, they make their own decisions; respect them and if you find that their decision is going to be different from yours, that means you have to bargain. I think he definitely learnt that people make different decisions, they come from different places and information is not everything, and even if they do make a different decision, so what?

Evidence for the failure of doctors to take this part of management seriously is found in statistics that reveal that up to 20 per cent of prescriptions given by GPs are never taken to the chemist, and of those that are, a significant percentage of patients do not take some or any of the medication as prescribed (Fry, 1993).

Typically, a negotiation about treatment with a patient means the doctor will present his or her assessment of the problem and proposed solution to it. The doctor may present alternatives and discuss with the patient the risks and benefits of each option, and will check the patient's understanding and views about the preferred form of treatment. Then the patient and doctor between them will come to an agreement about the treatment to be undertaken.

CASE STUDY 7.2 (continued)

Tests confirm that Mr G has moderately severe asthma and a number of allergies. You propose a regular steroid inhaler and beta-2 agonist as required. Mr G is unhappy with this; he has read about the side effects of steroids and anyway prefers to avoid drugs and favours homeopathy. You discuss with Mr G the lack of scientific evidence that homeopathy can be of benefit in this situation, but agree with him that he is perfectly at liberty to try this, if he should so choose.

You discuss the possibility of preventing his asthma by avoiding contact with allergens and conclude that, apart from avoiding his aunt's cats and reducing house dust mites at home, the effects of doing this are likely to be fairly limited. You discuss Mr G's fears of medication with him, and particularly corticosteroids when used in low doses in inhaled form. You eventually agree that Mr G will use a beta-2 agonist inhaler, will try to avoid contact with specific allergens and will continue to monitor his peak flow. He will also discuss things with his homeopath.

MONITORING PROGRESS

Having negotiated treatment and initiated it with the patient, the doctor needs to monitor its effectiveness. This may range from the very simple to much more highly organized schemes of testing and monitoring. At the simple end of the spectrum, the doctor who sees a child with an apparently uncomplicated upper respiratory chest infection will discuss with the mother the appropriate, usually non-prescription, remedies and will invite her to call the doctor or return to surgery if the child is not showing improvement within a certain time. The doctor may warn the mother of things to look out for which suggest something more serious is going on.

Even in this very simple example, the doctor has:
■ made a plan,
■ shared it with a patient,

■ set up criteria by which its success or failure will be judged,
■ considered arrangements for following up the patient.

In more complex situations, these same principles are followed, but in ways appropriate to the situation. For example, when a newly diagnosed diabetic is started on insulin, the doctor needs to know that the patient is able to measure and inject the dose of insulin. The patient needs to monitor his or her blood sugar using finger-prick samples. A specialist diabetes nurse can visit the patient at home to check how he or she is coping with these tasks. The patient needs an appropriate diet and is given brief advice on this in the surgery and an appointment is made with the dietician for more detailed advice. The doctor knows the appointment won't be for a number of weeks, which gives the patient time to learn about all the other aspects of treatment. Unlike the previous example where it was left to the mother to return if things weren't going well, here it is important that a definite meeting is arranged to review progress quite soon. The patient may have things that are important to discuss, the insulin dose will almost certainly need modifying, and the doctor will want to find out how the patient is getting on with the different aspects of treatment.

In these early days, there will be a number of meetings at frequent intervals. As the diabetes comes under control and the patient becomes more confident, so these intervals will be extended, and day-to-day responsibility for care may be taken over by the specialist nurse. When everything is stable, a different pattern of visits will be initiated at intervals of perhaps a year. The patient will be seen and checked for evidence of visual or renal impairment, the feet will be checked for vascular or neuropathic changes, and the patient and the doctor will discuss diet and medication. This pattern can be maintained for as long as the patient is well, but if the patient becomes acutely ill, the plan will change to allow effective monitoring and treatment of the condition.

Management by the whole primary care team

This section focuses on the role of the doctor; we have already mentioned the role of specialist nurses and the dietician in the patient's management. It is important to be aware that management is an issue for the care team as a whole and not just the doctor. Only by working together as a whole are the patient's best interests served. The relationship between the doctor and the primary healthcare team is discussed in Chapter 2.

CASE STUDY 7.2 (continued)

Mr G gets considerable benefit from his beta-2 agonist inhaler, but has frequent worsening attacks of asthma that result in two brief admissions. Partly as a result of the fright this gives him and partly through his good relationship with the practice nurse who runs the asthma clinic, he accepts the need for inhaled steroid therapy. Regular reviews in surgery are arranged by the nurse, but additionally the practice manager ensures that the receptionists are aware of the patient's need to be seen urgently whenever he requests it. Mr G avoids further admissions, but he continues to call out the doctors fairly frequently at night and makes considerable use of the practice nebulizer.

Thinking and Discussion Point

What further steps would you wish to take to improve Mr G's treatment? Discuss these with your tutor.

MAKING REFERRALS

REASONS FOR REFERRING

The GP has two main options in dealing with the problem that the patient brings: doing so alone or seeking assistance from other resources. It is impossible to give cut and dried rules about which is the 'correct' solution, as there are often a number of ways to deal with a problem, all of them equally valid and any of which may be chosen for a variety of reasons in different situations. Such reasons may emanate from the GP, the patient or the local situation.

- Different GPs' training, experience and personality will give them different approaches to the same problem.

- A patient may find one solution much more acceptable than another theoretically equally good one.
- Local facilities vary widely, and a service that may be well provided for in one area may be poor or non-existent in another.

Thus, a GP with experience of counselling or child psychiatry may be perfectly happy to tackle a complex psychological problem without outside help, but may refer to a specialist a child with something relatively straightforward about which the GP is uncertain for some reason. Allergy problems may be dealt with swiftly and efficiently by a special clinic in one area; in another there may be a virtual absence of such help, throwing the GP back on his or her own resources. A mother may be incapable of accepting reassurance about her child's condition until a specialist appointment is arranged in one situation, whilst another, similar situation is resolved by a brief chat with the doctor.

FEW REFERRALS GOOD; MORE REFERRALS BAD?

There is no straightforward relationship between the apparent abilities or training of a doctor and the number of referrals he or she makes. The assumption that better trained doctors refer less was challenged when it was found that GPs with specialist ear, nose and throat (ENT) training referred more ENT problems than those without. This may have been because of the need for specialist diagnostic equipment and operative surgery. We can hypothesize that GPs trained in specialties not requiring this sort of resource, such as dermatology, might refer less. Part of the explanation for different referral patterns amongst doctors lies in the ability of individuals to deal with uncertainty. The doctor who is comfortable living with a degree of uncertainty over diagnosis will refer less; the doctor who can't cope with uncertainty will refer more. For the patient, neither approach is without consequences. In the former case, it may mean not getting referred when it would have been advisable, and in the latter it may mean being referred unnecessarily. Secondary care depends upon primary care restricting the numbers presenting, so the GP is obliged to make a decision about what requires referral and what does not.

THE REFERRAL LETTER

A practical exercise in how to write a referral letter can be found in Chapter 6 of this book. However, in terms of what to say rather than how to say it, there are a number of points.

∎ Avoid long letters; few people read them. Choose only information that will be useful to the doctor receiving the letter.

∎ Be clear about why you are making the referral – what you hope to gain from it. There may be a number of factors:
  - you may need a service undertaken, such as an operation or an endoscopy;
  - you may require a second opinion to confirm an unclear diagnosis: you may feel happy about the diagnosis, but the patient may not, so the second opinion is for the patient's benefit;
  - you may be asking the specialist to take over the management of the patient problem, or one aspect of it – this may be appropriate for the patient who is moving from a chronic phase to an acute phase in an illness, such as someone with previously stable angina which has now become unstable and requires operative intervention.

It is important that the consultant should be aware of your reasons for the referral and what you expect to get back from him or her. The letter itself needs to be a coherent précis of the patient's condition, with relevant past, social and therapeutic histories. It is written to give the person to whom you are referring a clear view of the patient's problems rather than to show how clever you are. At the conclusion of this summary you will give your diagnosis, differential diagnosis or problem list.

Writing a referral letter is a useful exercise for a student, as it challenges you to produce a concise and accurate summary and think through the management of your patient, as well as helping you master the skill of writing the referral letter itself.

REVIEWING PATIENTS AFTER A REFERRAL

For the GP, the relationship with the patient is an ongoing one, so he or she will see the patient again after the referral has been made and will have to put into action any new plans that have been decided upon. In well-ordered circles, the specialist will write back to the GP with an opinion about the patient's problems and answering the questions the GP has raised. Things do not always work out like that, and the letter may not deal with the things that the referring doctor considered to be important and may not answer the questions that were raised. Occasionally, GPs may not have the courtesy of a reply at all.

When a reply has been received, it is a good time to review the patient and consider the various changes in his or her management. This is an important exercise to:

∎ check that the patient has understood what the consultant has proposed;

∎ ensure that new information has been added to the patient record, such as details of changes to medication;

∎ make sure that the management plan for the patient has been updated to take account of the changes.

The doctor must also consider how the management will be shared if the patient is to continue being seen by the specialist as well as by the GP. This is a critical area of communication and is frequently handled poorly. Mistakes and misunderstandings easily arise in areas such as changes of drugs and changes in dosage.

EVIDENCE-BASED MEDICINE IN GENERAL PRACTICE

Thinking and Discussion Point

Think about the last time you considered how to treat a particular patient; on what did you base your decision. Your own experience? Or perhaps you recalled the teaching of your GP tutor or hospital consultant. But on what did these 'oracles' base their teaching?

Medical practitioners have been criticized for basing decisions on patient care on their own personal experience and clinical judgement rather than on research evidence. The concept of **evidence-based medicine** refers to a process by which explicit use is made of research evidence in making medical decisions. This is not to say that clinical judgement is obsolete; evidence-based medicine should integrate best research evidence with clinical expertise and take into account individual patient circumstances and values.

The practice of evidence-based medicine can be divided into five steps (Sackett et al., 2000).

Step 1. Having identified a need for information (e.g. about diagnosis, causation, prognosis, therapy or prevention), frame it into an answerable question.

Step 2. Search for the best evidence with which to answer that question.

Step 3. Critically appraise that evidence for its validity (closeness to the truth), impact (size of the effect) and applicability (usefulness in your clinical practice).

Step 4. Integrate the results of the critical appraisal with your clinical judgement and with your patient's unique circumstances and values.

Step 5. Evaluate your effectiveness/efficiency in steps 1–4 and seek ways to improve next time.

Regarding the best information sources, you will find that most textbooks are already out of date and you will need to consult the research literature. The quickest way to do this is to look for evidence sources that have already been critically appraised. The *Cochrane Library*, ACP Journal Club and *Clinical evidence* are excellent sources of information (see 'Further reading' for more details). The electronic database *Evidence based medicine review* incorporates access to the *Cochrane Library* and ACP Journal Club and links to the *MEDLINE* database. Most universities subscribe. If you cannot find the necessary information in a pre-appraised source, you will need to do a *MEDLINE* search and critically appraise the data yourself. Try using the 'Clinical queries' tool in *PubMed*; this applies search filters to improve the yield of clinically relevant and scientifically sound articles. A detailed description of critical appraisal techniques is

beyond the scope of this book; you may have covered this topic elsewhere in your studies, if not, the book by Sackett et al. (2000) is an excellent guide.

Evidence-based medicine is becoming popular in many branches of medicine. Can it be applied in general practice? The answer is yes, but not without problems. Referring to the steps above:

1. In general practice, the clinical question is often not easily identified; patients frequently have multiple, ill-defined problems involving complex psychosocial factors, and a definite diagnosis may not be made.

2. Many general practice problems are poorly researched, and data from hospital studies may not be applicable in the general practice setting; in addition, the intensive follow-up given to participants in research studies cannot be provided in general practice.

3. GPs lack the time and sometimes the expertise to critically appraise published literature.

However, as more research is performed in the primary care setting, GPs are trained in critical appraisal techniques, and information technology advances allow on-line literature review in surgeries, it is possible that those more readily identifiable general practice problems will be amenable to an evidence-based approach (Fig. 7.1). Gill et al. (1996) have already shown that most interventions in a training general practice are based on evidence from clinical trials.

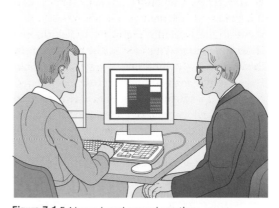

Figure 7.1 Evidence-based general practice.

Practical Exercise

❑ Choose a clinical problem and frame an answerable question. This should focus on a common problem, based on a patient you have seen in general practice. Possible examples might be: 'Should antibiotics be given for sore throats?' and 'Should patients in atrial fibrillation be anticoagulated?'

❑ Search the literature. If you do not know how to do literature searches, now would be a good time to learn; the library at your medical school will probably offer training.

❑ Critically appraise the literature. When you have collected a sheaf of references, you will need to evaluate the validity, impact and applicability of their results.

❑ Integrate the evidence with your clinical expertise and your individual patient's unique circumstances and values.

❑ Discuss your findings with your GP tutor. Does the existing patient management plan fit with that suggested by your research? If not, should it be altered? What factors other than the research evidence affect that particular patient and how should treatment be individualized?

GUIDELINES AND PROTOCOLS

Guidelines can provide further help with diagnostic and therapeutic decisions. These are written statements providing 'extensive, critical and well balanced information on the benefits and limitations of various diagnostic and therapeutic interventions' (WHO-ISH Mild Hypertension Committee, 1993). Good-quality guidelines should consist of two components: an evidence section (based on an up-to-date literature review with the level of evidence made explicit) and a detailed instruction section (with grades of recommendations tagged to the level of evidence available). In reality, many clinical issues, especially in primary care, have been inadequately researched and guidelines are then based on a consensus view of experts.

Sources of guidelines include expert panels from the Royal Colleges, professional associations and medical audit advisory groups. An example of guidelines that have been adopted widely is that of the British Thoracic Society on asthma management (revised 2003).

Guidelines are only useful if they are of high quality and if they can be applied to your particular patient population. In deciding whether to use a particular set of guidelines, it is therefore essential to assess their quality and to consider whether they are appropriate to your local population and resources. Where guidelines are based on the consensus view of experts rather than research evidence, consideration should be given as to how expert these experts are and upon what they are basing their advice. Additionally, in some cases experts agree on so little that such guidelines are not sufficiently comprehensive to be of use.

Many general practices have developed protocols or set ways of dealing with particular conditions, such as asthma and diabetes, often based on a detailed development of existing guidelines. The advantage of such protocols is that they help ensure uniformity and quality in patient care, especially where many different health professionals are involved.

For further information on guidelines and protocols, see the chapters on clinical audit (Chapter 13) and chronic illness (Chapter 9).

Practical Exercise

❑ Choose a topic based on a patient you have seen in general practice.

❑ Find out whether any guidelines exist on this topic and whether copies are available in the practice.

❑ Does the practice have a protocol for dealing with patients with this condition?

❑ How was this protocol developed?

❑ Interview a selection of the GPs and nurses in the practice to see whether they use these guidelines/protocols and their views of them (and of guidelines/protocols in general).

SUMMARY POINTS

To conclude, the most important messages of this chapter are:

- patients choose whether to see their doctor: the reasons vary greatly and are not necessarily medical;
- diagnoses exist at various levels: a firm diagnosis may be impossible to reach initially, and the early management of your patient may involve clarifying the diagnosis by various means; a firm diagnosis is not always required for good management;
- most diagnoses are made through the careful use of basic clinical skills: taking a history, making an examination and performing investigations are the starting point and basis of all patient management;
- investigations contribute to your patients' care when they are relevant, sensitive and specific: batteries of random investigations provide little additional information and may mislead;
- good patient management is your overall goal: it is not intrinsically difficult; the diagnostic information you have gathered is integrated into a detailed picture of your patient's problem; having developed this, you are able to develop a management plan that allows you to inform, reassure, treat and, where necessary, refer your patient;
- making a referral is an important communication between primary and secondary care: this chapter has considered the decision to refer and the objectives of a referral;
- decisions on patient care should be based on a combination of clinical judgement and research evidence and should take into account individual patients' unique circumstances and values;
- guidelines containing information on the benefits and limitations of various interventions are available for a range of conditions and can be a useful aid to patient care.

REFERENCES

British Thoracic Society/Scottish Intercollegiate Guidelines Network (BTS/SIGN) 2003: British guideline on the management of asthma. *Thorax* 58(Suppl. 1), i1–94. (The advice given is summarized in the *British National Formulary*.)

Fitzpatrick, R. 1996: Telling patients there is nothing wrong. *British Medical Journal* 313, 311–12.

Fry, J. 1993: *General practice: the facts*. Abingdon: Radcliffe Medical Press.

Gill, P., Dowell, A., Neal, R., Smith, N., Heywood, P. and Wilson, A. 1996: Evidence based general practice: a retrospective study of interventions in one training practice. *British Medical Journal* 312, 819–21.

Hoffbrand, B.I. 1989: Away with the systems review, a plea for parsimony. *British Medical Journal* 298, 817–19.

Ross, P.W., Christy, S.M. and Knox, J.D. 1971: Sore throat in children: its causation and incidence. *British Medical Journal* 2(762), 624–6.

Royal College of Radiologists 2003: *Making the best use of a department of clinical radiology: guidelines for doctors*, 5th edn. London: Royal College of Radiologists.

Sackett, D., Straus, S., Richardson, W., Rosenberg, W. and Haynes, R. 2000: *Evidence based medicine: how to practice and teach EBM*, 2nd edn. Edinburgh: Churchill Livingstone.

Stoate, H.G. 1989: Can health screening damage your health? *Journal of the Royal College of General Practitioners* 39(322), 193–5.

Thurber, J. 1965: The secret life of Walter Mitty. In *The Thurber carnival*. London: Penguin Books.

WHO-ISH Mild Hypertension Committee 1993: *Guidelines for the treatment of mild hypertension*. Memorandum from a WHO-ISH meeting. Geneva: World Health Organization.

Wilson, A. 1991: Consultation length in general practice: a review. *British Journal of General Practice* 41, 119–22.

FURTHER READING

DIAGNOSIS

Epstein, O., Perkin, G.D., Cookson, J. and de Bono, D. 2003: *Clinical examination*. Edinburgh and New York: Mosby.

Gray, D. and Toghill, P. (eds) 2000: *Introduction to the symptoms and signs of clinical medicine*. London: Arnold.

MANAGEMENT

Mead, M. and Patterson, H. 1999: *Tutorials in general practice*, 3rd edn. London: Churchill Livingstone. This book gives practical examples of problems in general practice and shows how to work through them using approaches to clinical reasoning similar to those described in this chapter.

Souhami, R.L., Hanna, M. and Holdright, D. 2003: *Tutorials in differential diagnosis*, 4th edn. London: Churchill Livingstone.

This book gives a series of tutorials on different clinical problems. It is not intended for undergraduate students, but for the MRCP (UK) examination. However, on its way to the (often rare) syndrome that is the final diagnosis, it works through all the important common ones. It provides an excellent way to learn medicine and challenge your own diagnostic thinking. The book is currently out of print but is likely to be available in your medical school library.

Souhami, R.L. and Moxham, J. 2002: *Textbook of medicine*, 4th edn. London: Churchill Livingstone. A good knowledge base is essential to clinical practice. Your understanding must be broad rather than deep. This is an excellent book, which spans the whole of medicine at an appropriate depth.

EVIDENCE-BASED MEDICINE

ACP Journal Club: American College of Physicians and BMJ Publishing Group.

A regularly updated electronic database that provides access to all issues of the ACP Journal Club and back issues of the *Evidence-Based Medicine Journal*. These summarize individual studies and systematic reviews from a large range of medical journals. Studies are selected according to explicit criteria for scientific merit and clinical relevance. Your library may subscribe; see http://www.acponline.org for more information.

Clinical evidence 2003: London: BMJ Publishing Group.

A compendium of evidence which provides a precise account of the current state of knowledge, ignorance and uncertainty about the prevention and treatment of a wide range of clinical conditions based on thorough searches of the literature. It is updated every 6 months. Print and on-line versions are available; see http://www.clinicalevidence.com for more details. Available free through the National Electronic Library for Health: http://www.nelh.nhs.uk

Cochrane Library. Oxford: Update Software.

A regularly updated source of information on systematic reviews of trials of healthcare interventions. Available free through the National Electronic Library for Health: http://www.nelh.nhs.uk

MEDLINE

The world's leading general biomedical research literature database. Available free from many sources, including its makers, the US National Library of Medicine; see http://www.ncbi.nlm.nih.gov/Entrez

National Electronic Library for Health: http://www.nelh.nhs.uk

Developed by the NHS Information Authority, this web-based resource provides free access to a range of high-quality evidence sources, including *Clinical evidence* and the *Cochrane Library*.

Ridsdale, L. 1995: *Evidence-based general practice: a critical reader*. Philadelphia: W.B. Saunders Co. Ltd.

This summarizes the research literature on a number of general practice problems such as minor illnesses and psychological distress. It also contains information on how to appraise scientific papers.

Sackett, D., Straus, S., Richardson, W., Rosenberg, W. and Haynes, R. 2000: *Evidence based medicine: how to practice and teach EBM*, 2nd edn. Edinburgh: Churchill Livingstone.

An excellent introduction to evidence-based medicine, it uses a case-based format focusing on general medicine, but the accompanying CD-ROM contains cases relevant to general practice. The book has a regularly updated website at http://www.cebm.utoronto.ca/

GUIDELINES AND PROTOCOLS

British Thoracic Society/Scottish Intercollegiate Guidelines Network (BTS/SIGN) 2003: British guideline on the management of asthma. *Thorax* 58(Suppl. 1), i1–94.

Royal College of General Practitioners 1995: *The development and implementation of clinical guidelines*. Report from general practice 26. London: RCGP.

This is a summary of the current thinking on the role of guidelines in general practice.

There are many useful websites providing details of clinical guidelines: The National Electronic Library for Health (http://www.nelh.nhs.uk) Guidelines Database has key national guidelines from the National Institute for Clinical Excellence (NICE), Royal Colleges and national professional bodies.

British Society of Gastroenterology Guidelines: http://www.bsg.org.uk/clinical_prac/guidelines.html

RCOG Clinical Guidelines: http://www.rcog.org.uk/guidelines/c_guidelines.html

National Guidelines Clearing House (USA): http://www.guideline.gov/

CMA Infobase (Canada): http://mdm.ca/cpgs/index.asp

PRESCRIBING IN GENERAL PRACTICE

The scale of medication use in the UK is enormous and the problems caused by side effects, drug interactions and drug errors are a major cause of illness for patients and a significant burden to the health service. This chapter outlines these problems and discusses a number of strategies to ensure you develop good prescribing habits.

LEARNING OBJECTIVES

By the end of this chapter you will be able to:

- understand the scale of medication usage in the UK;
- develop good prescribing habits;
- find sources of help with prescribing in primary care;
- write a prescription;
- understand how computers in primary care are used to aid acute and repeat prescribing;
- understand the importance of communications about medication between primary and secondary care;
- understand the legal and practical approaches to prevent the problems of drug abuse;
- understand self-prescribing and over-the-counter medication and the role of the community pharmacist and other healthcare professionals in prescribing.

INTRODUCTION

Miss Molly had a dolly, who was sick, sick, sick,
So she called for the doctor to come quick, quick, quick.
The doctor came with his bag and his hat,
And he knocked on the door with a rat a tat tat.

He looked at the dolly and he shook his head,
He said, Miss Molly, put her straight to bed,
He wrote on the paper for a pill, pill, pill,
I'll be back in the morning with my bill, bill, bill.

An old skipping song, its origins clouded with time, reveals an iconic view of the general practitioner (GP). Whilst hospital doctors may be associated with the stethoscope, GPs are identified by their bag, their bill and their prescription pad. Of these, the bill has gone, the bag is fading, but the prescription pad remains a pervasive symbol. This is not necessarily a positive image: 'The moment I sat down he started writing out a prescription' is a well-aired complaint.

Prescribing is a major part of general practice, but as this book reveals, it is far from the only aspect, neither is it the only approach to patient therapy and management. Nevertheless, it is important to understand the range of issues involved in prescribing medication and how to do so effectively.

THE SCALE OF MEDICATION USE IN THE UK

The scale of medication usage is vast. Two-thirds of the population are taking some kind of medication at any time, whether prescribed, purchased over the counter from a chemist or from alternative therapists (Fry, 1993):

■ At any one time, 66 per cent of the population is taking some form of medicine; half of this medicine is prescribed and half purchased 'over the counter' (Kohn and White, 1976).

■ A prescription is issued in 66 per cent of general practice consultations and a similar volume is generated using the repeat prescription system.

■ The average person receives eight prescription items per year.

■ The most widely prescribed drugs are cardiovascular, dermatological and anti-asthma preparations, and antibiotics. The most widely purchased 'over-the-counter' (OTC) drugs are analgesics, vitamins and cough medicines.

■ Drug costs consume 10 per cent of the total National Health Service (NHS) budget, of which 18 per cent is spent in hospitals and 82 per cent in general practice.

■ Up to 20 per cent of patients do not take their prescription to be dispensed.

In summary, the scale of prescribing is large and the costs are high. Drugs are beneficial in many conditions, but can also have side effects. How can you ensure that you prescribe effectively and safely?

GUIDELINES FOR GOOD PRESCRIBING

Good prescribing is not a particularly difficult task. It relates more to attitude: fastidiousness in considering a series of questions each time a drug is prescribed and a desire to do the best for each individual patient. Whilst as a student the list of drugs to learn about seems endless, in practice most doctors use only a limited number of drugs, which they therefore get to know well. This list is often based on a local formulary (see below).

The following guidelines for good prescribing have been adapted from the *British National Formulary* (*BNF*; 2003) and Palmer (1998). They are discussed in more detail in the succeeding paragraphs.

Every time you reach for your prescription pad consider the following.
1. Is a drug necessary?
2. Is the drug effective?
3. Is the drug safe?
4. Is therapy economical?
5. Do you and your patient agree on your management plan?
6. Does your patient understand how and when to take the medication?
7. Is there a long-term plan?

IS A DRUG NECESSARY?

Have you made a diagnosis?

In Chapter 7 ('Diagnosis and management in general practice') we considered how management decisions can be made with and without a diagnosis. Ideally, in choosing therapy you will have a diagnosis, but life is not always ideal.

Treatment may be initiated:
■ on a firm diagnosis,
■ on a provisional diagnosis,

- to relieve undiagnosed symptoms,
- as a trial of therapy (helping confirm the diagnosis if it works).

The less certain you are of what you are treating, the less chance you have of successful treatment. At the same time, the risk of adverse effects from your chosen medication is not diminished.

Symptomatic treatment

There are many situations in which it is entirely appropriate to treat the patient's symptoms. For instance in acute myocardial infarction, the pain requires treatment in addition to treatments to limit infarct size or deal with resulting rhythm problems. Symptomatic treatment is of particular importance when there is little that can be done for the underlying disease. The symptomatic relief of pain and breathlessness in lung cancer offers a major contribution to the patient's quality of life. For many self-limiting conditions seen in general practice, symptomatic treatment, often as self-treatment, is all that is appropriate (see below).

Remember that the same considerations of necessity, effectiveness, safety, economy and patient review apply to symptomatic treatments as to other therapeutic interventions.

Self-limiting conditions

Many of the patients seen by GPs present with self-limiting conditions. These are minor conditions that will resolve by themselves without necessarily requiring the GP's intervention.

It is the GP's role:

- to educate patients about the nature of their condition and how to recognize it themselves next time;
- to empower patients to deal with the problem by themselves and without recourse to medical services.

In doing so, the GP is not only helping the patient, but also aiming to manage demand for consultations. If patients deal with the problem by themselves next time, it contributes to reducing the burden on the surgery and other health-care services.

Upper respiratory tract infections (URTIs) in adults and children are very common examples:

the doctor's aim should be to help patients recognize the symptoms and treat themselves. The doctor will need to become involved if the illness becomes protracted or severe or unexpected complications arise, and will need to discuss with the patient the safe boundaries for patient self-management.

The increasing number of former prescription drugs now available over the counter has increased the range of conditions patients can treat themselves. For instance, topical anti-fungal treatments are available over the counter for candidal and fungal infections.

Whilst a condition may be self-limiting, it may not be common (so there is little point in teaching patients to recognize it themselves); the symptoms may be disturbing and merit treatment in their own right. Moreover, appropriate medication may only be available on prescription. For example, acute vestibuloneuronitis presents with dramatic vertigo, sometimes leading to falls and injury. Although it rarely lasts more than a few days, accurate diagnosis, symptomatic treatment (with vestibular sedatives) and appropriate advice from the GP (e.g. avoiding driving) are usually required, despite its being a self-limiting condition.

IS A DRUG THE RIGHT CHOICE?

We are fortunate to practise in an age in which numerous highly effective medications are available and in a country where they can be afforded. Doctors have a particular expertise in using drugs and it is therefore not surprising that they turn to them frequently. However, drug treatment is often not the only option, and often not the option of first choice. Although this chapter is principally about prescribing drugs, the section below reviews some of the non-drug approaches that the GP and his patient may turn to.

Options for non-drug therapies in practice

Physical therapy

- *Physiotherapy.* Physiotherapists are practitioners in their own right. A physiotherapist will not merely carry out a request for treatment, but will make his or her own assessment of the patient's condition and treat accordingly.

Generally, physiotherapists are based at hospital or in community clinics. Some are practice based by local arrangement.

■ *Osteopathy and chiropractic* are usually not available through the NHS, except by local arrangement. The GP is often asked to advise on their usefulness or otherwise.

■ *Alternative physical therapies, such as Alexander technique, reflexology*, may be available by local arrangement within the NHS. The GP's role is usually to counsel on availability and suitability.

■ *Exercise* is now seen as having a critical role in health, from maintaining bone mass in the postmenopausal and cardiovascular well-being to treating depression. GPs may be able to 'prescribe' exercise through local links with a fitness centre or similar.

Psychological therapy

■ *Counselling* is frequently available as a service within a practice. Counselling services are also widely available in the community as local-government-run services, run by voluntary groups such as the church, and private counsellors. There is a wide variation in the qualifications of counsellors, and the GP has a role advising on reputable sources of help.

■ *Specialist counselling*, for alcohol, smoking, drugs etc., often operates as an extension of local psychiatric services, and may be through self-referral or GP referral. The GP has a vital role in knowing about the availability of such services and directing patients to them.

■ *Psychotherapy* is widely available privately, from many different theoretical foundations, from Freudian psychoanalysis to behavioural approaches, and shading at the edges into alternative therapies and religious-type cults. Of the more orthodox therapies, the theoretical approach seems to have less bearing on outcome than the individual qualities of the practitioner. Mainstream psychotherapy is usually available within the NHS, although cost constraints may allow only a limited number of sessions for a patient and delay in getting a first appointment.

■ *Support and counselling from the GP*. The GP him/herself is a source of emotional and psychological support for patients. Many consultations with a partly or wholly psychological basis are dealt with by the GP in everyday consultations. Some GPs undergo additional training in counselling and psychotherapy and offer this as a service to their patients.

Psychological issues in general practice are discussed in Chapter 5.

Self-help

Many patients attempt, often successfully, to sort themselves out through their own efforts. The GP may act as a source of support and encouragement, may help the patient find self-help groups, and advise on the course of actions they propose. The Internet is now a major source of advice for patients. Advice ranges from the excellent to the ravings of the certifiably insane. To the patient, it may not be immediately obvious which sort they have discovered.

Alternative therapies

A huge variety of alternative or complementary practices is available to patients. It is important for the GP to be aware of the claims each makes and the evidence to support them. Because of the nature of complementary practices, many have little formal scientific evaluation. The dictum 'first do no harm' is of prime importance. Harm can be caused by the effects of a therapy (it is worth remembering that orthodox therapies have much greater potential for harm than most complementary therapies) and by using an ineffective remedy and refusing an effective one. Tragic and unnecessary deaths have resulted from an insistence on a particular type of therapy. Many therapies that started life as 'alternative' have moved, as prejudices have changed and evidence emerged, into the mainstream. Osteopathy and acupuncture are examples. Homeopathy has a strong following amongst doctors (and an equally vociferous medical opposition). The Alexander technique lacks much of an evidence base, but has sensible-sounding ideas about posture and voice training. Yoga and Transcendental Meditation are amongst a variety of Eastern-style philosophies that help patients relax (trials have shown them to be effective in lowering blood pressure, for example). Others, such as elimination diets and those to treat *Candida albicans*, are based on corrupted versions of Western science.

Lifestyle change

We are becoming increasingly aware of the effects of lifestyle on illness, and changes in lifestyle may provide a better remedy than medication. Some of the factors are listed below.

- Smoking remains a massive cause of ill-health of many kinds. Britain is doing relatively well compared to the rest of Europe, but the mortality and morbidity remain appalling.
- Alcohol may be a bigger problem than smoking. Alcohol-related problems cost an estimated 95 million pounds to the Scottish NHS in 2001, and a billion pounds to Scotland as a whole in that period (Catalyst Health Economics figures).
- Sexual activity: not only acquired immunodeficiency syndrome (AIDS) but also other sexually transmitted diseases are increasing, including hepatitis B.
- Sedentary lifestyles: we have become used to such sedentary lifestyles that very modest exercise can have enormous health gains. Cycling for 40 minutes a day (in other words about 3 miles to work and back again) reduces the risk of ischaemic heart disease by 50 per cent. Bone mass is increased more by exercise than by any other treatment of osteoporosis. Jogging, via endorphin release, is an effective treatment for mild and moderate depression.
- Work: working long hours under pressure puts a strain on relationships and may cause sleep and psychiatric problems. The physical working environment at the office may result in repetitive strain and back injuries, and worse at the factory. Changing working patterns may not be easy but may bring significant health benefits.
- Obesity: factors are often interrelated. Obesity relates to sedentary living and bad diets secondary to long working hours – and that includes middle-class fast food such as microwaveable tagliatelle, with its excess fat and salt (which enhances flavour at low cost to the manufacturer), just as much as burger and chip diets.

IS THE DRUG EFFECTIVE?

Always consider whether there is evidence that the particular drug you choose is of proven benefit in the condition you propose to treat.

The rise of evidence-based medicine has made available to the GP a large and accessible body of evidence for the effectiveness of many treatments. (See the section on evidence-based medicine in Chapter 7). This evidence is often used to provide guidelines and protocols for the management of a condition. Applying such guidelines in everyday practice is a major challenge of contemporary general practice. Guidelines do not negate the need for clinical judgement. Each patient's situation is different, and the challenge is to provide the best care for the individual patient based on the best available evidence.

Remember that indications for the treatment of any condition may differ with age, sex and other factors. For example, an elderly smoker with chronic obstructive pulmonary disease (COPD) who presents with influenza may very justifiably be given antibiotics to prevent secondary bacterial infection. There would be little reason to do the same for a fit 25 year old.

IS THE DRUG SAFE?

Adverse reactions

All medications carry a risk of adverse reactions. These may be of several kinds. Rawlins and Thompson's (1977) useful classification of drug side effects included *predictable* (type A); *idiosyncratic* (type B); *continuous reactions* (type C) from long-term drug use, such as the tardive dyskinesias related to neuroleptic use; *delayed reactions* (type D), such as the potential for carcinogenesis from alkylating agents; and *end-of-use reactions* (type E) where problems arise on discontinuing therapy, such as withdrawal symptoms following discontinuation of benzodiazepines or addisonian symptoms after the withdrawal of steroids. You will meet patients who have experienced all of these reactions in general practice, but types A, B and E are particularly common. Also important is the wrong attribution of adverse reactions to medication, and this is discussed in the next page.

Predictable reactions

Some side effects are entirely predictable as a consequence of the actions of the drug. For example, broad-spectrum antibiotics frequently produce diarrhoea in children and adults (5–30 per cent) through effects on normal bacterial flora (Editorial, 2002). In the debilitated, this can produce the life-threatening pseudomembranous colitis. I recently talked with parents whose 2-year-old child required admission and intravenous rehydration for antibiotic-related diarrhoea. The antibiotics were given for a simple URTI that was of likely viral origin.

Non-steroidal anti-inflammatory drugs (NSAIDs) are useful as painkillers in a range of situations, but are a major cause of upper gastrointestinal inflammation and bleeding, and elevate blood pressure through salt and water-retaining properties. Other drugs (such as paracetamol in combination or alone) are often equally effective.

Some drugs require more careful monitoring because of the risks of serious side effects, e.g. monitoring of prothrombin time during warfarin therapy, or for agranulocytosis with carbimazole.

Idiosyncratic reactions

Idiosyncratic reactions are not predictable, not dose related, and may be severe. Individual reactions are uncommon, and inevitably the doctor cannot be aware of all the many types and potential for idiosyncratic reactions of the drugs he or she uses. As elsewhere in general practice, prevention is much better than cure, reinforcing the importance of not prescribing drugs except when explicitly indicated.

Examples of idiosyncratic reactions include thrombocytopenia from quinine (commonly prescribed to the elderly for leg cramps) and Stevens–Johnson syndrome from sulphonamide antibiotics ('hidden' in combinations like co-trimoxazole, and in Flamazine cream, which is commonly used in treating burns and leg ulcers, from which systemic absorption can be high).

The *British National Formulary* (*BNF*) is the most useful everyday source of information about the reactions that may be associated with any particular drug or class of drugs.

General practitioners need a good working knowledge of the commoner predictable side effects of the drugs they use. This is an argument in favour of practice formularies (see p. 150), which restrict the number of drugs used in the practice and so give the opportunity for better understanding of this more limited range.

In addition, the GP should always be aware that a patient's symptoms may result from drug side effects, and a thorough review of the patient's medication is an essential part of the patient's assessment. This medication may be unknown to the GP at the time of presentation. The possibility of a reaction from an OTC remedy or a new prescription from a recent hospital appointment must always be considered.

Serious side effects of established drugs and all side effects of newer drugs should be reported to the Committee on Safety of Medicines using the yellow card system.

End-of-use reactions

Withdrawal reactions from the discontinuation of a drug can produce a variety of symptoms. Benzodiazepine withdrawal may result in anxiety and muscle cramps, confusion, convulsions or frank psychiatric illness if not carefully managed. Abrupt withdrawal of long-term steroids will produce addisonian symptoms. A more common and insidious scenario is a patient who, some months after discontinuing steroids, develops an intercurrent infection and becomes unexpectedly ill. It may take a year or more for the adrenal glands to recover fully after steroid withdrawal, and the patient, whilst able to maintain a basal cortisol output, is unable to respond to the increased glucocorticoid needs brought about by the infection. The patient may present, not with classic addisonian symptoms, but merely as being unexpectedly unwell. Oral steroids need to be reintroduced to provide cover over this period and then quickly tailed off again.

Wrongly identified side effects

When patients report side effects of a medication, it is important to take a history of the alleged reaction and attempt to establish whether or not it was a true side effect. Many patients will tell you they are 'allergic to penicillin'; often, on further questioning, the drug turns out not to have been penicillin. The reaction may be that it 'made me feel sick' or 'gave me diarrhoea'. Assessing the likelihood of a reaction may prove very difficult: when a rash follows an antibiotic prescription it is often not clear whether it was due to the antibiotic or to the viral illness for which it was inappropriately given. This serves as a further warning against prescribing antibiotics when the indications are not clear. It is important to discuss with patients whether or not they should avoid that drug in future. Confirming that they may take penicillin when they initially believed themselves to be allergic to it may save their life at some time in the future.

Drug interactions

Interactions between drugs are common, are a frequent cause of morbidity and sometimes mortality and are often avoidable. The elderly are particularly at risk, often having multiple pathologies, and may be particularly sensitive to the effects of any medication (see the section on the elderly, p. 148). Not all interactions are adverse. Synergistic effects of drugs in combination can be very useful, such as combining diuretics and angiotensin-converting enzyme (ACE) inhibitors for both heart failure and hypertension. Indeed, using lower doses of two drugs may be more therapeutically effective, whilst lowering the likelihood of dose-related side effects of the individual drugs. Interactions may be deliberately sought to offset the side effects of one drug with another, for instance the potassium-leaching effects of frusemide (furosemide) are countered by potassium-sparing amiloride, whilst increasing the overall diuretic effect.

Drug interactions arise through a number of mechanisms. Those mechanisms particularly encountered in general practice settings are discussed below; the reader is encouraged to consult a textbook of pharmacology to gain a broader overview.

Drug interactions are classified as:
■ pharmaceutical,
■ pharmacodynamic, and
■ pharmacokinetic.

We might add a further, behavioural, category of:
■ 'pharmaconfusion', where, as the number of medications increases, the chance of any being taken correctly decreases; this is perhaps the commonest and most important 'class' found in general practice (and see p. 145, 'A negotiated approach to therapy (concordance)').

Pharmaceutical reactions are rarely encountered by GPs. They occur when mixing drugs before they get to the patient; for example, diazepam injected into an infusion bag precipitates. Pharmacodynamic and pharmacokinetic reactions are discussed below.

Predictable (pharmacodynamic)

Interactions arise as a predictable consequence of the normal effects of the drugs. They are thus very common and frequently encountered in general practice. For instance, tricyclic antidepressants and alcohol both cause drowsiness. The effect of taking both is for one to augment the other. It is important to make a patient you are putting on tricyclics aware of this effect and its implications for safety, whilst driving for example. The NSAIDs are freely prescribed as analgesics, but their well-known salt and water retaining properties will diminish the effect of diuretics and anti-hypertensives.

Pharmacokinetic

Interactions occur when one drug affects the plasma levels of another. These work through a number of mechanisms.
■ *Absorption*. Interactions may occur through effects on drug absorption, for instance tetracyclines are chelated by aluminium (perhaps being taken by the patient as an OTC indigestion remedy) or milk (not a drug, but no less important as an interaction). Oral contraceptives are excreted conjugated in bile. They are deconjugated by bacteria in the gut, which enables them to be re-absorbed and maintains effective therapeutic drug levels. Broad-spectrum antibiotics kill the bacteria and disrupt the process, decreasing blood levels of hormone and increasing the potential for pregnancy.

■ *Metabolism.* Drugs may stimulate or inhibit liver enzyme production, resulting in the enhanced or diminished breakdown of other drugs. Erythromycin inhibits enzymes metabolizing theophyllines; treating an acute exacerbation of COPD with this antibiotic could precipitate theophylline toxicity. Anticonvulsants induce the enzymes that metabolize oral contraceptives; the increased rate of breakdown of oestrogen and progestogen is predictable, and an effective response may therefore be to increase the strength of the pill – typically increasing the oestrogen component from 30 to 50 micrograms (μg).

■ *Excretion.* The well-known potassium-leaching actions of loop and thiazide diuretics are often countered by combining them with a potassium-sparing diuretic such as spironolactone or amiloride. In this common example, the interaction is used to the patient's benefit. However, other interactions, such as the increased re-absorption of lithium when diuretics are given, will increase the blood levels to produce serious toxicity.

General practitioners use a huge spectrum of drugs, both those they prescribe themselves and continuing those prescribed by the hospital. If a patient is attending several clinics, the risk of adverse interactions multiplies, and the GP is best placed to overview the entire prescribing strategy. GPs need to be aware of the potential for interactions and actively monitor the overall prescribing pattern; they may be assisted by computer prescribing programs that can be set to warn automatically of potential interactions. Awareness of the potential for interactions, keeping up to date with new medications and vigilance with individual patients are crucial aspects of the GP's role (Fig. 8.1).

Many medications are initiated in hospital and the GP subsequently takes responsibility for continuing to prescribe them. The importance of adequate and accurate communication between hospital and general practice *and vice versa* cannot be over-emphasized. Unfortunately, it is still commonplace for patients to be discharged from hospital with inadequate or no information. Similarly, many GP referrals do not contain

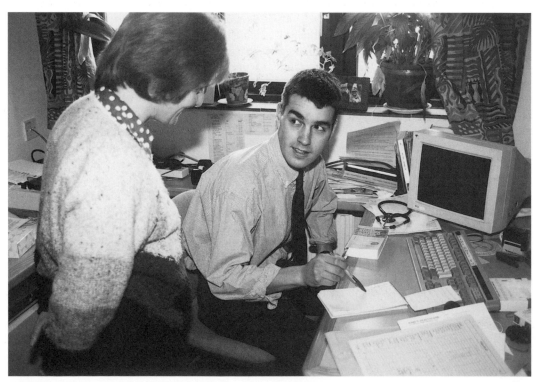

Figure 8.1 Would that be safe?

adequate information about patients' medication, even though this can usually be readily obtained from the practice computer system.

IS THERAPY ECONOMICAL?

Always prescribe drugs by generic name rather than by proprietary (brand) name. Generic drugs are of the same quality as proprietary drugs and prescribing generically ensures that the cheapest preparation is dispensed. The exceptions to this rule are discussed under 'Generic prescribing' on page 150.

AGREEING MANAGEMENT WITH YOUR PATIENT

There is evidence that only one-third of patients comply with recommended treatment; another third sometimes comply, and the remaining third do not comply at all (Fedder, 1982). Up to 20 per cent of patients do not take their prescriptions to be dispensed, and a sizeable proportion who do so do not subsequently take it (Fry, 1993). It has been estimated that, at most, only 50 per cent of people with chronic disease comply with their doctors' recommendations, irrespective of disease, treatment or age (Sackett and Snow, 1979; Dunbar-Jacob et al., 2000).

Patients may choose not to take prescribed medication for a variety of reasons.

- *Fear of taking a drug*: 'It's not natural … messing up my body with chemicals'.
- *Unconvinced about the need for medication*: the asymptomatic hypertensive patient will be understandably reluctant to engage in a lifetime of treatment with potential side effects.
- *Concern about side effects*: e.g. measles, mumps and rubella (MMR) vaccination and autism fears.
- *Inconvenience*: taking aerosol inhaler devices to school or work.
- *Cost*: significant in the UK, at £6.30 per item at the time of writing, and often prohibitive in countries where the full cost has to be borne by the patient.
- *Lack of confidence in the doctor*: if patients feel their doctor has not understood their problem, they are less likely to comply with the suggested treatment.

- *Stigma of illness*: this may make diagnosis difficult to accept for the patient – e.g. depression or other psychiatric problems – and hence there is a reluctance to take the appropriate treatment.
- *Risks outweigh benefits* in the patient's eyes.
- *Cultural values and health beliefs*: some patients have little faith in prescribed medication.
- *Complex drug regimens*: multiple drugs, different dosing regimens.

A negotiated aproach to therapy (concordance)

The extent to which patients conform to the doctor's plan is termed compliance. However, compliance is now seen as a very doctor-centred approach to therapy: it is about the doctor instructing the patient, who is expected to obey. This paternalistic view of therapy is thought to be part of the reason why compliance is so poor. A more recent and successful approach is to see therapy as a shared responsibility of patient and doctor, each of whom has a responsibility to understand the other's viewpoint (www.medicines-partnership.org). This 'concordance' between doctor and patient over therapy is discussed below.

Often, such a discussion will be a very straightforward affair, with the patient keen to receive the medication and little discussion required. But sometimes detailed discussion and negotiation are required, for instance in starting a trial of high-dose oral steroids in a patient with suspected temporal arteritis who has well-founded concerns about the side effects of such medication.

In order to understand the patient's possible concerns about therapy, their views need to be actively sought. In the same way that in Chapter 7 we discussed the importance of eliciting patients' concerns, ideas and expectations concerning their illness, it is not difficult to see why this must be extended to patients' ideas concerning treatment. This can then be the basis for a sharing of views between doctor and patient, out of which can come a negotiated approach to therapy that is acceptable to the patient and doctor alike.

An approach to reaching concordance with a patient might run as follows.

- The doctor presents the diagnosis and proposals for treatment.
- The patient is encouraged to talk about his or her ideas, concerns and expectations regarding the diagnosis and proposed treatment.
- The patient and doctor discuss their respective views of the illness and its treatment to reach a shared understanding.
- Based on this shared understanding, a treatment plan is agreed.
- The doctor gives clear instructions about the dose, frequency and duration of medication and checks the patient understands.
- A plan is agreed to review progress.

HELPING THE PATIENT TAKE MEDICATION CORRECTLY

Besides discussing and negotiating therapy, there are a number of ways in which the doctor can help the patient to take medication correctly.

- Give clear instructions and check the patient has understood them (perhaps by getting the patient to explain them back to you). Write them down if necessary.
- Prescribe as few medications as possible.
- Keep the dosing schedule simple:
  as few times a day as possible,
  if using several drugs, the same regimen for each (e.g. all twice daily).
- Avoid drugs likely to produce side effects; discuss any likely side effects and what to do if these arise.
- Stop drugs that are ineffective or no longer required.
- Tell the patient how long they are expected to continue the medication.
- Ensure your instructions to the pharmacist are clear and congruous with your instructions to the patient.

REVIEWING YOUR PATIENTS' PROGRESS AND USE OF MEDICATION

Discussing medication use should be part of your regular review of your patients. Your review must be able to tell you the following.

- *If the medication is having the desired effect*: this will come from your discussion with the patient, backed up by appropriate investigations. These investigations will take whatever form is appropriate, e.g. cardiovascular assessment in the patient with heart failure, reviewing the peak flow diary in the asthmatic patient, or laboratory measurement of thyroid-stimulating hormone levels in the treated myxoedemic patient.

- *Whether the medication is causing side effects*: likely side effects should be explicitly inquired about. Patients may not realize that new symptoms represent side effects or may be reluctant to discuss them (such as the impotence produced by many anti-hypertensives).

- *Whether the patient is taking the medication regularly*: besides developing a relationship of trust with your patient, medication usage can be assessed by monitoring how often the patient collects prescriptions, which may suggest either over-use or under-use of medication. Measuring blood levels of drugs gives indirect evidence of compliance, for instance a fall in serum anticonvulsant levels may mean your patient is becoming forgetful about taking the tablets, and should be the starting point for a discussion about compliance rather than eliciting a knee-jerk increase in dosage.

PRESCRIBING FOR SPECIAL GROUPS

The 'special groups' of children and elderly are actually the commonest groups to be seen in general practice and each, in its own way, is particularly vulnerable to medication. General practitioners need to take particular care when prescribing for these patients.

CHILDREN

The questions above of necessity, effectiveness and safety are of particular importance to this age group. The majority of children presenting in general practice have self-limiting illnesses for which simple supportive or symptomatic treatment only is required. Children are not merely small adults and may respond differently from adults to medication.

Making a firm diagnosis is difficult for a miserable child who is unable or unwilling to give a history or be examined. Differentiating the genuinely sick child from the merely miserable is a critical skill. Sick children need careful assessment and often re-assessment by a paediatrician. Antibiotics are often given to such children 'just in case' of bacterial infection. There is *some* justification for this approach: the child is sick, the illness might be bacterial, the diagnosis may not be provable, or proving it may require unjustifiably invasive investigations, and the illness is potentially worse than the side effects of the antibiotics.

Necessity

The majority of children seen in general practice have viral URTIs. There is no justification for treatment with antibiotics, even though there may be pressure from parents to provide them. There is no evidence that cough mixtures are effective. Miserable children with URTIs need rest, fluids, judicious doses of paracetamol and clear instructions to their carers about what would raise the threshold of concern and when to return. Unexpectedly protracted illnesses produce parental concern, often manifested in an insistence on antibiotics; this will often not be appropriate. For instance, asthma arising as a complication of a URTI is common and presents as a protracted and mainly nocturnal cough.

Effectiveness

Even those who present with likely bacterial infections are often not helped by antibiotics. For instance, there is little evidence that antibiotics change the history of otitis media; the majority of cases resolve spontaneously. Better public health means that progression to acute mastoiditis or chronic suppurative conditions that used to be common is now rare. Similarly, although pharyngitis is mainly viral, even the 40 per cent of cases that are not are only marginally helped by antibiotics. (One study demonstrated that giving antibiotics reduced the duration of symptoms by just 8 hours.)

Safety

Safety is a major concern in prescribing for children. Children metabolize certain drugs differently from adults, their relative body proportion of fat is different (changing the drug's volume of distribution) and certain drugs behave in inexplicable ways (for instance, amphetamine is *sedating* in children and used to treat hyperactivity syndromes).

Relatively minor side effects with antibiotics, such as diarrhoea, may settle quickly, but, given the often-limited justification for prescribing them and the relatively minor conditions for which they may have been prescribed, it is difficult to justify this sort of prescribing. Moreover, occasional children develop severe diarrhoea and dehydration, which may even be fatal in the case of antibiotic-related pseudomembranous colitis.

Calculating children's doses

Doses are often most accurately calculated from the child's surface area, itself estimated from nomograms relating to weight and height (Barrett et al., 2002). More commonly, dosage is calculated by body weight, which is less accurate and may give too large a dose in an obese child, for example. The *BNF* gives dose ranges for children based on age. This imprecise approach is reasonable for 'ordinary' doses of 'safe' drugs given to 'normal' children and is suitable for most drugs given to children in general practice. However, if a high dose of a drug is required, if the therapeutic window is narrow (i.e. the drug is not 'safe') or if the child is not of 'normal' height or weight, the more precise approaches must be adopted.

Compliance

Getting children to take the drug you have prescribed is fortunately delegated to the parents! The doctor can help by providing the drug in the most acceptable (or at any rate, least unacceptable) form to the child. Children are usually prescribed medication in liquid form, but may prefer tablets, so it is worth asking. If a dose of less than 5 mL is prescribed, an oral syringe must be supplied by the chemist; however, in practice, a syringe may be a far easier tool to use than the traditional teaspoon whatever the dose. A familiar form of the drug may be more acceptable, so the child may be persuaded to take proprietary Calpol but not a strange-tasting generic paracetamol.

THE ELDERLY

Whereas 15 per cent of the population is over the age of 65, around 40–45 per cent of prescriptions are for this age group. The elderly are at particular risk from the effects of drugs and poor prescribing practices.

Elderly people in particular may:

■ *have multiple pathologies*: elderly people often have several illnesses that potentially require intervention;

■ *be less able to cope*: the patient's mental faculties may make him or her less able to cope with the drug regimen;

■ *have altered metabolism* that may give rise to slower absorption, different distribution (for instance because of reduced serum albumin), and reduced excretion by the kidneys or metabolism by the liver. Generally, these factors tend to enhance the normal actions of a drug and increase the risk of dose-related adverse reactions.

A review of medicines as part of the National Service Framework (NSF) for Older People (Department of Health, 2001) identified a number of issues in prescribing particularly related to the elderly.

■ *Adverse reactions could be prevented*: between 5 and 17 per cent of hospital admissions are related to adverse reactions (Mannesse et al., 2000).

■ *Under-use of medications*: there is evidence that medications are under-used in areas such as stroke prevention, asthma and depression.

■ *Polypharmacy*: taking four or more medications is a particular risk factor for older people. There is clearly a conflict between the problems of polypharmacy and those of under-utilization of medication.

■ *Poor use of repeat prescribing*: whilst automated repeat prescribing has many benefits, it needs careful monitoring to ensure medications are up to date and are being taken as intended. Perhaps 50 per cent of elderly people do not take their medications as intended (Royal Pharmaceutical Society of Great Britain, 1997). Inconsistent quantities prescribed on repeat prescriptions result in waste and confusion. It is estimated that 6–10 per cent of the total prescribing budget is wasted in this way (Davidson et al., 1998).

■ *Changes in medication after hospital discharge*: many unintentional changes are made in medication following discharge from hospital. This partly relates to poor communication between primary and secondary care. (See p. 158 on communication between primary and secondary care.)

■ *Inadequate dosage instructions on labels*: 'as directed' is unhelpful if the directions are not remembered.

■ *Carers*: informal carers are often underused and under-supported in helping elderly patients take medicine correctly and appropriately. In care homes, numerous problems have been identified, from continued prescription of unnecessary drugs and prescription of drugs for which no indication was recorded, to frank abuse, with residents being excessively sedated with inappropriate neuroleptics.

Principles for prescribing for the elderly are essentially the same as any principles for good prescribing, but need to be even more fastidiously observed.

■ Assess your patient and his or her medication carefully; do not rush to treatment.

■ Negotiate your proposed treatment carefully with the patient, ensuring he or she understands what is involved and is happy to comply.

■ Be realistic with the patient about what you can and cannot treat. Do not get drawn into chasing minor symptoms with drugs. Remember that depression is common in the elderly and often presents with physical rather than psychological symptoms.

Necessity

Only treat those conditions which are important, for which treatment can change the natural history or which give relief from intolerable symptoms. These concerns may be particular to your elderly patients: for instance, there is no point in treating mild hypertension or raised cholesterol in an elderly individual who is unlikely to live long enough to benefit. Indeed, the side effects of the drugs may be fatal (e.g. a fall related to anti-hypertensive-induced postural hypotension).

Effectiveness

Effective doses may be much lower in the elderly. Half the normal adult dose may be effective and is a sensible dose to start at.

Safety

Try to avoid medications with frequent side effects: these will be worse in your elderly patients. For example, NSAIDs are prescribed in vast quantities for mild osteoarthritis in the elderly; there is little evidence that they are more effective than simple paracetamol for mild disease and they are a major cause of gastrointestinal bleeding.

Compliance

Keep treatment regimens simple: as few drugs, as few times a day as possible, preferably all with the same frequency (i.e. if a drug must be three times daily, make everything thrice daily). Long-acting preparations and combined tablets (e.g. Frumil) can be used to keep things simple. Write down the regimen for your patient and ensure that he or she has understood it. For patients who have limited understanding or for a necessarily complicated regimen, the 'dosette' box can be very helpful (Fig. 8.2). This is a box divided into sections for the days of the week and into subdivisions for morning, noon, afternoon and evening. The community pharmacist loads the box once a week and the patient then takes the contents of each section at the appropriate time each day. This is not foolproof: a dosette box was recently organized for a patient with learning difficulties and a complex drug regimen. The patient was delighted, swallowed the entire contents of the box on returning home and slept for 48 hours!

Review

Review your patient regularly, ensuring your treatment is doing what it is meant to, and be alert to side effects and adverse interactions. If

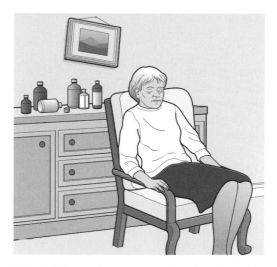

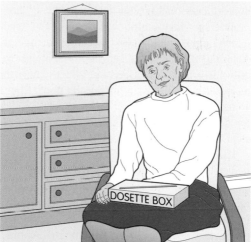

Figure 8.2 Improving compliance with complex drug regimens by the use of a dosette box.

your patient is also attending other clinics, review the prescription carefully after each visit in the context of the whole. As a GP, you need to overview the prescribing pattern, which can easily become confused if a number of clinics are involved. The NSF review recommends a detailed annual medication review, or more often if the patient is at higher risk, i.e.:

- taking multiple medications (more than four),
- recently discharged from hospital,
- living in a care home,
- having known medicine-related problems,
- following an adverse change of health (to identify potential drug contributors to the change).

'Brown bag' reviews

Get your patient to bring in all the medication he or she is currently taking. This allows you to assess the patient's understanding of what is being taken, any drugs you did not know about, any drugs being taken incorrectly, and outdated or obsolete medications hanging around in the cupboard and potentially causing confusion. It has been suggested that community pharmacists should take on this role in the future.

GENERIC PRESCRIBING

Most drugs have a generic name, usually an abbreviated version of their chemical name and a proprietary or trade name. For instance the beta-blocker metoprolol is available as non-proprietary metoprolol and under the trade names of Lopresor and Betaloc. Doctors are encouraged to prescribe generic formulations, not only for economic reasons but also to allow the pharmacist flexibility in purchasing drugs from a wider range of sources. It is also better practice for doctors to become familiar with one generic stem name rather than several trade names.

There are two exceptions to this. Certain modified release preparations, such as some anti-epileptic drugs and calcium channel antagonists, have different bio-availabilities with different formulations. Such drugs should be prescribed by proprietary name. Some preparations contain several drugs and are known as compound preparations. It may be impracticable to write out all the constituents, and confusing for the pharmacist. In these cases it is permissible to use the trade name, for example with combined oral contraceptives. Recently, generic names have been developed for the commoner combinations, such as co-codamol (paracetamol and codeine) and co-amilofruse (amiloride and frusemide). Never be tempted to 'invent' generic names or abbreviate drug names on prescriptions: confusion and dispensing errors will result.

PRESCRIBING SUPPORT IN PRIMARY CARE

To help GPs make appropriate and accurate prescribing decisions, a variety of sources of support are available to them. These can be broadly classified into paper, computer and human, and in different ways provide drug information and prescribing support to primary care.

PAPER REFERENCE SOURCES

The *BNF* is a condensed, practical textbook of the drugs currently available in Britain. It is, in effect, the drug handbook for the NHS and indicates which drugs may and may not be given on NHS prescriptions. It is an invaluable brief overview of individual drugs and notes on approaches to the treatment of a wide variety of common conditions. As part of its remit, it lists every member of a class of drug (for instance it lists 16 beta-blockers and 14 NSAIDs), most of which have very similar actions.

It is better for the individual doctor to become experienced with one or a few examples of each class of drug. Doctors working in groups (such as general practices) can help themselves by agreeing on which drugs they will choose to focus on. This is the basis for producing local *practice formularies* of agreed drugs that aim to promote rational, safe and cost-effective prescribing. Local formularies usually specify a limited choice of drugs to use in any particular condition, chosen for their effectiveness, safety and cost.

The choice of drugs can be linked to *local protocols* and *guidelines*, ensuring the most appropriate drug is available in any given situation. Whilst this is a good foundation for rational and safe prescribing, it does not replace the need for clinical judgement. Guidelines give general advice that may not be appropriate to the particular circumstances of your patient. Departing from established guidelines should, however, be a conscious and carefully justified decision by the GP.

Costs can also be controlled by ensuring that after taking considerations of effectiveness into account, the formulary contains the cheapest acceptable preparations in that class. These will often be generic versions.

Whilst general practice formularies allow GPs to initiate prescriptions from a limited and well-understood list, they often find themselves continuing prescriptions from other sources which are not within their chosen formulary. The GP has to decide whether it is in the patient's interests to change to a drug in their formulary or (more usually) to continue with the drug as originally prescribed.

The *Drug and Therapeutics Bulletin* is sent free to all GPs (and hospital doctors) and provides short reviews of medications and the therapy of conditions. The Medicines Resource Centre produces similar material in its 'MeReC' reviews.

The *Monthly Index of Medical Specialties* (*MIMS*) is a brief guide to medications produced by the drug industry and circulated to GPs. Being updated monthly, it contains details of new medications and other information that has not yet reached the *BNF*.

A wide variety of other publications (much of it drug company sponsored) swells the in-tray of the GP.

COMPUTER-BASED SOURCES

Information technology (IT)-based sources of information are becoming progressively more common and more useful. The *BNF* and *MIMS* are both available electronically in forms easily accessible from the doctor's desk. General practice computer databases not only allow computer-based prescribing, but can also link to databases, automatically producing drug interaction alerts and even sophisticated decision support tools capable of extracting data from patient records and suggesting ranked lists of suitable drugs with appropriate doses. The use of computers in prescribing is dealt with on page 154.

PRESCRIBING ADVISORS

In the UK, primary care trusts have designated prescribing advisors who have specialized knowledge of drug and prescribing issues in primary care. Their role includes the development of prescribing policies in primary care and direct support of GPs in prescribing matters.

COMMUNITY PHARMACISTS

These professionals are highly trained and knowledgeable about drug matters and an excellent source of information. Further information on community pharmacists can be found on page 157.

Practical Exercise

❏ Find out what sources of information on prescribing are available in your practice. Ask your GP tutor and practice manager to help you.
❏ Is there a practice formulary? Is it used?
❏ Consider with your GP tutor the advantages and disadvantages of a practice drug formulary.

WRITING A PRESCRIPTION

HOW TO WRITE A PRESCRIPTION

A prescription is a written instruction to a pharmacist to dispense a drug. Historically, prescriptions were only written by doctors; more recently, nurses with specialist training are now also allowed to prescribe from a limited list. Only registered doctors can write a general practice prescription – so pre-registration house officers (PRHOs) in general practice are not allowed to do so. The legal responsibility for the prescription lies with the doctor who signs it. A prescription is therefore a legal document.

Most general practices use computer systems to produce acute prescriptions during the consultation and to generate repeat prescriptions. The format of a prescription is the same whether it is handwritten (Fig. 8.3) or computerized (Fig. 8.4). All prescriptions, however produced, must conform to prescribing regulations and be signed by a doctor. Additional requirements apply to the prescription of controlled drugs (CDs), for example morphine and barbiturates (see p. 155).

In Britain, NHS prescriptions are issued from general practice on a form known as an FP10 (these are not used for non-NHS prescriptions). When writing a prescription, you should follow the guidelines set out by the Department of Health, which you will find in the *BNF*.

A prescription should be written legibly in ink or other indelible substance and should include the following.

■ *The name and address of the patient.* Always confirm the patient's address during the consultation. A wrong address could result in the patient being untraceable which, in the event

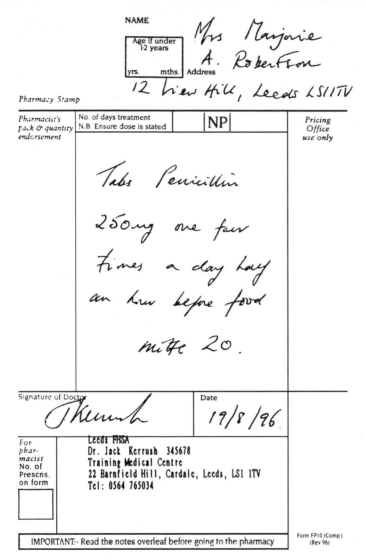

NAME

Mrs Marjorie
A. Robertson

Age if under 12 years

yrs.   mths.   Address

12 View Hill, Leeds LS11TV

Pharmacy Stamp

Pharmacist's pack & quantity endorsement	No. of days treatment N.B. Ensure dose is stated	NP	Pricing Office use only

Tabs Penicillin

250mg one four
times a day half
an hour before food

mitte 20.

Signature of Doctor

J Kerrush

Date

19/8/96

For pharmacist No. of Prescns. on form

Leeds FHSA
Dr. Jack Kerrush 345678
Training Medical Centre
22 Barnfield Hill, Cardale, Leeds, LS1 1TV
Tel : 0564 765034

IMPORTANT:- Read the notes overleaf before going to the pharmacy

Form FP10 (Comp.)
(Rev 96)

Figure 8.3 Specimen prescription on form FP10, handwritten.

of a prescribing, dispensing or collection error, could have disastrous consequences.

- ■ *The patient's age* (a legal requirement in children under 12 years).
- ■ *The number of days' treatment* in the designated space. If several items with different lengths of treatment are to be prescribed, specify each separately (see below under 'The total quantity to be dispensed').
- ■ *The drug name.* Use the generic name unless there are good reasons not to. (See 'Generic prescribing' above).
- ■ *The drug formulation*, e.g. capsules, tablets, suppositories, syrup, ampoules, etc.

- ■ *The drug dosage*:
  - quantities of one gram or more should be written as 1 g, 2 g etc.;
  - quantities less than one gram should be written in milligrams, as 1 mg, 2 mg etc.;
  - quantities less than one milligram should be written in micrograms, e.g. 50 micrograms – 'micrograms' should not be abbreviated;
  - decimal points should be avoided; when this is not possible, the decimal point should be preceded by zero, e.g. 0.5 mg;
  - with liquid preparations, millilitre, ml or mL is used, e.g. 5 ml (and not cubic centimetre or cc).

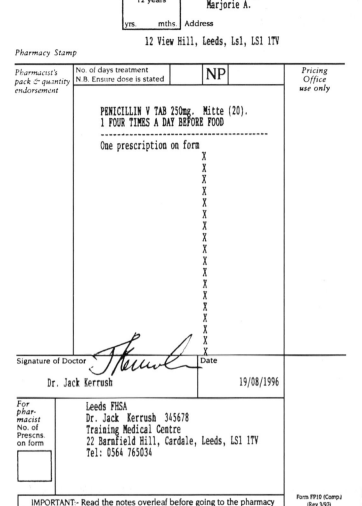

NAME

Age if under 12 years
yrs.   mths.

Mrs. Robertson
Marjorie A.

Address

12 View Hill, Leeds, Ls1, LS1 1TV

Pharmacy Stamp

Pharmacist's pack & quantity endorsement

No. of days treatment
N.B. Ensure dose is stated

NP

Pricing Office use only

PENICILLIN V TAB 250mg. Mitte (20).
1 FOUR TIMES A DAY BEFORE FOOD

One prescription on form

Signature of Doctor

Dr. Jack Kerrush

Date

19/08/1996

For pharmacist No. of Prescns. on form

Leeds FHSA
Dr. Jack Kerrush 345678
Training Medical Centre
22 Barnfield Hill, Cardale, Leeds, LS1 1TV
Tel: 0564 765034

IMPORTANT:- Read the notes overleaf before going to the pharmacy

Form FP10 (Comp.)
(Rev 3/97)

Figure 8.4 Specimen prescription on form FP10, computer generated.

■ *The dose frequency*, e.g. three times daily or eight hourly. If a medication is to be taken symptomatically, you may state 'as required', but the minimum dose interval should be specified. You will sometimes see Latin abbreviations used on prescriptions (e.g. b.d., t.d.s. – see the back page of the *BNF*), but English is to be preferred. Computer prescribing software automatically converts instructions entered in Latin abbreviations into English for prescription printing.

■ *Advice about how to take the drug*, e.g. whether it should be taken before food, as with a tetracycline, or after food, as with a NSAID, or at night, for hypnotics. The pharmacist may add written or oral precautionary warnings to your own instructions when dispensing medication and these may appear on the drug name label.

■ *The total quantity to be dispensed*. If the number of days of treatment has been indicated (see above), the quantity is not required, as this can be calculated by the pharmacist. However, when several drugs of different durations are prescribed on one prescription form, this is inappropriate and the total quantity to be dispensed or number of days of treatment should be written after each item.

- *Limit the number of items to three* on any prescription form. The pharmacist will dispense more if included, but the more congested the prescription, the greater the risk of error.
- *Sign* or, as you are not yet medically qualified, ask your tutor to sign, and date the prescription.
- *The name and address of the GP* and *the doctor's prescribing number* will normally be pre-printed at the bottom of the prescription, but must be added if absent.

PRESCRIBING BY COMPUTER

Most prescriptions in general practice are now produced by computer. In the UK, 98 per cent of practices use computers to generate repeat prescriptions, 80 per cent of GPs use computers to prescribe during consultations, and 26 per cent of GPs use computer software to support prescribing decisions (Franke et al., 2000). Handwritten prescriptions are still used on home visits, are needed when the computer goes down, and remain in use amongst the diminishing band of GPs not yet computerized. Prescriptions for controlled drugs have to be partially or wholly handwritten.

Prescribing by computer has a number of advantages.

- Prescribing is from a database of recognized drugs in recognized doses, improving drug choice and dose accuracy.
- The computer will not allow the prescription until all key information has been included.
- The computer automatically records the prescription to the patient's record.
- The prescription data are stored in a form that can be readily audited.
- The computer automatically includes correct patient details (name, age and address).
- The output is a printed and therefore legible prescription.
- Computers can semi-automatically produce generic prescriptions and so increase generic prescribing.
- Some systems provide immediate warnings of potential *adverse reactions* based on past drug histories stored on the system, and *adverse interactions* with other drugs the patient is taking.

- Computers can be set to produce repeat prescriptions, which can be produced by practice staff (though all have to be approved and signed by a doctor) – see 'Repeat prescribing' below.
- Computers provide an accurate printed record of repeat medications for the patient.

Together, these factors reduce the potential for errors by the GP and dispenser and produce an accurate prescription very rapidly.

However, computers do not remove the need for skill or vigilance in prescribing and are only as good as the drug and patient information stored in the computer's database.

REPEAT PRESCRIBING

Half of all prescriptions issued in the UK are 'repeats' (Fry, 1993). In repeat prescribing, the GP makes a decision that a particular drug needs to be continued long term; the patient is then allowed to request further supplies without needing to see the doctor each time. Usually the system is computerized and the patient has a list of the drugs allowed. Requests are handed in to the reception staff, who check with the computer database and generate a computer script if the request is appropriate. The doctor then checks and signs the script, which is collected by the patient one to two days later.

Repeat prescribing can save time for patients and doctors, but it can lead to problems. Patients may not be reviewed regularly by their doctor, which could result in their underlying disease not being monitored, drugs being continued when no longer needed, side effects being missed or compliance not being assessed. It is therefore important to ensure that a patient recall facility is built into any repeat prescription system, such that each patient is only allowed a certain number of repeats before being reviewed by the doctor. It is also essential to ensure that the system is accurate.

Any repeat prescribing system (computer or manual) should:

- provide only the medications and doses agreed with the doctor;
- monitor patient compliance by providing a warning if patients are taking too much or

too little of their medication (by giving a warning if the prescription is collected before or after it is due);

- not allow a prescription to be produced if the regular review of the patient has not taken place;
- be flexible: a patient should not be deprived of treatment because he or she has missed an appointment, but any deviations from the agreed protocol must be with the doctor's permission and appropriate review agreed.

Practical Exercise

Find out about the repeat prescribing system in your practice. Ask one of the reception staff to explain the system to you. Consider the advantages and disadvantages of repeat prescribing and discuss these with your GP tutor.

ABUSE OF DRUGS AND CONTROLLED DRUGS

Whilst drug abuse is a major problem in society, very few illegal drugs derive from pharmaceutical or healthcare sources. Nevertheless, stringent precautions are taken to ensure that potential drugs of abuse are not accessible illegally.

These precautions include the physical security of the practice and legal requirements to store drugs securely, and controls over the prescribing of certain potential drugs of abuse.

Many GPs in inner cities, where drug problems are widespread, have an interest in addiction management and take an active part in harm reduction programmes and the management of addiction.

PRESCRIBING CONTROLLED DRUGS

In order to control the availability of particular drugs, the various Misuse of Drugs Acts specify certain drugs as 'controlled drugs', to which particular prescribing requirements apply. Prescriptions must be handwritten by the prescriber and include:

- the patient's name and address,
- the form and strength of the preparation,
- the total quantity of the preparation in both words and figures,
- the dose (e.g. one tablet three times a day),
- the date and prescriber's signature.

These requirements apply to schedule 2 and 3 drugs, which include the morphine derivatives and cocaine. Schedule 3 includes the barbiturates, which are now little used and to which the above rules apply, with the exception that the prescription does not have to be handwritten (though the date does!). Temazepam, which recently enjoyed a vogue for being injected intravenously, and flunitrazepam (Rohypnol), infamous for its drug rape connotations, are also in schedule 3 but no restrictions apply to these or to the other benzodiazepines that are in schedule 4. Schedule 1 contains drugs such as LSD and cannabis, which are not used medicinally and so cannot be prescribed.

THE DOCTOR'S BAG

Usually GPs prescribe, but are not allowed to dispense medications. The exceptions to this are drugs for emergency and on-call use, and in some rural practices that dispense all their patients' drugs (see below). GPs on call have to treat emergencies and urgent problems and are permitted to carry and dispense appropriate drugs in order to do so. They also carry small quantities of basic drugs that they are allowed to dispense to patients to avoid delay in starting medications at night and other times when community pharmacies are closed. This is particularly important in rural areas, where the pharmacies and hospital resources may be at some distance. It carries dangers in urban areas, where often doctors are assaulted by drug users trying to obtain supplies.

WHAT IS IN THE DOCTOR'S BAG?

On call, GPs will carry a selection of drugs to deal with the situations they are most likely to meet. This varies with individual preference and the needs of different practices, e.g. city versus rural (Anonymous, 2000).

The following list is based on that used in a city practice; a rural list would usually be more extensive.

Analgesics

– Mild paracetamol tablets.
– Moderate co-codamol tablets, dihydrocodeine tablets, diclofenac injection, tablets and suppositories.
– Strong diamorphine.
– Naloxone (opiate antagonist).

Antibiotics

– Benzylpenicillin injection.
– Amoxicillin, flucloxacillin, trimethoprim and erythromycin as tablets/capsules and paediatric elixir.

Respiratory

– Prednisolone tablets.
– Hydrocortisone injection.
– Salbutamol, ipratropium and beclomethasone inhalers (high doses can be given via a spacer device with results comparable to that of a nebulizer).
– Nebulizer solutions of the above.

Cardiovascular

– Aspirin 75 mg tablets.
– Glyceryl trinitrate (GTN) spray (a better choice than tablets because of its long shelf life).
– Fibrinolytics, which have major benefits if started early but carry serious side effects. There is a case for GPs initiating these in isolated areas.
– Frusemide tablets and injection.
– Atropine injection.
– Adrenaline injection.

Obstetric

– Ergometrine injection.

Psychiatric

– Temazepam tablets.
– Diazepam tablets.
– Chlorpromazine tablets and injection.
– Haloperidol injection.
– Procyclidine injection (for drug-induced dystonic reactions).

Neurological

– Diazepam, intravenous and rectal preparations.
– Flumazenil (benzodiazepine antagonist).

Paediatric

– Antipyretics/analgesics, paracetamol, ibuprofen.
– Paediatric preparations of antibiotics (above).

Allergic

– Adrenaline.
– Chlorphenamine (Piriton) injection and tablets.
– Cetirizine tablets.

Gastrointestinal

– Metoclopramide injection and tablets.
– Prochlorperazine tablets and elixir.
– Hyoscine butylbromide injection and tablets.

Endocrine

– Glucose injection.
– Glucagon injection.

DISPENSING PRACTICES

In the UK, practices are allowed to dispense drugs for those patients on their practice list who live more than 1 mile from a pharmacy. To make this worthwhile for a practice, it needs to apply to a sizeable proportion of patients and usually this is only the case in rural practices. Dispensing practices act as pharmacies, buying drugs in, dispensing them and claiming payment from the NHS. This is a useful service for patients and can generate income for the practice. Possible drawbacks are the need for extra security in the practice if stocks of drugs are kept on the premises and the need for specialized knowledge on the part of the GP. The practice may employ a pharmacist or trained dispenser.

PRESCRIBING BY NURSES IN PRACTICE

Nurse practitioners are trained to diagnose and treat a range of ailments. They are allowed to prescribe a limited range of simple medications on their own initiative, including emollient creams, nicotine preparations and some aperients. A full list can be found in the *BNF*.

THE ROLE OF THE COMMUNITY PHARMACIST

Community pharmacies (usually known to the public as 'the chemist') dispense the majority of the drugs prescribed in general practice as well as OTC remedies, as discussed in the next section.

Community pharmacists are highly trained and knowledgeable about drug matters, but are currently under-utilized in primary care. In the UK there is a move towards extending the role of community pharmacists and integrating them into the primary healthcare team.

Potential areas of collaboration between pharmacists and GPs include (Bradley et al., 1997):

- repeat prescription review,
- total medication 'brown bag' review (where the patient brings *all* medication, prescribed or not, for review),
- Prescribing, Analyses and Cost (PACT) data analysis (see below),
- development of practice formularies,
- development of prescribing policies, e.g. for antibiotics,
- prescribing audits.

Such joint working could benefit GPs, pharmacists and patients.

Community pharmacists are also an important source of advice to the general public on health issues generally and on the treatment of minor ailments in particular. Community pharmacists are trained to advise on minor illnesses and to recommend non-prescription medications. A pharmacist who is concerned that the illness is more serious or beyond his or her abilities to advise will recommend the patient attends their GP.

OVER-THE-COUNTER MEDICATION

For every prescription medicine consumed there is probably at least one non-prescription medicine taken. In the UK, the Medicines Control Agency is responsible for classifying drugs as prescription only (PoM), pharmacy only (P) – sold only in pharmacies under the supervision of a registered pharmacist but without the need for a prescription – or general sales list (GSL) – available from a wide range of retailers (e.g. supermarkets) and including cough mixtures, throat pastilles and indigestion remedies.

Recent national and international developments have led to many drugs previously designated as prescription only being reclassified as pharmacy only and thus available 'over the counter'; examples include antihistamines, hydrocortisone cream, H_2 blockers for dyspepsia, 'morning after' contraceptive pills, and small quantities of analgesics such as paracetamol and ibuprofen. Criteria for such a change include the need for a proven safety record, low toxicity in overdose and use for the treatment of minor self-limiting conditions.

Potential advantages of such an increase in OTC preparations include promoting individuals to take more responsibility for their own health, decreasing the need for GP appointments (less inconvenience for the patient and saving time for GPs), less financial cost to patients (often OTC preparations are cheaper than the prescription charge), and removing some of the financial burden for the NHS. Potential disadvantages include the fostering of a 'pill for every ill' mentality among the public, an increased risk of interactions and side effects (some OTC preparations can have serious side effects – Clark et al., 2001), less feedback to the regulatory authorities on adverse drug reactions, patients taking the wrong preparation or in the wrong way, and patients self-medicating

Practical Exercise

Local pharmacists have an important role to play in the primary healthcare team. In addition to dispensing prescribed drugs, they sell drugs 'over the counter' and give advice on health and drug matters.

- ❑ Ask your GP tutor to arrange for you to spend some time in a local pharmacy.
- ❑ Find out about the role pharmacists play and their training.
- ❑ Observe how prescriptions are dispensed.
- ❑ What kinds of advice do pharmacists give patients?
- ❑ Are there rules governing the sale of OTC drugs?

for a serious condition requiring medical attention (Bradley and Bond, 1995).

Doctors need to take into account any non-prescription medicines their patients may be taking (the *OTC Directory* lists 95 per cent of the market); OTC preparations could interact with prescribed drugs and could cause adverse drug reactions. For medico-legal reasons, if a GP recommends a patient to purchase an OTC preparation, he or she should document the preparation recommended and advise the patient to confer with the pharmacist before purchase and to follow the information leaflet carefully.

COMMUNICATING ABOUT MEDICATIONS BETWEEN PRIMARY AND SECONDARY CARE

Sometimes it seems that the only things reliably transferred between primary and secondary care are the patients themselves! Poor communications have a deleterious effect on care generally and, for medication, may be disastrous. Unintentional changes in medication following discharge from hospital to primary care have been identified in half the patients discharged (Duffin et al., 1998).

Many medications are initiated by the hospital, and the GP subsequently takes responsibility for continuing to prescribe them. Unfortunately, it is still commonplace for patients to be discharged from hospital with inadequate or no information. Similarly, many GP referrals do not contain adequate information on the patient's medication, even though this can usually be readily obtained from the practice computer system.

As a student who will in time become a PRHO, you can have a major impact in this area by providing accurate discharge notifications or summaries. An accurate summary of medication is often the most important part.

A discharge notification should be legible and prompt (often, handing it to the patient at discharge is the best way of ensuring the GP receives it). The medication details are best written as a prescription (indeed, in most trusts the medication details are also used as prescription instructions to the hospital pharmacy). It should also specify the expected duration of treatment for each drug. This is important, as most hospitals only give a 2-week supply of discharge medications. The GP needs to know what the longer-term intentions for each drug are.

The discharge notification should also contain:

■ the patient's details: name, address, date of birth and hospital number (a label may be used);
■ admission and discharge dates,
■ the reason for admission (e.g. 'unable to stand following fall', 'inferior MI');
■ the outcome of admission (e.g. 'right hip replacement', 'uneventful recovery');
■ outstanding problems and a plan to deal with these;
■ home care arrangements (e.g. district nurse, meals on wheels, specialist nurse to visit);
■ follow-up arrangements (e.g. hospital doctor or other service).

PRESCRIBING COSTS AND MONITORING

In the UK, primary care trusts set budgets for prescribing costs for individual general practices. Factors taken into account when setting these budgets include historical prescribing patterns, average prescribing costs locally, list size and age profile, and special factors identified by the practice or primary care trust. Practices are encouraged to stay within, or save on, their budget by incentives such as bonus amounts that can be used in other areas, e.g. service development. In addition, sanctions may be applied in the case of an over-spend. Detailed information on prescribing in primary care is available in the form of PACT data (similar systems exist in Scotland and Wales). PACT data contain information on prescribing costs, the number of items prescribed and the level of generic prescribing at individual GP level, health authority and national level. Unfortunately, PACT data cannot be linked with demographic or clinical patient information. They can be used by the NHS to set prescribing budgets for health authorities, by health authorities and primary care trusts to set and monitor GP prescribing budgets, by health service researchers and by individual GPs to audit and improve their prescribing (Majeed et al., 1997). GPs receive quarterly PACT reports that include a comparison with local and national averages.

Practical Exercise

Ask your GP tutor to go through his or her PACT data with you. (If you are studying outside the UK, find out if similar data exist locally.) What are the benefits and limits of such data?

SUMMARY POINTS

To conclude, the most important messages in this chapter are:

- the scale of prescribing is large, costs are high and drugs have both beneficial and harmful effects; you must therefore prescribe effectively and safely;
- in order for the drugs that you prescribe to be taken by the patient, agreement must be reached with the patients that the drugs are necessary, the patient needs to understand what the drugs do and how to take them correctly, and the patient's use of the medication and progress must be reviewed regularly;
- children and the elderly are particularly vulnerable to medication, and care needs to be taken when prescribing for these patients;
- paper references and computer-based prescribing sources, prescribing advisers and community pharmacists are all helpful in providing support for prescribing.

REFERENCES

Anonymous 2000: Drugs for the doctor's bag revisited. *Drug and Therapeutics Bulletin* 38(9), 65–8.

Barrett, T., Lander, A. and Diwaker, V. 2002: *A paediatric vade-mecum*, 14th edn. London: Arnold.

Bradley, C. and Bond, C. 1995: Increasing the number of drugs available over the counter: arguments for and against. *British Journal of General Practice* 45, 553–6.

Bradley, C., Taylor, R. and Blenkinsopp, A. 1997: Primary care – opportunities and threats: developing prescribing in primary care. *British Medical Journal* 314, 744–7.

British National Formulary 2003: London: The British Medical Association and the Royal Pharmaceutical Society of Great Britain.

Clark, D., Layton, D. and Shakir, S. 2001: Monitoring the safety of over the counter drugs. *British Medical Journal* 323, 706–7.

Davidson, W., Collett, J.H., Jackson, C. and Rees, J.A. 1998: An analysis of the quality and cost of repeat prescriptions. *Pharmacology Journal* 260, 458–60.

Department of Health 2001: *Medicines for older people: implementing medicines-related aspects of the NSF for Older People 2001*. London: Deparment of Health. Also available at http://www.doh.gov.uk/nsf/olderpeople/pdfs/medicinesbooklet.pdf

Duffin, J., Norwood, J. and Blenkinsopp, A. 1998: An investigation into medication changes initiated in general practice after patients are discharged from hospital. *Pharmacology Journal* 261 (Suppl.), R32.

Dunbar-Jacob, J., Erlen, J., Schlenk, E., Ryan, C., Sereika, S. and Diswell, W. 2000: Adherence in chronic disease. *Annual Review of Nursing Research* 18, 48–90.

Editorial 2002: Managing antibiotic-associated diarrhoea. *British Medical Journal* 324, 1345–6.

Fedder, D.O. 1982: Managing medication and compliance: physician–pharmacist–patient interaction. *Journal of the American Geriatric Society* 30, S113–17.

Franke, L., Avery, A., Groom, L. and Horsfield, P. 2000: Is there a role for computerised decision support for drug dosing in general practice? *Journal of Clinical Pharmacy and Therapeutics* 25(5), 373–7.

Fry, J. 1993: *General practice: the facts.* Oxford: Radcliffe Medical Press.

Kohn, R. and White, K. 1976: *Health care.* Oxford: Oxford University Press.

Majeed, A., Evans, N. and Head, P. 1997: What can PACT tell us about prescribing in general practice? *British Medical Journal* 315, 1515–19.

Mannesse, C.K., Derkx, F.H., de Ridder, M.A., Man in't Veld, A.J. and van der Cammen, T.J. 2000: Contribution of adverse drug reactions to hospital admission of older patients. *Age and Ageing* 29, 35–9.

Palmer, K.T. 1998: *Notes for the MRCGP*, 3rd edn. Oxford: Blackwell Science.

Rawlins, M.D. and Thompson, J.W. 1977: *Pathogenesis of adverse drug reactions*, 2nd edn. Oxford: Oxford University Press.

Royal Pharmaceutical Society of Great Britain 1997: *From compliance to concordance – achieving partnership in medicine-taking.* London: RPSGB.

Sackett, D.L. and Snow, J.C. 1979: The magnitude of compliance and non-compliance. In: Haynes, R.B. and Sackett, D.L. (eds). *Compliance in health care.* Baltimore: Johns Hopkins University Press, 11–22.

FURTHER READING

British National Formulary. London: British Medical Association and the Royal Pharmaceutical Society of Great Britain.

This is an invaluable source of information on prescribing. Your medical school may arrange for you to receive your own copy; use it frequently. It is also available on CD-ROM and online at http://www.bnf.org/

Drug and Therapeutics Bulletins. London: Which? Ltd.

MeReC Bulletins. Liverpool: Medicines Resource Centre.

These organizations publish monthly bulletins summarizing prescribing information on various topics.

www.concordance.org

This website discusses a variety of issues related to concordance and compliance.

CHRONIC ILLNESS AND ITS MANAGEMENT IN GENERAL PRACTICE

Most chronic illnesses present the patient with a tough challenge. Usually the challenge can be lived with; less often can it be overcome. The task that faces the doctor is also challenging. It requires technical expertise, a personal partnership with the patient, and acknowledgement of the need to deliver a service to all the patients registered with the GP.

The treatment of chronic illness is helped by a keen grasp of the complex effects the illness has on the individual. It also requires a clear structure within which effective and predictable long-term care can be provided.

LEARNING OBJECTIVES

By the end of this chapter you will be able to:

- understand the nature of chronic illness;
- understand the impact of chronic illness;
- describe five different illness models;
- know the prevalence and workload associated with the common chronic illnesses;
- understand the role of screening for chronic illness;
- construct a programme for the long-term management of common chronic illnesses

A TRIPARTITE APPROACH TO CHRONIC ILLNESS CARE

The commonest cause of the deaths of most people alive today will be a chronic illness which could have been postponed, at least, if not prevented. Most chronic illnesses should be better managed. The key to improving chronic illness management lies in systematic structured care or what has recently been proposed

as the Chronic Care Model (Wagner et al., 2001). The risk of ill-health or death from chronic illness varies amongst different groups in a population. It makes sense, therefore, to target efforts to improve the care of diseases such as ischaemic heart disease, diabetes mellitus and chronic obstructive pulmonary disease as closely as possible to those at greatest risk. Chronic illness care presents a dilemma for general practitioners (GPs) and primary care teams.

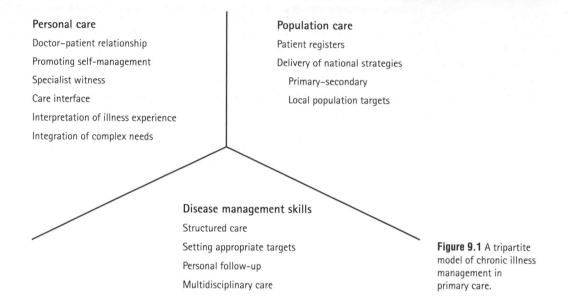

Personal care

Doctor–patient relationship

Promoting self-management

Specialist witness

Care interface

Interpretation of illness experience

Integration of complex needs

Population care

Patient registers

Delivery of national strategies

Primary–secondary

Local population targets

Disease management skills

Structured care

Setting appropriate targets

Personal follow-up

Multidisciplinary care

Figure 9.1 A tripartite model of chronic illness management in primary care.

Can the ethos of personal care, which has been at the core of general practice throughout the twentieth century, be maintained in an environment that also demands precise disease management skills and the delivery of national strategies to local populations? A tripartite approach to the care of chronic illness is now essential in primary care (Fig. 9.1). Personal care must be integrated with a population strategy. In both of these the achievement of high-quality chronic illness management depends on excellent disease management skills.

In this chapter, the management of chronic illness is considered first from the point of view of the person with the disease. The population statistics of the major chronic illnesses and their impact are then examined. The chapter ends with a detailed presentation of structured care and the strategies available to GPs in delivering high-quality chronic illness care to all the patients registered with them.

THE PATIENT

WHEN CHRONIC ILLNESS PRESENTS

When a chronic illness is diagnosed, the possible consequences of the illness and of its treatment will be apparent to the doctor. The patient may have little sense of what lies ahead. Although chronic illnesses become chronic with time, they often start out as 'chronic' to the doctor. Asthma, diabetes and hypertension are good examples. For the patient, on the other hand, most illnesses generally start as acute illnesses. Indeed, most people would prefer that their illnesses stayed acute and limited. So the realization that the illness might be here to stay or might come and go is one of the first hurdles to address in coming to terms with chronic illness. 'Surely, with the right treatment this illness can be cured?' the rheumatoid arthritis patient might reasonably ask. 'After all, if you doctors can transplant hearts, and diagnose heart valve disease in babies in the womb, you must be able to treat my simple, ordinary arthritis' sounds reasonable enough.

The major advances of modern medicine have done more to help us understand chronic illnesses than to relieve or cure them. This is a bewildering fact to many patients who develop a chronic illness. They may have to compare the relative impotence of modern medicine in the face of their illness with the dramatic improvements achieved in such fields as coronary artery bypass surgery or the chemotherapy of the lymphomas. They have to face the fact that chronic illnesses remain a common burden in our society. Doctors can help them to understand chronic illness, and can help to limit its intrusion into their lives, but for the most part chronic illnesses cannot be cured, and it is one of the duties of doctors to help patients to come to terms with their illnesses, rather than to reject or deny them.

THE NATURE OF CHRONIC ILLNESS

One of the defining features of many common chronic illnesses is that they are often diseases of process or processes rather than disorders of structure. Typical examples of this type of chronic illness include *asthma, hypertension, rheumatoid arthritis, inflammatory bowel disease* and *schizophrenia*. A shared aspect of these diseases is the diffuseness of the disordered process in the tissue or system. In asthma there is a complex inflammatory response in the airways that may continue long after symptoms appear to have resolved. In hypertension there is a generalized over-pressurizing of the arterial system that may be chemically or humorally mediated through the central barometer of arterial pressure or through the peripheral baroreceptors. In rheumatoid arthritis there is an over-reaction of the immune system that fails to identify the synovium of the joint as self and starts to attack joints as foreign matter. In inflammatory bowel disease the immune system again reacts inappropriately and attacks the bowel endothelium as though it were a foreign intruder. In schizophrenia there appears to be a diffuse deficiency or imbalance in one or more neurotransmitters in the brain, with resulting disorganization of intellect and emotion.

In each of these diseases, the process whose failure is causing the signs and symptoms of the disease is spread throughout the tissue or system. It cannot be removed through a cut or series of cuts, and cannot easily be overridden through a chemical or humoral switch. In all of them the underlying disorder is complex and usually beyond the reach of the drugs at our disposal. But in all of them we can exert some influence on the disease in most patients.

These illnesses contrast with another group of illnesses which are also chronic either in their development or in their impact but which are more amenable to treatments offering long-term relief. These more 'amenable' diseases are distinguished by either the relative simplicity of the disease process or their limited extent within the body. Examples include *atheroma of the coronary arteries, benign hypertrophy of the prostate, cataracts of the eyes, osteroarthritis of the hips* and *peptic ulceration*. The approaches outlined in this chapter may be suitable for these diseases also. However, where there is a realistic and reasonable hope of cure or sustained remission following a course of treatment, the approach and attitude of the doctor and the patient are likely to be influenced by this expectation.

Between these two poles of chronic illness lie a number of illnesses for which there are effective treatments but whose treatments need to be taken continuously. Examples of these are *Addison's disease, hypothyroidism, idiopathic atrial fibrillation, myasthenia gravis* and *pernicious anaemia*. The treatment of these diseases is more predictably effective. The diseases mentioned in this group are specific deficiency or function disorders that can be treated either by replacing the deficiency or by correcting the disordered function. By comparison with the first group of diseases, they are simple diseases.

Three categories of chronic illness have been identified here, according to responsiveness to treatment. The three categories are used in Table 9.1 to classify some of the more common chronic illnesses seen in Western Europe.

THE IMPACT OF CHRONIC ILLNESS

The development of a chronic illness may have a profound effect on the patient's life through morbidity (symptoms and interference with the activities of daily living), disability, handicap, impairment, interference with personal relationships, loss of confidence, loss of earnings, loss of self-image, and stigma. In order to be able to respond appropriately to the needs of the patient, the doctor has to understand how the illness is affecting the particular patient and how the patient sees the problem. Mrs B's situation is a good example.

Table 9.1 Common chronic illnesses categorized by responsiveness to treatment

Difficult to treat	Treatable – one stop	Treatable – continuous
Asthma	Coronary atheroma	Addison's disease
Chronic obstructive pulmonary disease	Cataract of eye	Depression
Diabetes mellitus	Osteoarthritis of hips/knees	Epilepsy
Hypertension	Peptic ulceration	Hypothyroidism
Inflammatory bowel disease	Prostate hypertrophy (benign)	Idiopathic atrial fibrillation
Multiple sclerosis		Manic–depressive psychosis
Osteoarthritis		Myasthenia gravis
Parkinson's disease		Pernicious anaemia
Rheumatoid arthritis		
Schizophrenia		

CASE STUDY 9.1

Mrs B is the head teacher of a primary school in Central London. She is 52 years old and has smoked all her adult life. Last year she came to see her GP, Dr A, with a bad attack of bronchitis and was told by her doctor that she suspected she had asthma in addition. Dr A prescribed an antibiotic for the bronchitis and an inhaler for the asthma. Mrs B disagreed with her diagnosis of asthma and so took the antibiotics only. Within about 2 weeks, she was much better and felt vindicated in her opinion about the asthma. She continued to have difficulty climbing the stairs to the third floor at the top of the school but put it down to the ravages of age and cigarettes. Her peak flow when Dr A measured it in her surgery was 240 L/min. It should have been 480 L/min.

When Dr A saw Mrs B 6 months later with osteoarthritis in her knee, she took the opportunity to repeat her peak flow test. This time it was 375 L/min and Dr A was now convinced that the diagnosis of asthma was correct.

useful to ask ourselves what we would want if we were in the patient's shoes. Sometimes the answer to that question is that the doctor should take over and simply tell the patient what to do. In acute appendicitis, for example, the patient does not usually want to get into much discussion about what should be done. More often than not, however, patients would like to have the opportunity to express their own views and to have those views taken into account in the doctor's decision making. This is especially true in chronic illness.

CASE STUDY 9.1 (continued)

Dr A told Mrs B that she was very pleased that the peak flow test was now much better and asked Mrs B how the inhaler had worked. Mrs B blushed and said that she had not used the inhaler but that the antibiotics had made her chest much better in a matter of 10 days. Dr A then asked Mrs B if her chest caused her any difficulty now. Mrs B said, 'None at all except that I get short of breath climbing the stairs at

Thinking and Discussion Point

What do you think Dr A should do now? Should she tell Mrs B that she has asthma? How would Mrs B best be helped in her current situation?

Thinking and Discussion Point

Dr A is in a bit of a dilemma. Should she pursue the issue of the asthma now or wait until the problem recurs and deal with it then? Dr A decided to leave the asthma for now and get on with the management of the arthritis in Mrs B's knee.

If we are ever in doubt as to how we should approach a tricky situation with a patient, it is school'. Dr A said she thought that might be due to her asthma. Mrs B frowned and said that she didn't have asthma. She said she knew what asthma was from her own daughter and she certainly did not have that.

When there appears to be a conflict between the view of the patient and the view of the doctor, it is sometimes because each is approaching the problem from a different perspective. Patients' priorities are often different from those of doctors. The patient may accept different degrees of illness or disability depending on what has to be gained or sacrificed in undertaking a particular treatment. For example, a doctor's desire to control hypertension by prescribing drugs to be taken every day may be unacceptable to a man for whom illness represents moral frailty and for whom medication represents capitulation to that frailty.

Patients sometimes feel isolated by their illnesses. They may feel isolated because family and friends do not or cannot understand what it is like to have the illness, or they may feel stigmatized by their disability or appearance. The doctor may be in a special position with the patient with a chronic illness, acting as what Heath (1996) has called a 'specialist witness' and also as a specialist 'interpreter' of the illness experience. The experience of chronic illness provokes complex reactions. The feelings and ideas generated sometimes have to be worked through carefully in order that emotional blocks to effective treatment can be overcome and that action to avoid secondary complications can be taken.

THE POPULATION

MODELS OF ILLNESS

Five different illness models have been proposed by Memel (1996) to explore the experience of chronic illness and the role and function of doctors who work with people who have chronic diseases. These models demonstrate how the perception of chronic illness can vary, and how the patient and the doctor may often approach the problem of chronic illness very differently (Table 9.2).

Thinking and Discussion Point

As you read the short summaries of each model, reflect on your own viewpoint. Is there anything new here? Are you thinking on more than one level at any time? What is the patient's angle, and is it reflected in the model?

The *medical model* is the traditional starting point of doctors. This model assumes that the main variable in a chronic illness is the disease itself and that all patients are much the same when it comes to considering the disease. The medical model has been essential to the development of medical science. It encourages the recognition of patterns of disease and patterns of response to treatment. If there are differences between patients, then, according to the medical model, the differences that count are more likely to be aspects of the disease than aspects of the patient or his or her environment. The

Table 9.2 Attributes of the five illness models

	Models of illness				
	Medical	**Functional**	**Social**	**Sociological**	**Biopsychosocial**
Doctor centred	▓			▓	
Patient centred		▓		▓	
Multi-dimensional					▓
Technical	▓	▓		▓	▓
Professional	▓				▓

chief concerns within this model of seeing illness are medical and technical. The patient's presentation and experience are interpreted in terms of disease patterns. In medical practice, the effect of this model can make patients feel like outsiders to the management of their own illnesses.

The *functional model* of illness is concerned with how the patient copes with his or her everyday life. This model contrasts with the medical model in being person orientated rather than disease orientated. Its aim is to look at functional ability such as mobility, self-care, social integration and independence, and to consider the impact of symptoms. However, it is similar to the medical model in being centred on the concerns of the professionals, because the assumption inherent in this model is that the definition of functional ability is a technical one. Nonetheless, functional scales provide an assessment of the illness that is patient centred in its orientation, and that assessment may be more accessible to the patient than one based purely on the medical model.

The *social model* considers the disease from the viewpoint of social organization and the society in which the individual resides. It is concerned with the influences of society on the individual. It interprets the illness and its consequences in terms of the limitations which society imposes on the individual. Thus the social model addresses the effects of chronic illness in terms of social disadvantage. The dimensions of the social impact of chronic illness are broad and include financial penalties for individuals and their families, access to employment, access to education and training, and access to recreation and the arts. A particular advantage of this model is the emphasis it places on the patient's viewpoint. In most areas of public and social service, and increasingly in the commercial world as well, there is an awareness of the needs of people with disabilities. Customers and clients with disabilities are not only catered for, but their needs and opinions are sought out. One problem associated with the social model of chronic illness is the tendency to adopt a global view of disability and impairment and handicap. The effect of such simplification is to emphasize the visible elements of disability such as paralysis, blindness or deafness, and to underestimate the less visible aspects of chronic diseases such as chronic schizophrenia and learning disorders.

The *sociological model* of chronic illness contrasts with the first three models described here in being concerned with observing and describing the experience of people with chronic illness rather than defining a specialized framework within which to categorize chronic illness. Medical sociologists have explored both the meaning and themes evident in the life experience of people with chronic illness and the perspectives of the professionals who work with sufferers. Bury has proposed the idea of 'biographical disruption', which follows the onset of chronic illness. The patient has to review his or her identity that has been so altered by becoming someone with a disease or disability. The concept of biographical disruption is a powerful aid to doctors, who are usually the ones who have to label the onset of the chronic illness. By being sensitive to the potential disturbance and disorientation that can follow the diagnosis of a chronic illness, the doctor can promote the acknowledgement and resolution of some of the conflicts that the onset of the illness will inevitability provoke. It was the sociological model that encouraged the exploration of the way in which the doctor–patient relationship can promote or hinder effective diagnosis and treatment. The sociological model is a model for understanding chronic illness, not for managing or controlling it.

The *biopsychosocial model* was developed to explain how the impact of chronic illness can operate at several levels at once. It embodies a holistic approach that encourages the doctor and the patient to look at the process of the disease and its physical, psychological and social effects simultaneously. Since the publication of the General Medical Council's document *Tomorrow's doctors* in 1992, every medical school in the UK has been charged with the task of examining their curricula to ensure that the holism of the biopsychosocial model is demonstrable throughout undergraduate medical training. If this is achieved, the medical, functional and social models of illness will become less conspicuous in the teaching and practice of medicine.

These models of illness provide a key to analysing how patients, doctors and society might respond to chronic illness. In Mrs B's case, there was a clear difference between the patient's and the doctor's views.

CASE STUDY 9.1 (continued)

Six months later, Mrs B developed another attack of bronchitis and came to see Dr A again. This time her peak flow was 200 L/min and she was having considerable difficulty climbing the stairs at school. Even before the infection, she had been scheduling her visits to the classrooms on the top floor so that she could get up there in stages. Dr A prescribed the antibiotics again and once more raised the question of asthma. Mrs B was adamant that it was not asthma. She did agree to try to stop smoking. Dr A persuaded her to use a steroid inhaler for her chest. 'I don't mind what I take so long as you don't call it asthma', Mrs B declared.

Dr A never found out why Mrs B was so adamant to avoid the diagnosis of asthma. She was prepared to work on Mrs B's terms so long as she could get Mrs B to try the asthma treatment. Mrs B found the inhaler a great help.

There are several advantages to the position adopted by Dr A. She has made it clear to Mrs B that she was on her side and prepared to compromise in tackling the illness. It may be that the prospect of the diagnosis of asthma was unacceptable to Mrs B for what it meant to her self-image as a headmistress or for its implications about her future health. Whatever the reason, Dr A succeeded in prescribing the treatment and engaging Mrs B in a dialogue about her breathlessness. In the longer term, this approach will have given Mrs B confidence in raising other difficult health issues. The disadvantage of not naming asthma is that it may lead to delay in obtaining the right treatment when attacks occur in the future and may make subsequent discussion of Mrs B's breathlessness unduly complex. It is sometimes difficult to be sure about the diagnosis of asthma in older people and in children. Having the label of asthma can get patients onto the fast track to treatment.

CHRONIC ILLNESS FACTS AND FIGURES

Chronic illnesses are relatively common and comprise a substantial part of the work of GPs (see Chapter 4, 'Common illnesses in general practice'). They are also major components of the work of specialists in internal medicine, where in some areas such as rheumatology they are the backbone of the discipline.

There are three main sources of our knowledge of the prevalence and impact of chronic illnesses in the UK. The first is the General Household Survey, which is conducted by the Office for National Statistics – formerly the Office of Population Censuses and Surveys – and is reported annually (Office for National Statistics, annual). The second source is the National Morbidity Survey in General Practice (NMSGP), which is carried out jointly every 10 years by the Office for National Statistics and the Royal College of General Practitioners (McCormick et al., 1995). The final source of epidemiological data on chronic illness comes from specific epidemiological studies. These are carried out in distinct populations such as people with a specific disease in a particular area whose names are drawn from the electoral register or from GPs' patient lists. Specific diagnostic definitions and tests are used to identify 'cases' and determine prevalence and severity.

The following general and specific observations help to paint the picture of chronic illness as a common significant problem experienced throughout the population in all ages and social groups.

- The following questions were asked in the *General Household Survey* in 2000 (Office for National Statistics, 2002) – 13 000 addresses, 19 266 people aged 16 years and over in 9852 households, response rate 67 per cent.
  - 'Do you have any longstanding illness or disability or infirmity? (By longstanding I mean anything that has troubled you over a period of time or that is likely to affect you over a period of time.)': *Yes: 32 per cent.*

- 'Does this illness or disability (these illnesses or disabilities) limit your activities in any way?': *Yes: 19 per cent.*
■ A clear description of the place of chronic illness in the work of GPs is provided by the Fourth NMSGP (McCormick et al., 1995). It was conducted in 1991/92 in 60 practices comprising 480 000 people and representative of the population of England and Wales. It recorded and analysed every consultation between GPs, practice nurses and patients in the practices taking part. Its results were expressed as the number of cases or consultations per person consulting per year. It did not report the prevalence of conditions in the population. The Fifth National Survey of Morbidity Statistics from General Practice is currently in preparation.
■ In Table 9.3, we have compared the 'prevalence' figures derived from the consultation data in the Fourth NMSGP with prevalence figures derived from a variety of epidemiological studies. These studies reported the prevalence of the diseases referred to in different areas of England and Wales and in different population groups.

Thinking and Discussion Point

❑ Do these figures contain any surprises?
❑ Did you think ischaemic heart disease was more common?
❑ Did you expect asthma to be the commonest of the chronic diseases?
❑ It is clear from Table 9.3 that in every disease noted the true prevalence is higher than the prevalence estimated from consultations. There seems to be a number of patients who do not consult their GP at all in every category of disease. What explanations could there be for this discrepancy? (See the next section in this chapter.)

Practical Exercise

If you are currently attached to a primary care team, you may wish to discuss with your tutor the following exercise, which should be carried out within the practice. It requires you to investigate the practice disease register, which may be a computer list or a manual card index. You should

Table 9.3 Consultation prevalences of chronic illnesses from consultation data in the Fourth National Morbidity Survey in General Practice (NMSGP) compared with prevalence data from specific epidemiological studies

Disease	Consultation prevalence (%)	Epidemiology prevalence (%)	Cases/GP per year
Asthma	5.4	6.5+	86
Hypertension	4.2	10	200
Backache	4.0	–	80
Osteoarthritis	3.0	–	60
Ischaemic heart disease	1.7	3.5	34
Chronic obstructive pulmonary disease	1.2	–	24
Diabetes mellitus	1.1	3.0	22
Cerebrovascular disease	0.66	1.0	20
Epilepsy	0.36	0.6	8
Alcohol-related disorders	0.13	0.2	4
Schizophrenia	0.11	0.15	5
Multiple sclerosis	0.07	0.09	2

Number of cases likely to be registered with a GP in 1 year are computed from epidemiological studies where available or from the Fourth NMSGP.

also investigate a prescription listing from the computer to identify patients whose names have been missed from the disease register.

How many patients are listed in your practice with asthma? How many patients are listed in your practice with epilepsy? If your practice is computerized, ask the practice manager or computer manager if lists can be generated based on these two diagnoses. Ask also for a list of all patients for whom an asthma drug has been prescribed and a list of all patients for whom an anticonvulsant has been prescribed. Use the two lists of drugs for asthma and epilepsy below. Your tutor will tell you which drugs are never prescribed for the practice's patients and which therefore can be ignored. Don't forget to add to the list the brand names for these drugs if they are supported by your computer. Check in your local formulary (e.g. *British National Formulary*, *BNF*) and branded product list (e.g. *Monthly Index of Medical Specialities*, *MIMS*) for new medications not included in these lists.

❑ *Asthma*: aminophylline, bambuterol, beclomethasone, budesonide, cromoglycate, eformoterol, formoterol, fenoterol, fluticasone, ipratropium, ketotifen, montelukast, nedocromil, oxitropium, pirbuterol, reproterol, rimiterol, salbutamol, salmeterol, terbutaline, theophylline, tiotropium, tulobuterol, zafirlukast.

❑ *Epilepsy*: carbamazepine, clobazam, clonazepam, ethosuximide, gabapentin, lamotrigine, phenytoin, phenobarbitone, primidone, topiramate, (sodium) valproate, vigabatrin.

When you have obtained the lists, calculate the total number of patients with each disease by cross-checking between the disease register list and the prescription list. What percentage of the total practice patient list do the two total numbers of asthmatics and epileptics make? Do they differ from the percentages in Table 9.3? What explanation can you offer for the differences?

UNDETECTED AND UNSEEN CHRONIC DISEASE

A reasonable interpretation of the discrepancy between the consultation prevalence figures and the epidemiological prevalence figures in Table 9.3 is that some people with chronic illnesses

either do not attend their GPs at all in the course of a year or have never had their disease detected. In the cases of diabetes and epilepsy, this figure would seem to be nearly 50 per cent (Jacoby et al., 1996; King et al., 1998). What does this mean? There are a number of possible explanations. Some patients attend hospital clinics and never see their GP. Some patients have diseases that are asymptomatic. Some patients would rather have symptoms than have any contact with doctors and their devices! And some patients think that nothing can be done about their symptoms so why attend the GP anyway?

A GP is likely to see about 78 per cent of the patients registered on his or her list in one year, according to the Fourth NMSGP (McCormick et al., 1995). This means that about 25 per cent of patients will not attend in any one year. Because patients with diagnosed diseases are more likely to attend than those without, the proportion of people who do not attend is probably much less than 25 per cent in the case of most people with *known* chronic illness. However, some patients with chronic illness who do attend their GP may not attend to discuss the chronic disease in question, and therefore the disease may not appear in the consultation statistics.

There is a problem in addition with the detection of certain chronic illnesses. Some chronic diseases are symptomless throughout their course until complications occur. Two examples of this problem are hypertension and non-insulin-dependent diabetes mellitus. Almost all published studies of hypertension prevalence have shown that hypertension is detected in only 50 per cent of those people who actually have hypertension for which treatment is indicated. Recently, there has been a marked increase in the recording of blood pressure in primary care in the UK, due to the linking of GPs' incomes with specific chronic disease service targets. So the detection of raised blood pressure may have increased. Meantime, the low detection rates up to now serve to show that it cannot be left entirely to the individual to request screening tests for symptomless diseases if we want to reduce the morbidity which these diseases cause. To complicate matters further, there is now concern that hypertension is over-diagnosed by physicians because of isolated elevations of blood pressure in their consulting rooms – called 'white coat hypertension'. It is not yet clear if white coat hypertension (where 24-hour ambulatory blood pressure is normal) carries added cardiovascular risk, but the diagnosis of hypertension does require surveillance of asymptomatic adults using explicit guidelines (see British Hypertension Society at http://www.hyp.ac.uk/bhs/). Diabetes is another disease that is asymptomatic in the early stages and in which early treatment can forestall the onset of complications. In both of these diseases, the rewards of effective detection are tangible. This is the argument for screening in chronic illness and it is why the UK National Health Service (NHS) has made part of the GPs' income dependent on them achieving certain minimum targets in the care of ischaemic heart disease, hypertension, diabetes and asthma.

Epilepsy is a little different. Epilepsy is not asymptomatic, yet it is easy to ignore for both patients and doctors. Take the case of Mr O, a fourth-year medical student.

CASE STUDY 9.2

Mr O, a 24-year-old medical student, had had epilepsy since he was 18 years old. On the night he had his first fit he had just finished his 'A' level exams and had driven two of his friends to an end-of-year party. He only had his driving licence for 4 months. It was an all-night party, but because Mr O was driving, he didn't drink any alcohol. At about 5 in the morning, Mr O was dancing when he had a grand mal fit that lasted for about 2 minutes. Following assessment at an accident and emergency department that night, he attended the neurology outpatients. Six months later, he had two further fits and was started on phenytoin capsules. No cause was found for the fits and Mr O was in every other way in good health.

Mr O attended the neurology clinic regularly for the first 2 years, but he continued to have a fit once every 6 months or so and got fed up seeing the doctors. He simply obtained his prescription from his GP and kept taking the tablets regularly. At this stage he had finished his first 2 years in medical school. His GP assumed he was still attending the neurologists and he assumed the GP knew he wasn't.

There is good evidence that both patients and doctors have low expectations of epilepsy, even though research has shown that it can be completely controlled in more than 80 per cent of patients by taking only one drug (Shorvon et al., 1978). It may be an aspect of the stigma associated with epilepsy that sufferers do not attend doctors, for they do not attend neurologists any more than they attend their GPs.

CASE STUDY 9.2 (continued)

It came as something of a surprise to Mr O, when he was placed finally in the neurology department of his medical school, to learn that his epilepsy treatment had been poor. To be taught by the medical school's neurology consultant that the great majority of epileptics should be controlled free of fits was galling. On the one hand, he was his own worst enemy by not attending the clinic, but he could not recall hearing that his epilepsy should be completely controlled. Mr O was effectively treated eventually and regained his driving licence. Without a driving licence, he would have been prevented from becoming a GP, which is what he chose to do.

Thinking and Discussion Point

As a GP, how could Mr O go about ensuring that other sufferers from epilepsy had a better deal than he did?

SCREENING AND SURVEILLANCE OF CHRONIC DISEASE

Screening

It is apparent from the unsatisfactory detection of hypertension and non-insulin-dependent diabetes mellitus that screening of these diseases is needed. But how should this be carried out? Two principles are paramount (Hart, 1975; Sackett and Holland, 1975).

1. The screening test should be specific enough to ensure that the number of false positives (positive test but no disease) is manageable, and sensitive enough to give confidence that most actual cases are detected.

2. The disease or risk factor detected should be amenable to prevention or treatment.

There are two approaches to screening in general practice – population screening and opportunistic screening.

1. In *population screening*, the screening test is offered to the whole population being screened (e.g. letters of invitation for cervical smear to all women aged 18 to 65 years).

2. In *opportunistic screening*, the test is offered to members of the group to be screened who happen to present at the surgery (e.g. cholesterol testing of all adults with a family history of ischaemic heart disease who happen to attend for whatever reason).

In most chronic illnesses, population screening is not carried out because the resources to do it are simply not available. Furthermore, it is not clear that the rewards to patients and society would justify the inconvenience and costs. In a disease such as hypertension, for which up to 50 per cent of cases go undetected, a more acceptable approach is to screen once a year all adults over the age of 30 who attend the surgery. Since about 75 per cent of people attend their GP once a year and 97 per cent attend every 5 years, this seems to most GPs a more suitable way of screening for hypertension.

Most chronic illnesses cannot be detected by screening because there is not a screening test for the disease which is specific and sensitive enough. Chronic diseases or chronic disease risk factors for which effective screening can be carried out include *diabetes mellitus, hypertension, hyperlipidaemia* and *chronic renal failure.*

Thinking and Discussion Point

Asthma is a common disease, affecting more than 25 per cent of the population in the course of their lives and more than 6.5 per cent of the population at any point in time. Can you think of a screening test for asthma? This test, if it is to be used, has to be sensitive enough to detect most cases of asthma (e.g. at least 75 per cent) and specific enough not to have too many false positives (e.g. 25 per cent or more). (See the end of the chapter for the answer.)

Surveillance

Having detected hypertension, what should the GP or practice nurse do?

Practical Exercise

If you are currently attached to a primary care team, you might discuss the following exercise with your GP tutor. Compare your findings with the advice given by the British Hypertension Society in their guidelines for the management of hypertension (http://www.hyp.ac.uk/bhs/).

Ask your tutor to identify for you five patients with established hypertension. Obtain the medical records for these patients and record for each of them the following information:

- date of detection of hypertension,
- reason for recording of blood pressure at time of detection,
- date of commencement of treatment,
- number of blood pressure recordings between first detection and start of treatment,
- number of changes of treatment since first detection,
- number of blood pressure recordings per year since detection,
- investigations carried out since first detection.

Discuss the findings with your tutor and ask his or her opinion on how representative your findings are of blood pressure management in the practice.

In addition to the 50 per cent of hypertensives who are undetected, only about 50 per cent of those with detected hypertension for which treatment is indicated are actually on treatment. Furthermore, only 50 per cent of those on treatment are on adequate treatment. These three observations make up what has become known as *the rule of halves* in hypertension. Their significance is in showing that not only is it necessary to detect hypertension, but also that its ongoing treatment demands careful surveillance by the primary care team. It is hard to decide whether this performance in hypertension care is simply the best that can be achieved in a symptomless condition in which patient motivation is low, or whether it reflects poor management by the primary care team. It is up to primary care teams to ensure that they provide the highest possible quality of care. If patient attendance and uptake of the service remain low despite the best efforts of the primary care team, there is no cause for self-reproach.

THE DISEASE

AGREEING THE MANAGEMENT PLAN

How far doctors and nurses should go in ensuring patients attend for treatment and comply with the treatment advised is a matter for debate. At the beginning, the patient with a chronic illness should be asked what he or she expects from the primary care team and be told what the primary care team expects from him or her. There should follow a degree of negotiation in which a plan is agreed between the patient and the primary care team and, if possible, this should be written down. If the primary care team has a structure for managing chronic illness, the patient should be informed about it. Without a structure, the management of chronic illness is very much a hit-and-miss affair. How would you approach Mrs G, whose story follows?

CASE STUDY 9.3

Mrs G is 71 and has had insulin-dependent diabetes mellitus for the last 10 years. She lives alone in sheltered accommodation, all the rest of her family having moved to the USA. She has recently developed a neuropathic ulcer in her right foot and is unable to come to the surgery. She has macular degeneration of the retina and her visual acuity is limited to 6/12 on both sides. Her diabetes is poorly controlled and her last glycated haemoglobin (HbA1c) was 12.2 per cent (normal 4.4–6.7 per cent).

Thinking and Discussion Point

How would you organize Mrs G's care? What services should be provided at home and what should be provided in hospital or other health service centres?

The main challenge in Mrs G's case is to provide effective care at home. She has advanced diabetes, with probable involvement of the vasa nervorum of her foot causing her neuropathy. Her diabetes is out of control and she is entering a rapid downward spiral. It is likely that in becoming housebound she has lost contact with the services for her diabetes and is now at risk of a major infection or acute ischaemia of her feet or vital organs.

Does she need to see a diabetologist to get advice on her insulin? Is the chiropodist attending her at home? Should she have the advice of a neurologist about her peripheral neuropathy? What about her eyes? Will active surveillance of her eyes prevent the additional insult of diabetic retinopathy to add to her senile macular degeneration? Is she able to draw up her own insulin? Who is dressing her ulcer? What aids would help at home? When was the last time her renal function was checked? Is she getting meals on wheels? Could she attend a day centre for elderly people?

Mrs G's situation is not unusual. The role of the primary care team is to co-ordinate her care, and one member should take the lead. A case conference with other members of the community health and social services, if not also the diabetic team, may be especially useful. Many diabetic teams have the capacity for nursing outreach to support people like Mrs G, but there is no reason why she should not attend the diabetic clinic in the first instance if she is not already doing so.

Mrs G needs an explicit plan of care in which the roles of the various healthcare professionals are stated and she knows what to expect from whom. The primary care team should be able to assess their own performance in delivering services to people like Mrs G to ensure that patients do not fall through the net of services. What is required is structured care of her illness.

In major psychiatric illness, formal care in the community occurs under the title of The Care Programme Approach (CPA; Department of Health and Social Security, 1990). The CPA was introduced in the UK in 1991 in response to growing concern about the care of mentally ill people in the community. It promotes interprofessional collaboration and ensures that both psychiatric and social needs are addressed.

A key worker is appointed, who may or may not have a role in the treatment of the patient. This person is responsible both to ensure decisions made within the CPA are carried out and to act as the main point of contact of the patient with the care team. The CPA is now enshrined in UK government statute. There is much about the CPA which is reflected in formal, structured care of chronic illness in general practice, but the principle behind both is simple: people with chronic illness need clear objectives, clear leadership and a clearly identified key worker in the management of their illness.

STRUCTURED CARE OF CHRONIC ILLNESS

In the section that follows, the various elements of the structured care of chronic illness are outlined. It is not necessary for all elements of this programme to be included in every case of chronic illness care. It would be wise to ask: 'If they are not included, would the care be better with them than without?'

The goal of providing high-quality care to a population of patients should not conflict with the GP's primary aim of serving patients within a personal relationship that extends over time and across consultations. In a now celebrated study in diabetes care, Kinmonth and colleagues (1998) found specific disease-related outcomes were worse among GPs in their trial who had undertaken training in a more person-centred approach than among those who continued with routine care. They pointed out the need for those who are committed to more person-centred consulting also to keep their focus on disease management. Structured care of chronic illness is designed to ensure that disease management goals are kept to the fore.

The idea behind structured care is that of a safety net which operates at a number of different levels. It begins at a population level, promoting a systematic approach to the population or disease group under consideration. It should define the goals of management, who is responsible for carrying it out and what the management approach will consist of. It should address the resources that are required, the impact on other aspects of the service, and the systems that will be used to serve the programme. Finally, it should include a process for reviewing the effectiveness of the programme and for making changes in response to that review.

What population?

- What disease? This could be set by diagnostic criteria such as level of blood pressure or by specific prescription such as anticonvulsant.
- What target population? Identify all those known with the disease criterion.
- Are the patients at risk being identified? Compare the number known with the disease with the number predicted from national figures for the practice population size.

What goals are set?

- Individual: what each patient should expect from the treatment. For example, a hypertensive might expect to have blood pressure controlled according to the guidelines of the British Hypertension Society, or according to a practice agreed derivative of those guidelines.
- Group: what should be achieved with all known members of that disease group. For example, the aim might be to review all asthma patients on inhaled steroids at least once a year.
- Practice: what the practice should achieve in its administration and management programme for the disease. In epilepsy, the aim might be to conduct a practice audit of epilepsy once a year, to review the epilepsy guidelines and protocol every 3 years, and to establish effective liaison with the local neurologist.

How will the programme be delivered?

- Advertisement within the surgery: how patients will be informed of the service.
- Organization: whether to run a service as part of normal surgery consulting or to provide special disease-oriented sessions such as a diabetic clinic.
- Clinical leadership: should this service be led by one of the doctors or one of the nurses or the manager or another team member?
- Clinical care: should the service be provided by all doctors and nurses (probably essential

in asthma due to the numbers) or by one or two interested clinical staff (a more practical requirement for a less common disease such as epilepsy)?

- Administration: who will be responsible for maintenance of the disease and prescription registers, and the recall system?
- What clinical disciplines should be involved? A dietician and chiropodist might be essential for diabetes mellitus.

What resources are needed?

- Personnel: doctor and nursing time, administrative support.
- Time: impact on existing general medical services.
- Accommodation: e.g. room for nurses to run special clinics.
- Equipment: e.g. blood glucose monitoring equipment, placebo devices in asthma, choice of cuff sizes for sphygmomanometry.
- Finance: cost of providing special equipment, carrying out audit (potentially very expensive, depending on the extensiveness of data collection and the existence of computerized clinical records).

What information will be kept?

- Computer systems: almost a prerequisite for structured care of chronic illness. The manual recording of disease and prescription registers is almost unbearably tedious.
- Manual systems: it can be done, but it is essential in establishing any programme of clinical care to ensure that the administrative system serves the clinical objectives. If the system is manual, it has to be kept as simple as possible so that accurate and complete recording can be achieved.

How will the patients be reviewed?

- Establish a disease register: cross-check against prescription register.
- Establish a prescription register: cross-check against disease register.
- Formal annual review: this may not be possible for all patients, so prioritize patients.

- Recall systems: either from set recall mechanisms within a computerized record or from a manual card index or from repeat prescriptions. Computerized repeat prescriptions may provide the easiest and most efficient access to patients who need recall. Most NHS practices operate a repeat prescription system in which patients are given access to a limited supply of repeat medication. The amount is determined by the prescribing doctor during a clinical consultation. Requests for repeat prescriptions that have not been authorized bring to the attention of the practice staff patients who should have attended but who have not. Reluctant patients can be encouraged by the issuing of limited supplies of their drugs!

Summarize into a protocol

- Team meetings: structured care is best provided by a team in which each discipline can play to its strengths – doctors concentrate on medical care, nurses on nursing, managers on managing, and clerical staff on appointment systems, records and filing. If structured care is to work, all the desired action points have to be agreed by the relevant team members.
- Written protocols: plans that are written down are likely to be clearer and more realistic. Agreements that are recorded can be challenged and developed. Audit is made considerably easier if the basis of what is being assessed has been recorded. New members of the team will find it easier to take part in an enterprise which requires collaboration if the purpose and method of the work have been written down.

Ensure standards

- Audit: self-review by the practice team of its performance in the structured care of chronic illness is the best way of ensuring that change and development take place. Audit requires adequate resources to be carried out effectively. Under-resourced, it becomes a source of irritation. Properly prepared, it is encouraging and promotes high quality.

SUMMARY POINTS

The most important messages of this chapter are:

- chronic illness is a major element of most areas of clinical medicine;
- chronic illness is often detected or diagnosed late and then often under-treated;
- the impact of chronic illness is complex, and understanding chronic illness requires a model of illness that takes into account the medical, functional, social and sociological aspects of the disease;
- screening is essential in chronic illnesses such as diabetes and hypertension, but does not have a place in the detection of most chronic illnesses;
- the proper long-term management of all chronic illnesses requires a programme of formal structured care involving multidisciplinary members of primary and secondary care teams.

SCREENING IN ASTHMA – YES OR NO? THE ANSWER!

The diagnostic criterion for asthma is variability (or reversibility after administration of a bronchodilator) in peak expiratory flow rate (PEFR) or in forced expiratory volume in the first second (FEV_1) of at least 20 per cent. Asthma cannot be diagnosed on a single test. A screening test would therefore have to be applied either on two separate occasions or before and after the administration of a bronchodilator. While it is unlikely that all symptomatic asthmatics are currently taking treatment, the first two principles of screening would nonetheless have to be met. And since there is as yet no evidence that screening for asthma would detect disease for which treatment would be worth prescribing, there could be no justification for screening for asthma.

REFERENCES

Department of Health and Social Security 1990: *The care programme approach for people with a mental illness referred to the specialist psychiatric services*. HC(90)23/LASSL(90)11. London: HMSO.

Hart, J.T. 1975: Screening in primary care. In: Hart, C.R. (ed.) *Screening in general practice*. Edinburgh: Churchill Livingstone, 17–29.

Heath, I. 1996: *The mystery of general practice*. Oxford: Nuffield Provincial Hospitals Trust.

Jacoby, A., Baker, G.A., Steen, N., Potts, P. and Chadwick, D.W. 1996: The clinical course of epilepsy and its psychosocial correlates: findings from a UK community study. *Epilepsia* 37(2), 148–61.

King, H., Aubert, R.E. and Herman, W.H. 1998: Global burden of diabetes, 1995–2025: prevalence, numerical estimates, and projections. *Diabetes Care* 21(9), 1414–31.

Kinmonth, A.L., Woodcock, A., Griffin, S., Spiegal, N. and Campbell, M.J. 1998: Randomised controlled trial of patient centred care of diabetes in general practice: impact on current wellbeing and future disease risk. *British Medical Journal* 17(7167), 1202–8.

McCormick, A., Fleming, D., Charlton, J., Royal College of General Practitioners, Office of Population Censuses and Surveys, and Department of Health 1995: *Morbidity Statistics from General Practice. Fourth National Survey 1991–1992*. London: HMSO.

Memel, D. 1996: Chronic disease or physical disability? The role of the general practitioner. *British Journal of General Practice* 46, 109–13.

Office for National Statistics (annual): *General Household Survey*. London: HMSO. Also available online at: http://www.statistics.gov.uk/lib/resources/fileAttachments/GHS2002.pdf

Sackett, D. and Holland, W.W. 1975: Controversy in the detection of disease. *Lancet* ii, 357–9.

Shorvon, S., Chadwick, D., Galbraith, A. and Reynolds, E. 1978: One drug for epilepsy. *British Medical Journal* 1, 474–6.

Wagner, E.H., Austin, B.T., Davis, C., Hindmarsh, M., Schaefer, J. and Bonomi, A. 2001: Improving chronic illness care: translating evidence into action. *Health Affairs* 20(6), 64–77.

FURTHER READING

Anderson, R. and Bury, M. (eds) 1988: *Living with chronic illness, the experience of patients and their families.* London: Unwin.

    This is an authoritative and highly informative account of the meaning of chronic illness from the perspective of the sufferer.

Littlejohns, P. and Victor, C. (eds) 1996: *Making sense of a primary care-led health service.* Abingdon: Radcliffe Medical Press.

    Littlejohns and Victor have gathered together a group of authors who have a good grasp of the main issues facing GPs as purchasers of health care. The book is relevant to this subject in describing how GPs might respond to rising demand, because rising demand is the central issue now in chronic illness care.

Wagner, E.H., Austin, B.T., Davis, C., Hindmarsh, M., Schaefer, J. and Bonomi, A. 2001: Improving chronic illness care: translating evidence into action. *Health Affairs* 20(6), 64–77.

    This paper summarizes the challenges of delivering care for chronic illness in healthcare systems that remain predominantly orientated towards acute illness care.

Treating people in their own homes provides GPs with a fascinating and privileged insight into their lives. It often reveals important elements of their medical problems. It is also time consuming. Doctors have to consider carefully who needs to be seen at home and who can actually get to the surgery in order to use the doctor's time most effectively. People who are housebound are often treated at home by a variety of health professionals. New approaches to the management of illness, including so-called 'hospital at home', can enable people to be discharged early from hospital and can allow highly dependent patients to be managed at home with a mixture of high-tech medicine and intensive social care.

LEARNING OBJECTIVES

By the end of this chapter you will be able to:

■ understand the reasons for treating patients in their homes;
■ understand the role of home visiting in the work of a general practitioner (GP);
■ describe the workload related to treating people at home;
■ discuss the variety of arrangements for treating patients out of hours;
■ list the services available for housebound patients.

HOME CARE BY GPs

In the British Isles, the GP is often identified as the doctor who comes to the house when a member of the family is ill. This view is surprisingly common, even though home visits make up only a small fraction of the work of the GP. It is confirmed in popular television and stage drama and in literature, where much of the emotion-laden encounters between GPs and their patients is recounted in the setting of the patients' homes. In most other parts of the world, home visiting by doctors is even less common, although whichever the country, consulting with a patient in his or her own home is a highly significant event for both the patient and the doctor, and is likely to be remembered by both.

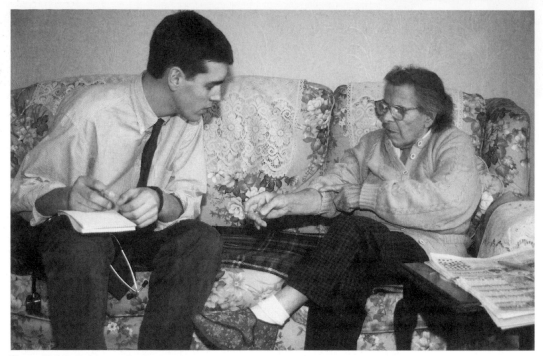

Figure 10.1 The home examination couch.

Home visits afford the GP a privileged insight into the personal life of the patient, and they give the patient exceptional access to the GP. Moreover, information obtained at home may be crucial to the management of the illness. Consider the case of Mr F.

CASE STUDY 10.1

Mr F, a 63-year-old unemployed widower, had chronic venous ulceration of both lower legs that required twice-weekly compression dressing by the practice nurse in the surgery. Despite this intensive treatment, the ulcers would not heal. Dr S had to see Mr F at home when he developed pneumonia. He was shocked to discover the poverty of Mr F's circumstances: he had no bed and slept every night in his armchair. He suffered terrible body odour that was not helped by his being unable to bath because of his dressings, and he was clearly depressed. By involving social services, Dr S enabled Mr F to get financial support to purchase a bed and bed coverings and sort out his social security benefits so that he could improve his circumstances at home. Within 4 weeks of him starting to sleep every night in bed, his ulcers healed and he was able to bathe. His mood improved considerably and he renewed contact with his son, whom he had not seen for more than 2 years.

DECIDING WHEN TO VISIT

Home visits are likely to take more than twice the time required for a surgery consultation (current average in the National Health Service (NHS) is approximately 10 minutes) when one takes into account the time for the journey there and back. Who should be visited, when and by whom are key issues for every GP who wants to manage his or her time effectively. How would you respond to the next case, in which the mother of a 3-year-old boy requests a visit for her son who has a sore throat?

CASE STUDY 10.2

Mrs M phones Dr S's surgery at 8.30 a.m. to request a home visit for her son, Jason, aged 3, who has been disturbed through the night with a sore throat.

Thinking and Discussion Point

Before reading the next part of the case study, think what questions you would ask Mrs M before deciding whether or not to visit her son at home.

CASE STUDY 10.2 (continued)

Mrs M says she does not want to bring Jason to the surgery because he has been awake all night and has a high temperature. She is worried it might develop into pneumonia if she takes him out.

Dr S explains to Mrs M that there is no risk to Jason of developing pneumonia by going outside and that his fever might even be helped by taking him out of doors.

There is a clash of beliefs here, with little research evidence to support the position of either Dr S or Mrs M. Dr S's belief is supported by his experience and his rationale that there is no pathological basis on which to suggest that short-term changes in ambient temperature might influence the progress of infection. Mrs M's belief is based on the authoritative opinion of her own mother and family that pneumonia is due to the cold temperature entering the body and allowing the infection to become deep seated. When she was a child, the doctor always visited the children when they were ill.

CASE STUDY 10.2 (continued)

Dr S tries to resolve the impasse by offering to see Jason as soon as he arrives in the surgery so that his mother can take him straight home without delay. Mrs M accepts the offer with great reluctance.

From the GP's viewpoint, there is the risk of setting a precedent here by visiting at home a child who in his view could come to the surgery safely. If he did visit the child at home, it could be seen to undermine the position of his receptionists. He had instructed them to discourage any home visiting except in an emergency. Home visiting is an aspect of general practice that affects the whole team and for which there should be a clear policy.

The situation in relatively minor self-limiting illness is made complex by differences between the expectations of doctors and those of patients. Nonetheless, it is more a matter of convention and etiquette than life and death. However, major life-threatening illness can also present difficult dilemmas, as the experience of Mr J demonstrates.

CASE STUDY 10.3

Mr J is a 52-year-old taxi driver who had a myocardial infarction a year ago. He made a good recovery and was able to resume his work after about 6 months. One weekday morning, he woke up feeling tired and weak. By 10.45 a.m., he was short of breath and called the surgery asking for a doctor to visit straight away. Dr S had attended Mr J during his heart attack the previous year and had come to know him very well since. He knew Mr J was an anxious man and that he had a deep fear that another heart attack would not be far off. Dr S recognized that this fear was quite reasonable in someone who had already had a heart attack at the relatively young age of 51. Dr S was himself in the middle of a busy morning surgery and was running about half an hour late. He still had eight more patients to see. Should he simply call the ambulance or should he visit Mr J at home himself?

Thinking and Discussion Point

What are the arguments for and against Dr S visiting Mr J at home immediately as against calling the emergency ambulance? Give this scenario to your GP tutor and find out how he or she would want to deal with it?

Mr J could be having another myocardial infarction with associated left ventricular decompensation. He might be suffering from one of a number of other causes of breathlessness completely unrelated to his heart. Could he be suffering acute anxiety with air hunger?

The dilemma facing Dr S is hard to resolve. He knows Mr J had an uncomplicated myocardial infarction with minor damage to the myocardium. He had streptokinase at the time and a subsequent angiogram was remarkably free of coronary disease, with the exception of the affected blood vessel. The doctor thinks a further myocardial infarction is unlikely. If he sends Mr J off to hospital in an ambulance, he will be reinforcing Mr J's belief that he is a man with precarious health which needs a dramatic response every time. If there is some other cause to his breathlessness, he may need to attend hospital anyway and Dr S will have added unnecessarily to the burden of his own morning's work. On the other hand, if the problem is simply an acute anxiety attack, it is in Mr J's and Dr S's interests to manage it at home. If the problem is respiratory rather than cardiac, it could perhaps be managed in an organized fashion from Mr J's home rather than by 'blue light' emergency, with all the stress and disruption that would ensue in the emergency department of the local hospital.

CASE STUDY 10.3 (continued)

Dr S decided to see Mr J at home straight away. Mr J was quite distressed by his breathlessness, with a respiratory rate of 32 breaths/min. He had slight pleuritic pain in his right lung base, and he had a tachycardia of 102 beats/min. His blood pressure was normal at 146/84 mmHg. Having ruled out a pneumothorax, Dr S thought he either had pleurisy or a pulmonary embolus. Mr J had just returned from holiday in Kenya and the journey had involved a 5-hour flight. He had swelling and redness in his left lower leg. Dr S decided a deep vein thrombosis (DVT) with pulmonary embolus was the most likely diagnosis and immediately sent Mr J by ambulance to see the medical registrar of the local hospital. Mr J was admitted to hospital, had a venogram that confirmed the DVT, and a lung scan that confirmed the pulmonary embolus. He was started on heparin intravenously and warfarin by mouth. He was discharged after 5 days with elastic compression hose on both legs, and a certificate to stay off work for at least a month.

Thinking and Discussion Point

Now that you know the outcome, has it influenced the way you see this case? Do you think Dr S was kicking himself when he got back to the surgery for not calling the ambulance in the first place? Or do you think he saw some value in the home visit?

The element of confidence and control which might have been imparted by the visit by Dr S is hard to measure. However, the overall experience of an arranged emergency referral to hospital with a tentative diagnosis is likely to be more constructive and acceptable than an emergency arrival at the accident and emergency department. The cost to Dr S is considerable in terms of both the personal stress and the impact of the event on his other patients. Was it worth it? This judgement is influenced by the doctor's feelings towards the patient and the relationship they have together. It is affected also by the support the doctor receives from his or her colleagues and staff on return to the surgery. Some GPs feel such home visits are not justified and resent colleagues who embark on what they themselves see as futile mercy errands leading to unacceptable stresses back in the surgery while the on-call GP is out on the emergency. This is a good reason to have protocols for the conduct of home visits, both in an emergency and otherwise.

The basic principles governing home visits by GPs have been considered by the National Association of GP Co-operatives (NAGPC) in the UK. This is an organization of which most GP out-of-hours co-operatives in the UK are members. The NAGPC states that, 'general practice has never been and can never be an emergency service along the lines of the police or ambulance'. While it recognizes that there may be occasions when the GP will attend an acute emergency, it stresses that it is unlikely to be in the interests either of the acutely ill patient or of those patients being treated in the surgery for the GP to attempt routinely to augment the care provided by the emergency services. There is a notable exception to this principle. In some locations, patients live very far from the emergency services and it is essential for their GP to be able to provide a relatively immediate response to most medical emergencies. However, most ambulance services in the UK now include highly trained paramedics who can assess and treat life-threatening arrhythmias, cardiovascular and respiratory emergencies and haemorrhages.

Some of the problems that might lead to a more easily defined rationale for home visiting are listed in Table 10.1.

Table 10.1 Reasons for visiting or for not visiting patients in their homes

---

Reasons to visit patients in the home

Some acute emergencies, e.g. acute left ventricular failure, acute abdomen

Patient too ill to travel, e.g. severe vertigo, advanced chronic obstructive pulmonary disease, terminal illness

Patient unable to travel, e.g. paraparesis, motor neuron disease, severe agoraphobia

Patients who should be able to attend the surgery

Almost all children

All ambulant patients

Most adults with viral illnesses

Sometimes, patients who request a home visit by the GP will happily travel to hospital by car or taxi if an urgent hospital assessment has to be made as a result of the visit. This willingness to travel to the hospital by car yet unwillingness to attend the GP's office may simply reflect a difference between the patient's view of the role of the GP and their view of the role of the hospital doctor. It may represent the patient's acceptance of the need to travel on learning that he or she is a 'hospital case', or it may represent the patient's horror of travelling in an ambulance.

Within the NHS, GPs are not obliged to attend patients in their home provided in 'the doctor's reasonable opinion' the patient's 'condition is such' that the patient should attend a doctor's premises. In the USA, Medicare, the national health insurance system, will support physician visits to the home if the services are reasonable and necessary and if a plan of care is established and reviewed. What is reasonable and necessary is defined in terms of observation and assessment, teaching and training of the patient, and therapy, management and evaluation of the illness (Oldenquist et al., 2001). Also, there is good evidence, for example, that home-based assessments improve the likelihood that elderly patients will remain at home.

There is information for medical students on how to do a home visit in Chapter 6 (p. 112).

HOME VISITS – FACTS AND FIGURES

The average home visiting rate in England and Wales in 1991/92 was 299 per 1000 patient-years, according to the Fourth National Survey of Morbidity in General Practice (Table 10.2; McCormick et al., 1995). This amounts to around 600 calls per GP per year. About one in nine of these calls took place between 10 p.m. and 8 a.m. On average, therefore, each GP in England and Wales can expect to do 1.5–2 home visits every day between 8 a.m. and 10 p.m. People over the age of 85 have a home visiting rate of 3009/1000 patient-years in comparison with a rate of 103/1000 patient-years in people aged 16–24 years and a rate of 477/1000 patient-years in people under the age of 5 years. People in social class V have higher rates of home visiting than those in social class I. However, home visiting rates can vary greatly between practices, even allowing for age and sex differences, so that in the study which recorded these figures, some practices had home visiting rates as low as 100 visits per GP per year (Aylin et al., 1996). This

Table 10.2 Home visit rates in England and Wales, 1991–92

	Home visits per 1000 patient–years	Number on average list	Average GP visits/year
All patients	299	2000	600
Patients under 5 years	477	138	66
Patients 16–24 years	103	256	26
Patients over 84 years	3009	28	84

The denominator '1000 patient-years' allows for patients who have moved away or died and is more accurate than '1000 patients'. Data from McCormick et al., 1995.

compares with practices at the other extreme, with a visiting rate of 1110 visits per GP per year. These differences cannot be explained solely by the ethnic or social structure of the practice populations. At least some of the variation is determined by practice characteristics. These could be as diverse as the structure of the appointment system (is there a facility for fitting in urgent consultations? can advice be obtained over the phone?), the willingness or otherwise of the doctors to do home visits (do the doctors accept all requests for home visits without question? do receptionists try to avoid home visits by fitting patients in as an emergency, or by getting the doctors to speak to patients requesting home visits on the phone?), or the advertising of practice arrangements (is it clear to patients what constitutes the need for a home visit in the eyes of the doctors?).

If you are currently attached to a primary care team, you might discuss the following exercise with your GP tutor. Having carried out the exercise, are there any other members of the team who could give you an opinion about the result? It might help to let them see the national figures compared to those of the practice.

Practical Exercise

How many home visits have been done in office hours in your tutor's practice in the past 3 months? Count the number of home visits in the period in question from the visit book, or its equivalent if computerized. Multiply that number by four. Divide the resulting number by the number of patients on the practice list and multiply by 1000. This is your tutor's practice daytime visiting rate per thousand patients per year. How does it differ from national figures? Can you offer any explanation for similarities or differences compared with the national figures given above?

OUT OF HOURS

Reliable data on the proportion of home visits made out of office hours are not available. There was a fall of 27 per cent in home visiting rates between 1981/2 and 1991/2. This was matched by a substantial rise in night visits during the same period. The results of the 2001/2 Fifth National Survey of Morbidity Statistics from General Practice are awaited and will show if this trend in falling numbers of home visits has continued. Recently, there have been great changes in the organization of out-of-hours care in Britain (Jessop ct al., 1997; Department of Health, 2002). Among the innovations that have taken place, there have been dramatic increases both in the number of GP out-of-hours co-operatives and in the number of out-of-hours primary care centres. A GP out-of-hours co-operative is a formal business arrangement amongst GPs within a particular area. The aim of the co-operative is to share in the provision of out-of-hours general medical services to patients registered with participating GPs so as to achieve maximum efficiency of service and minimum costs in manpower, time and expense. Out-of-hours primary care centres are local centres manned by primary care professionals providing out-of-hours services on behalf of local primary care teams. This service is usually an emergency service, but in some examples routine care is also provided in these centres. Within the NHS, a new plan for out-of-hours care called the 'Out of Hours Review' is currently being implemented (Department of Health, 2002). It proposes a fully integrated out-of-hours service by 2004 with a unified structure. Within this integrated service, all telephone calls out of hours will be received by NHS Direct, the patient telephone advice line. Where clinical care is required, it will be provided by existing GP services (e.g. out-of-hours co-operatives), but also by walk-in centres, primary care centres and accident and emergency centres. These services will be integrated with or have close liaison with minor injury units, social services, community nursing, the ambulance service and mental health and palliative care units.

A notable change in the pattern of out-of-hours provision is the increasing number of contacts that are being dealt with by telephone advice (Studdiford et al., 1996). Salisbury (1997) has reported that almost 60 per cent of contacts out of hours with one GP co-operative are conducted by telephone alone. The rate with which contacts are managed by telephone varies amongst out-of-hours co-operatives from 10 per cent to 65 per cent, according to Jessop and colleagues (1997). This differs strikingly from the rate of 1 per cent reported for GP deputizing services in 1994/5 by Cragg et al. (1997). The whole issue of telephone consulting is now receiving more attention in the UK, with special training programmes and research projects being developed in a number of different centres. By contrast, there has been a long tradition of telephone consulting in the USA, where up to a quarter of primary care contacts are by telephone (Studdiford et al., 1996). Telephone consulting allows assessments to be made and advice given to patients who are either unwilling or unable to come to the surgery. In many surgeries it is only when the doctor gets to the patient's home that he or she learns about the reason for the home visit request. My own experience suggests that it is not uncommon for the doctor to discover to his or her dismay that the home visit was not justified purely on clinical grounds. So the development of formal telephone consulting may well prove to be a major positive development in limiting the current expansion in demand for general medical services. It may also improve access to GP services and reduce the time and travelling costs for consumers. Telephone consulting has been used for chronic disease surveillance for which the patient carries out home monitoring. This can be useful in the care of hypertension or diabetes mellitus, for which the results of home tests done by the patient can be discussed with a doctor or nurse and appropriate advice given.

REASON FOR VISITS

Diseases of the respiratory system are the commonest diagnoses made during home visits (Aylin et al., 1996). These include upper respiratory tract infections, pneumonia, asthma and chronic bronchitis. Diseases of the respiratory tract account for 40 per cent of home visits for children and 20 per cent for adults. In 11 per cent of home visits, the category of diagnosis (drawn from the *International classification of diseases – Version 9*) was 'symptoms, signs, and ill defined conditions'. In people aged 65 years and over, respiratory diseases account for 17 per cent of home visits and diseases of the circulatory system account for 16 per cent.

TREATING AT HOME CAN CAUSE PROBLEMS!

In contrast with Mrs M's experience of Jason's sore throat is that of Mr V.

CASE STUDY 10.4

Mr V is 45 years old and has acquired immune deficiency syndrome (AIDS). He is now receiving terminal care at home and is being looked after by his partner and the local district nurses supported by the Macmillan team. Requests for a visit to Mr V are put in the home visit book by the receptionists without question.

But Mr V's situation led to other difficulties for Dr S.

CASE STUDY 10.4 (continued)

Mr V had a necrotic bedsore on his buttocks that was discharging heavily. Dr S visited him on Saturday morning. Mr V's pain was poorly controlled and the doctor decided to start him on morphine. Dr S is part of an out-of-hours co-operative, so between 1.00 p.m. on Saturday and 7.00 a.m. on Monday morning, emergency visits would have to be done by other local GPs in the co-operative. Dr S wanted to warn any doctors who might come to see Mr V about his condition so that they could be informed about how best to relieve his pain and also to ensure that they would protect themselves against contamination. Could Dr S tell the answering service that Mr V had AIDS (and tell the answering service to warn any doctors who might visit) without asking the patient's consent?

Thinking and Discussion Point

❑ What arrangements does your GP tutor use for out-of-hours cover?
❑ What are the arguments for and against disclosure of the information about Mr V?
❑ To whom can a doctor disclose confidential patient information?

A variety of arrangements are made by GPs for general medical services out of hours. Within the NHS, GPs are contractually obliged to provide services for their patients for 24 hours every day, although these are not necessarily provided in person by the GP with whom the patient is registered.

Patients who require treatment at home may not always be able to see the doctor they usually see at the surgery. They should nonetheless expect the same degree of confidentiality from the attending doctor. They should assume that their doctor will share information about them with other doctors either directly or through the medical record. However, just as a patient can rightly expect the doctor to hold medical information in confidence from other members of the primary care team such as receptionists, so it should be assumed that such confidentiality is observed with the telephonists and administrators of an out-of-hours service.

What are the issues in Mr V's case? Dr S may be concerned that a colleague in the co-operative who visits Mr V may take inadequate precautions on coming into contact with Mr V's body fluids. He may worry that Mr V or his carers will fail to communicate the nature of his disease, either because of embarrassment or because he is too ill or they are too distressed to do so. Dr S's anxiety for the safety of his colleagues is not adequate cause to disclose Mr V's diagnosis beyond his medical or nursing attendants without his informed consent. There are other actions that Dr S could take. He could discuss his dilemma with Mr V or Mr V's carer. He could leave a message in the home to be given to a visiting doctor on his or her arrival. The principal issue here is the patient's right to confidentiality and the doctor's duty to observe that right. This right is paramount, except where the risk of injury to others is such that breaching the confidence is the only way in which that risk can be avoided. The onus will then be on the doctor to prove that breaching the confidentiality of the doctor–patient relationship was justified. Because it is not ever possible to be certain that patients are free from infection, doctors are warned to assume that all body

fluids are contaminated until proven otherwise and to take appropriate precautions. By the same token, the risk of infection from contact with body fluids is not in itself adequate reason to breach patient confidentiality. However, doctors should always aim to reduce such risks by making information about infectivity as accessible as possible to patients, their carers and fellow professionals.

Home visiting often brings to the fore medico-legal and ethical issues that seem less pressing in the surgery office.

SERVICES FOR HOUSEBOUND PATIENTS

Some people become housebound in the course of their illness, so that they are unable to attend their GP or other health professionals in their offices. If they have carers who can look after their daily needs such as shopping, banking and cleaning, they may only require particular health services on an intermittent basis. If, on the other hand, they need daily nursing care, they are likely to require carefully co-ordinated services from district nurses, and may in addition need physiotherapy, chiropody and occupational therapy at home. The GP will have a key role in assessing the needs of housebound patients and obtaining the assessment of other professionals at the appropriate stage of the illness.

The cost of hospital admissions and the higher risk of accidents and infections for people in hospital have led to earlier discharge of patients from hospital and the development of 'hospital at home' services. 'Hospital at home' is defined as a service that provides treatment by healthcare professionals in the patient's home of illnesses that would otherwise require acute treatment in hospital. In a systematic review of randomized trials of 'hospital at home', Shepperd and Iliffe (2001) could not support its development as a cheaper alternative to inpatient care. However, more recent studies give cause for optimism and it is likely that attempts to reduce the length of hospital stay by providing high-tech medical services at home supported by intensive social services home care will continue.

A particular problem arises when the housebound patient has a chronic illness that requires ongoing surveillance. The elements of structured care that are described in the section on chronic illness apply equally here. However, account needs to be taken of the patient's ability to demand visits when they are required. Mrs W provides a good example of the problem.

CASE STUDY 10.5

Mrs W was 74 years old when she developed insulin-dependent diabetes mellitus. She had been admitted to hospital for a left knee replacement, as she had severe osteoarthritis in both knees and could not walk more than 10 metres without severe pain. She had hypertension, for which she took enalapril 10 mg daily, and she was hypothyroid, for which she took thyroxine 0.1 mg daily. She was partially blind and could not draw up her own insulin, although she did inject the insulin herself. The district nurse visited her every 3 days to draw up her insulin. Dr S would call about every 3 months to take her blood pressure. A year after the diagnosis, the practice nurse was carrying out a diabetic audit and noticed that Mrs W was on insulin but did not appear to attend either the hospital or the practice. It became obvious that no surveillance of her diabetes was taking place.

Thinking and Discussion Point

What should be done? Who should do it?

MANAGING HOUSEBOUND PATIENTS WITH TEAMWORK

It may prove embarrassing for patients such as Mrs W to ask the doctor or nurse to visit to take their blood pressure or to demand checks for their diabetes. Anyway, most patients will not have a detailed concept about what is required in chronic illness management. It seems reasonable to convene a meeting about Mrs W with all the team members involved in order to decide who should have responsibility for what element of her care. Such a meeting is likely to raise other issues such as the need for chiropody, which would be a key service for a diabetic of Mrs W's age. If the meeting is held with Mrs W, she will have the opportunity to say what way she would like her care to be organized. It is wise to determine who has the main overall responsibility to ensure the service is delivered effectively. The best person to do this may well be the district nurse rather than the GP, since it is the district nurse who is seeing Mrs W most frequently.

SERVICES DELIVERED AT HOME

In addition to the GP and district nurse, there is a wide variety of home services that are provided for housebound patients. These are listed in Table 10.3 in two categories – health services and social services.

Table 10.3 Health and social services provided in the home

Health services for the housebound	Social services for the housebound
General practitioner	Home care (personal care, meals, shopping, banking, laundry)
District nurse	Occupational therapist
Health visitor	Bathing attendant (some districts only)
Chiropodist	Meals on wheels
Nurse specialists (paediatric, diabetic, etc.)	Social worker
Early discharge teams	

SUMMARY POINTS

To conclude, the most important messages in this chapter are:

- home visiting offers a privileged insight into the lives of patients, but is time consuming and should be justified by the severity or urgency of the illness or by the immobility of the patient;
- within the NHS, each GP does 600 home visits on average each year, of which about 65 are done between 10 p.m. and 8 a.m; the rate of home visiting for people aged 85 years or more is 30 times that for people between the ages of 16 and 35;
- rates of home visiting in the NHS vary from 100 per GP per year to 1100 per GP per year, a difference that cannot be explained solely by patient need;
- respiratory diseases are the commonest diagnoses recorded on home visits, accounting for more than 20 per cent of diagnoses on visits to adults and for more than 40 per cent of diagnoses on visits to children;
- housebound patients are sometimes under-treated through their own unwillingness to demand appropriate treatment at home; a structured approach to their care such as that described in Chapter 9 ('Chronic illness and its management in general practice') may help to ensure effective continuing care of people who are confined to their homes through illness or disability.

REFERENCES

Aylin, P., Majeed, F.A. and Cook, D.G. 1996: Home visiting by general practitioners in England and Wales. *British Medical Journal* 313, 207–10.

Cragg, D.K., McKinley, R.K., Roland, M.O. et al., 1997: Comparison of out of hours care provided by patients' own general practitioners and commercial deputising services: a randomised controlled trial. I: The process of care. *British Medical Journal* 314, 187–9.

Department of Health 2002: *Raising standards for patients. New partnerships in out of hours care.* London: Department of Health. Also available online at: http://www.doh.gov.uk/pricare/imple-mentoohplanguide.pdf

General Medical Services Committee 1992: *Your choices: special report.* London: British Medical Association.

Hallam, L. 1994: Primary medical care outside of normal working hours: review of published work. *British Medical Journal* 308, 249–53.

Hallam, L. 1997: Out of hours primary care. *British Medical Journal* 314, 157–8.

Jessop, L., Beck, I., Hollins, L., Shipman, C., Reynolds, M. and Dale, J. 1997: Changing the pattern of out of hours: a survey of general practice co-operatives. *British Medical Journal* 314, 199–200.

McCormick, A., Fleming, D., Charlton, J., Royal College of General Practitioners, Office of Population Censuses and Surveys, and Department of Health 1995: *Morbidity Statistics from General Practice. Fourth National Survey 1991–1992.* London: HMSO.

Oldenquist, G.W., Scott, L. and Finucane, T.E. 2001: Home care: what a physician needs to know. *Cleveland Clinic Journal of Medicine* 68(5), 433–40.

Salisbury, C. 1997: Observational study of a general practice out of hours co-operative: measures of activity. *British Medical Journal* 314, 182–6.

Shepperd, S. and Iliffe, S. 2001: *Hospital at home versus in-patient hospital care.* Cochrane Review, Issue 2. Oxford: Cochrane Library.

Studdiford III, J.S., Panitch, K.M., Snyderman, D.A. and Pharr, M.E. 1996: Telephone in primary care. *Primary Care* 23(1), 83–97.

FURTHER READING

The references to the work of Aylin et al. and Hallam cover most of the key issues in this topic and are recommended further reading for this chapter.

HEALTH PROMOTION IN GENERAL PRACTICE

In this chapter the practice and theories associated with this contested field of study and work, referred to as health promotion, are discussed as they relate to the general practice context. Why is health promotion relevant to general practice? What is being understood by the term? What are the skills needed? What type of expertise, knowledge and skills inform practice and what evidence base is referred to? Perhaps the most important issues for this chapter relate to notions of successful, effective, efficient and pragmatic interventions and how to avoid harm. In addition, this chapter reflects on some ethical questions associated with health promotion interventions and the potential for harm.

LEARNING OBJECTIVES

By the end of this chapter you should be aware of:

- definitions of health, illness, determinants of health and disease and health promotion;
- the contested nature of health promotion;
- the main theories, models and concepts that inform health promotion practice;
- the skills associated with health promotion practice in the general practice context;
- what defines successful health promotion practice;
- what is the potential for harm and how ethics and moral philosophy can be used for guidance;
- health promotion beyond the medical arena.

BACKGROUND

The most frequently used definition of health promotion is from the World Health Organization (WHO) Ottawa Charter, 1986:

> Health promotion is a process of enabling people to increase control over and to improve their health.

Health promotion is one of the newest fields and professions within the broad genre of health. Despite the apparent simplicity of the WHO definition above, health promotion is contested, complex, eclectic, challenging, swathed in jargon, littered with acronyms, political in nature and open to abuse.

The very term is one that can have multiple meanings; it is not exclusive to any elitist group and is part of everyday language. What is meant by health – that which is to be promoted – depends on whom you ask and how you ask. The ethical issues relating to health promotion can be argued from different perspectives. The theories that inform those who are specialists within the field are drawn from many different 'feeder disciplines', such as psychology, sociology, education, epidemiology, politics and economics. Seedhouse not surprisingly refers to it as 'the magpie profession' (Seedhouse, 1997). Most activity that is defined as 'health promotion' is funded from the public purse and as such is associated with political agendas and ideology. So for the comment 'open to abuse', I refer to claims sometimes made about health promotion and the way people define their actions as health promoting. Claims such as health promotion 'does not work' or 'is a waste of resources' need to be challenged. Equally, those that classify their activities as health promotion when these activities are not based on, or informed by, theory, evidence or associated skills also need to be challenged.

Health promotion, for some, especially those in academia, is seen as a post-modernist discipline and a synergy of philosophies that can be applied in a variety of arenas. It is a young and emerging discipline, applied mainly outside the medical context, but it can and does have a place within the healthcare sector. In fact, within the context of general practice and primary care, health promotion has become an integral part of provision, and the growth of the discipline has been nurtured within general practice and primary care.

The other branch of medicine that is closely linked to health promotion is that of public health.

HEALTH PROMOTION AND PUBLIC HEALTH

The health promotion movement and public health have had some shared history. The famous cholera outbreak in London in the early nineteenth century was a classic public health issue. First, by plotting the details of the outbreak, it was clear that there was a location issue, and some link or association was made with a specific water pump. Although at this stage it could not be fully explained, the intervention

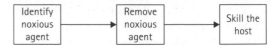

Figure 11.1 A trajectory of a public health intervention.

could be implemented – close the access to the contaminated water pump, inform the public and arrange alternatives. Figure 11.1 shows how others have seen this process.

The epidemiological data identified the noxious agent (i.e. the water pump); it was closed and people were given safe alternatives. But was this health promotion? If health promotion is defined as 'the study of, and the study of the response to, the modifiable determinants of health', this historical episode was both public health work and health promotion (Wylie, 2002). The public's health was at risk and, by an intervention or response, this risk was reduced. For a more detailed summary of the background and the development of contemporary health promotion practice, the book *Health promotion: foundations for practice* by Naidoo and Wills (2000) is recommended.

The health of the UK population started to improve towards the end of the nineteenth century, in terms of reduced morbidity and mortality. This was probably a result of improved sanitation and housing as well as access to education, safe food and social welfare. Individuals were the beneficiaries of these improvements with little effort on their part.

FROM COMMUNICABLE DISEASE TO CHRONIC DISEASE

These social and environmental improvements led to a reduction in communicable diseases. Although communicable diseases reduced, there was a rise in chronic disease in the mid-twentieth century, and with that came a shift in public health work. This shift looked at interventions that focused on the individual, whereby individuals might need to modify their behaviour to reduce risks and improve health. Doctors and healthcare professionals in the primary care context started to face the dilemmas of how to respond to patients whose own actions were deleterious to their health and where therapeutic interventions are limited, at best.

The first major dilemma that doctors, and especially general practitioners (GPs), encountered with health education and information was related to Doll and Hill's work on smoking behaviour in 1964 (Doll and Hill, 1964). They used epidemiological methods to establish a link between tobacco and lung cancer and their work identified 'modifiable' determinants of disease. Smoking was the modifiable determinant and if smokers ceased smoking or if non-smokers remained non-smokers, the disease (lung cancer) would be dramatically reduced. The dilemmas concerned how doctors should respond with regard to their own patients who smoked and how far government should lead on this. For themselves, doctors could make choices to smoke or not to smoke, but they also found that giving up smoking was no easy matter and other factors would dictate how successful they would be in becoming ex-smokers. It soon became evident that having the 'facts' and 'being informed' would not be enough for behaviour change, especially when the behaviour is related to addiction, habit and social norms. If smoking behaviour were to change in the population at large, strategic approaches would need to be developed.

Thinking and Discussion Point

- ❑ To what extent is the smoking behaviour of patients and staff the responsibility of the GP and the primary care team?
- ❑ Would patients expect their smoking behaviour to be addressed or commented on?
- ❑ Would colleagues within the practice who smoke expect their behaviour to be addressed or commented on?
- ❑ How have these expectations changed since 1964?

EXPLORING DEFINITIONS OF HEALTH, ILLNESS, DETERMINANTS OF HEALTH AND DISEASE AND HEALTH PROMOTION

The words used in the title of this section hardly need reference to a dictionary, but there are questions of semantics to be addressed. What is meant by the term health, for example, differs depending on who is using it and in what context. Illness also has multiple meanings but, like health, forms part of 'common speak' and everyday language. There is no professional monopoly or ownership of language, but a reminder here that when using these terms we may need to elaborate or ask patients to explain further rather than assume some shared understanding. The term 'determinants of health and disease' is perhaps not part of everyday language; however, it does enable some focused discussion about making sense of symptoms, cause and effect.

In the health promotion academic literature, two terms, proximal and distal, are sometimes used. Proximal refers to the more immediate and obvious cause-and-effect determinants of health and disease. For example, a sexually active teenager is exposed to the possibility of sexually transmitted infections, and pregnancy advice about the use of condoms may be seen as a proximal response. Distal refers to more in-depth and contested determinants of risk behaviours, predisposing factors, social and environmental factors, which inevitably are more complex. The sexually active teenager may be living in an abusive environment, may see this type of sexual behaviour as a norm and may have low education attainment or aspirations and low self-esteem. Addressing or responding to these distal determinants of health and disease usually takes the health promotion activity beyond the clinical arena.

Lalonde, in 1974, noted that people's health is influenced not just by, or even principally by, the availability of medical science and care. He was possibly the first to use the term health promotion when he was the Canadian Minister of National Health and Welfare. His report *A new perspective on the health of Canadians* was to have a major influence on the WHO building on his ideas and calling for a shift of emphasis from medical care to primary care in the pursuit of health. By the time of the WHO Ottawa Charter in 1986, health promotion had become established and was broad based.

Whilst Lalonde's statement is obvious today, at the time of writing medical science was in the ascendancy, developments and discoveries were high profile and there were few critics of medical progress apart from Illich (1976). Little attention in mainstream health journals was given to the non-biological factors influencing health. In fact, the term health has proved a challenge, but for many within the health sector health is frequently understood as being in a state of health as opposed to ill-health and the absence of disease. It is beyond the scope of this chapter to explore fully the vast literature on the concepts and values related to definitions of health, illness and disease, but it is incumbent on those who want to promote health or engage in health promotion activity to have cognizance of these challenges. These challenges are faced daily within the context of general practice, where patients may be free of morbidity but in need of health promotion, information or advice to maintain or improve their health. Examples such as antenatal care, travel advice and immunization provision are part of the work of general practice. Of course, patients are also seen with a lack of well-being and self-worth but no clear biomedical morbidity. The determinants of their health and disease status are more complex, encompassing psychological, sociological, environmental and demographic issues.

In fact, it was a decade after Lalonde's statement when the landmark publication of the Black Report in the UK highlighted the impact of inequality on health outcome (Townsend and Davidson, 1982). This report may have stated the obvious to some, especially those in general practice, but it was important for a number of reasons. It widened the definition of morbidity and enabled those who were disadvantaged, and the relevant health professionals, to see their ill-health or lack of well-being in the context of their social situation rather than just fate or bad luck. The social factors such as inequalities, housing and income could not be addressed by individuals alone but would need political change.

Jones and Douglas (2000) argue that health promotion does not have a single definition but is about working in new ways to address the determinants of health. In the UK, several cities joined the Healthy Cities Project 1987, recognizing that ambitious intersectoral action programmes would be needed to improve health. Liverpool was one of the first cities to attempt the notion of joint working in 1988 but was initially too ambitious, and it was 1994 before a more focused and realistic plan emerged.

The trajectory for progress at this time was slowed when the Government failed to put in the resources to support these new ways of working but put the emphasis for health back with the individual, as was evident in the publication of *The health of the nation* in 1992 (Department of Health, 1992). Despite this, the concept of the New Public Health and the need to identify and address the determinants of health and disease that are outside the control of the individual grew. Several influential reports asserted the link or association of poverty with health or its absence, their goal being to put poverty back on the political agenda as a major determinant of health and disease (Ashton and Seymour, 1988; Jones and Douglas, 2000).

> Just as in the last century it was in the interests of all to introduce public health measures to combat the spread of infectious physical disease fostered by poverty, so in this century it is in the interests of all to remove the factors that are fostering the social diseases of drugs, crime, political extremism and social unrest.
>
> *(Rowntree Foundation, 1995)*

Similar concerns, that the determinants of health go beyond the factors associated with biomedical cause and effect and the individual's actions, were expressed globally at the Jakarta Declaration in 1997. Poverty and the lack of social capital were above all the greatest threat to health. Neither poverty nor social capital is easily defined, but within the health promotion field, poverty is associated with income relative to the local norms, level of disposable income and relative deprivation. Social capital, however, relates to social assets and the ability to function within a community and beyond, to have social networks and to access social support when needed. For example, a medical student's income may be very low and his or her debt high, so poverty and deprivation may exist. However, the medical student probably has a high level of education, access to loans, personal advice and support and is able to relate to the wider community of medical school and university – thus a high level of social capital. In the presence of poverty and the absence of social capital, communities are more prone to loss of social order and crime that will impact on health and health-related behaviour.

> Health promotion, through investment and action, has a marked impact on the determinants of health so as to create the greatest health gain for people, to contribute significantly to the reduction of inequalities in health, to further human rights and to build social capital.
>
> *(World Health Organization, 1997)*

Since the Lalonde report, health promotion has developed as an academic discipline and professional field of practice. There are now four specialized peer-reviewed journals. Many universities offer master's courses specifically in health promotion. In the UK, specialists in the field are likely to belong to the Society of Health Education and Promotion Specialists (SHEPS), with its own principles of practice and code of conduct, and/or the Institute of Health Education and Promotion Specialists. There are currently changes in the field of public health whereby senior posts will now be available to non-medically qualified applicants who can demonstrate they meet the requirements. The first non-medically qualified appointments have been given to health promotion specialists.

This chapter explores what kinds of knowledge and skills are embodied in health promotion that can be relevant and applicable to the general practice context.

At the time of the Ottawa conference, when health promotion was given a definition, the New Public Health was emerging whereby the efforts of individuals to improve their health were of limited value unless other social changes were addressed.

What was 'modifiable' with regard to health determinants depended not just on the response of the individual, but also on the efforts and interventions of others, be they engineers or economists, educationalists or ecologists, politicians or political activists.

The Ottawa Charter for Health Promotion in 1986 advocated five areas for action:
1. build healthy public policy,
2. create supportive environments,
3. strengthen community action,
4. develop personal skills,
5. re-orient health services.

Thinking and Discussion Point

An elderly couple take up the offer of 'flu jabs', but are otherwise rare visitors to the practice. During the generic conversation, you become concerned about their well-being. They tell you the house is damp and in need of some repairs that are expensive, they find driving more trying and their son, who lives 200 miles away, jokes that they shouldn't still be driving! Both have been a little low since the cat, aged 17, died last month. They appear to like each other's company and no longer go out much apart from church, complaining that the library is always busy, so they don't like to ask for help, they can't use the computer there and their eyesight is not so good. They don't like the 'old people's' activities such as bingo. They used to be keen walkers but don't want to go with an organized group.

❑ Reflect on the five areas for action advocated by the Ottawa Charter in relation to the above couple and consider what role/action could be initiated within the context of primary care.

❑ What could be the 'modifiable' determinants of health?

❑ How have these changed since 1986 (i.e. the year of the charter)?

THEORIES AND MODELS

If health promotion is to have some credibility as an academic discipline, as a field of professional practice and as a contributor to health gain, some guidance as to theoretical frameworks and approaches to practice needs to be explored. As a young and emerging discipline, with a wide-ranging agenda, the theories, models and approaches that have been presented so far in its short history are numerous and constantly evolving. The complexity of these models increased as they evolved. Rawson reported that 17 distinct models were identifiable in 1992. This growth suggests a lack of consensus about the discipline and arguably reflects development and innovation, in part linked to political agendas. What matters, however, is that 'good practice' should be informed by one or more of these models, but no single model encompasses health promotion. What I have done in this section is to be a prudent, or possibly ruthless, editor and focused on a selection of models that help inform practice, especially within the context of primary care.

TONES

One of the most prominent writers in the field of health promotion during the latter part of the twentieth century has been Tones. Tones argues for the following equation:

Health promotion = health education
$$\times \text{ healthy public policy}$$

This equation suggests an ideology and justification for action or interventions (Tones, 1991).

We can illustrate this by referring to an issue of community safety, road safety. Traffic-calming measures times improved competence of the drivers could equate to the promotion of safer travel. Within the context of primary care, the meaning of health education may be limited to information giving, improving patient knowledge about a health-related issue and providing skill-based programmes such as antenatal classes about pain management in labour.

Healthy public policy may include government initiatives, local and national, such as developing and implementing health improvement programmes (HImPs), Sure Start and Healthy Action Zones (HAZ). Here we see examples of political agendas, jargon and acronyms dominating practice, but they are also part of the wider remit of the Government's approach to tackling inequalities and social exclusion.

These policies are currently well resourced and therefore attractive to the newly formed primary care trusts (PCTs), which now have significant public health responsibilities for local UK populations of approximately 100 000–170 000.

NORDENFELT

Nordenfelt may be less familiar than Tones to health promotion practitioners, but his model (Fig. 11.2) offers help with some parameters and complements his assertion that health is about being able to achieve vital goals (Nordenfelt, 1995; 1998).

It could be argued that, using this model, action defined as health promotion would need to lead to health enhancement and achievement of vital goals, yet be action that is different in essence from health care. It does not help so much with process as with outcome, that is what should be achievable by the intervention and why such action is worthwhile.

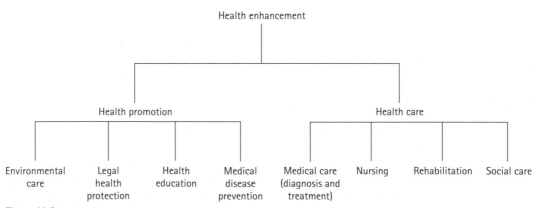

Figure 11.2 Nordenfelt's health enhancement model.

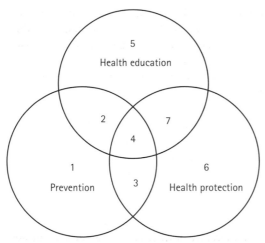

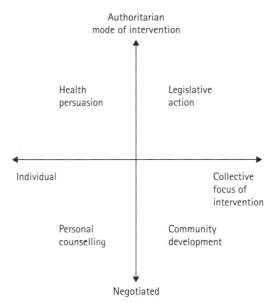

Figure 11.3 The Tannahill model. Reprinted from Downie, R.S., Fyfe, C. and Tannahill, A. 1993: *Health promotion models and values.* With permission from Oxford University Press.

Figure 11.4 Beattie's model (Beattie et al., 1993).

TANNAHILL

The Tannahill model (Fig. 11.3) is another way of explaining or justifying action that could be classed as health promotion (Downie et al., 1993). The three domains and the overlapping sectors provide seven options that collectively equate to health promotion. Within these broad public health measures are included such issues as fluoridation of water and lobbying for a ban on tobacco advertising. These activities, whilst important, may not be directly relevant for the primary care arena. In contrast, however, preventative services and preventative health education are relevant and part of the daily fodder of general practice.

BEATTIE

It is Beattie's model (Figs 11.4 and 11.5) that provides the potential practitioner with the clearest understanding of health promotion practice in terms of skills needed, setting goals and evaluating success (Beattie et al., 1993). Although this section explores the potential of Beattie's model for health promotion practice, it also represents ideologies and values that underpin health promotion practice.

Each quadrant requires its own skills base and evidence, but some interventions will have a strategic approach relating to all quadrants.

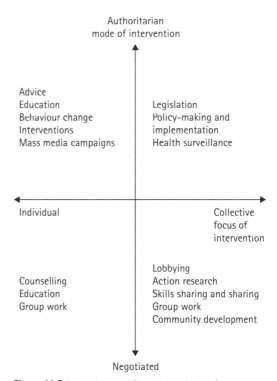

Figure 11.5 Beattie's model (Beattie et al., 1993).

Although health promotion practitioners would benefit from having an overview of the relevant strategy and how it was developed, it is possible to work within one quadrant. The following suggests how two examples may be informed by Beattie's model.

Example 1

A social issue such as road safety. The overall strategy could be reduction in the number of road traffic accidents (RTAs) associated with alcohol use.

The personal counselling quadrant draws on communication skills, listening and exploring, allowing people to reflect on their drinking patterns and the risks, what options they have and what help they may need. An action plan may result. The intervention could be to facilitate discussion, and success is related to that being achieved, with or without an action plan. Within the context of patient centredness, working within this quadrant is more likely to lead to concordance.

The health persuasion quadrant can be seen as more expert led, advice giving and information giving. There are two options within the general practice setting, the first being display of leaflets and posters as well as issuing information and/or showing videos. The second option is in the consultation setting. Patients are advised, whether or not they ask for advice. They may be referred to specific clinics or professionals within the practice to address their alcohol-related problems, warning them of the dangers and risks associated with driving and alcohol consumption. Within the context of duty, many health professionals would see this type of work as acceptable. Success here is related to having noted that the information/ advice was targeted and made available. There may be no evidence of behaviour change or knowledge about safe drinking levels, but if there were, that would be 'value added'.

The third quadrant, that of legislation, may have limited relevance to the primary care setting but it will juxtapose at times. Knowing the legislation will be important, as well as knowing how to support patients who may be affected as either the accused or the victims of alcohol-related RTAs. Increasingly, the courts are sending the convicted on specific courses to address their drinking behaviour. Some, as a result of these courses, will seek help via their GPs. You

are then back to the first quadrant! Victims, on the other hand, may seek your support with a criminal charge or compensation.

The final quadrant in Beattie's model may have had little to do with general practice in the past. Now, however, the community initiatives will be of increasing importance with the advent of PCTs. Local self-help groups may be suitable for referral of clients, and other community initiatives may link into campaigns for better local transport, increasing the options for drinkers to leave their cars at home. The indicators of success could be the improved transport provision or the setting up of a community group itself in the first instance to look at local issues and consider local solutions. There are few examples of general practices getting involved in this type of community development, although this will increasingly be expected. Fisher was a pioneer with the initiation of bus provision for his patients in 1994 (Fisher, 1994). Other examples have been poorly documented, but include the initiation of local walking groups and increasing local physical activity provision at low costs to local residents as well as practice patients.

Example 2

A settings issue such as Healthy Schools Awards.

A major aspect of health promotion specialists' work is often focused on the school setting. Within this environment, there are many health promotion opportunities and interventions within curriculum as well as extra-curricular activities and for the benefit of pupils, staff, parents and local community. Within this context, all four quadrants in Beattie's model are useful for developing strategy and defining the role of the various protagonists. School nurses increasingly offer drop-in facilities where pupils and staff can discuss health-related issues with the nurse. The nurse will be a skilled listener, enabling the client to set the agenda.

The health persuasion quadrant is very pragmatic, with pupils being given instructions, for example about response to head lice infestation, contents and use of vending machines, and availability of drinking water. As well as health-related school rules, this will be included in some of the curricular content, with importance given to health-related topics and activities. Much of school life is governed by legislation, but within the community quadrant there are increased opportunities to work with parents and local communities on issues such as sex education and using the school facilities for the benefit of the local community outside school time.

It would be unusual for one person to excel in all these different areas, but within the context of general practice, quadrants 1 and 2 will probably be the most relevant for day-to-day work.

Thinking and Discussion Point

A young woman has, for the second time in 6 months, asked for emergency contraception. Which of Beattie's quadrants would help you most in deciding how to respond?

EWLES AND SIMNETT

We can now turn to approaches such as those described by Ewles and Simnett (1999) and commonly used in primary care, explicitly or implicitly (Table 11.1).

Ewles and Simnett offer ways of working in practice, suggesting there is no right aim for health promotion, and describe five approaches that a practitioner can consider, deciding on the merits of each within the context of a given situation. They also acknowledge that practitioners will not necessarily be confined to working with one approach, but may use a combination (see Table 11.1). It is probable that much of the day-to-day work classified as health promotion within general practice and primary care adopts one of these five approaches, probably more usually the medical, behavioural and educational approaches. The empowerment approach is usually the preferred choice of community

Table 11.1 Ewles and Simnett approaches and health promotion

Approach	Aims	Methods	Worker/client relationship
Medical	To identify those at risk from disease	Primary healthcare consultation, e.g. measurement of body mass index	Expert led Passive, conforming client
Behaviour change	To encourage individuals to take responsibility for their own health and choose healthier lifestyles	Persuasion through one-to-one advice, information, mass campaigns, e.g. 'Look after your heart' dietary messages	Expert led Dependent client Victim-blaming ideology
Educational	To increase knowledge and skills related to healthy lifestyles	Information Exploration of attitudes through small group work Development of skills, e.g. women's health groups	May be expert led May also involve client in negotiation of issues for discussion
Empowerment	To work with clients or communities to meet their perceived needs	Advocacy Negotiation Networking Facilitation, e.g. food co-operative, fat women's group	Health promoter is facilitator Client becomes empowered
Social change	To address inequalities in health based on class, race, gender, geography	Development of organizational policy, e.g. hospital catering policy Public health legislation, e.g. food labelling Lobbying Fiscal controls, e.g. subsidy to farmers to produce lean meat	Entails social regulation and is top-down

workers and self-help groups, but the concept of empowerment is difficult. With the first three approaches, empowerment as a concept may be more easily understood by its absence (rather like the relationship of health to disease), and it is possible that professionally led actions using these three approaches could lead to disempowerment or, as Ewles and Simnett suggest, 'victim blaming'. This is also the concern of others, with such action resulting in harm or potential harm. Coercion or victim blaming is unacceptable, breaching the code of practice for the SHEPS. By referring to the earlier definition of health promotion – the study of, and the study of the response to, the modifiable determinants of health – it is important to explore what is modifiable for the client/patient to reduce the possibility of harm. Graham's work on women living in deprivation and reviewing their smoking behaviour advanced our understanding of this notion of 'modifiable'. In such circumstances, reference to smoking may alienate the woman from the health sector, reduce her self-esteem and self-worth and disempower her (Graham, 1988; 1993).

The fifth approach offered by Ewles and Simnett, the social change approach, has resonance with Beattie's model and the legislative action quadrant, with the dominating values related to the greater good. Their social change approach relates to activities working for social change rather than focusing on the individuals, and they include legislative changes such as fiscal policy to address inequalities. The impetus for change may come from campaigning groups and/or community development initiatives, but if successful, the dominating values are then imposed on the majority. A recent example is paternity leave in the UK, which requires employers to accommodate leave for new fathers. Such ideology may seem to be 'good' for the majority of fathers, mothers and infants. It may, however, be difficult for some employers and unwelcome to some fathers.

'STAGES OF CHANGE'

The final model, the 'Stages of change' model (Fig. 11.6), provides a more structured way of working, taken from the psychologists who claimed success when using this with alcohol-dependent

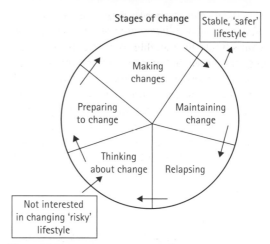

Figure 11.6 'Stages of change' model (Health Education Authority, 1993).

patients. This is a behavioural approach to health promotion, which gained popularity within primary care when the Health Education Authority (HEA) developed a course, *Helping people change*, specifically to address lifestyle change issues such as weight loss and smoking cessation (Health Education Authority, 1993). They reported that a high proportion of people trusted their GP's advice and so developed this course to give GPs the tools, skills and resources to approach lifestyle change with their patients. This model was widely adapted within primary care and the development of resources, such as leaflets and training packs to address smoking, used a similar approach.

The model is dependent on the facilitator being able to establish a working relationship with the client and explore where, in the process of change, the client is in order to focus appropriately. Those clients 'outside the circle' are not yet ready for change and there may be little that health professionals within the context of primary care can do. However, whether due to media campaigns, ill-health or death of a significant other, when clients 'enter the circle' they are said to be modifying their attitude to their behaviour. This phase may last for many weeks, months or even years. A skilled facilitator reinforces their new attitudes, enabling them to reflect on the personal benefits if they are to modify their behaviour, providing evidence of health gain or financial gain. Gradually progress is evident when they start to want to explore how to change, what are the challenges, what support is available. With regard to smoking, this may be nicotine replacement, telephone help lines, self-help groups, leaflets and tips for success. Once the client is in this phase, progress to the next should be fairly rapid and constructive. This is a dynamic phase and one that can rapidly bring success. One day without a cigarette could be defined as success, the next phase being the most difficult – that of maintaining change. It would be unusual for a person to progress without relapse, and this model accepts that. Whilst clients are in the relapse phase, and they may visit this many times, they can reflect on the success they had, how they coped, what actions were helpful, and where and what are the identified weaknesses. Understanding the model and its principles is a prerequisite to enabling the 'right' or 'appropriate' action to be taken by the facilitator to maintain motivation and target resources.

However, the model has its critics, from essentially two camps. First are the philosophers with regard to the ethical principles, and second the positivists, who want evidence from randomized controlled trials (RCTs) that the intervention is effective. Duncan and Cribb set out their arguments about the ethics of the 'Stages of change' model with regard to questions of autonomy (Duncan and Cribb, 1996). Hilton et al. are seeking to test the effectiveness of the intervention via a RCT (Hilton et al., 1999).

Whilst definitions concerning the field of health promotion may be helpful, theoretical models provide a conceptual framework that can inform practice. They also represent the ideologies and values associated with health promotion. As can be seen, a number of theoretical models have emerged to further our understanding of the processes, identify the skills required and clarify expectations, especially with regard to notions of success.

SKILLS FOR HEALTH PROMOTION IN GENERAL PRACTICE

How are the aspirations associated with health promotion interpreted and acted upon? Key theorists presented models of health promotion that could inform or govern practice. These models would provide the basis for new strategies and interventions as well as the process for defining the aims of an intervention and therefore the factors that can be relevant as indicators of success. From these models not only could the aims be defined, but also the skills identified for the specific intervention or strategy. What types of evidence and disciplines are relevant, and how the interventions are to be evaluated become more explicit when models are used.

When trying to assert that one was 'doing' health promotion, we might like to reflect on exactly what it was that we were doing – listening, advising, informing, using a leaflet, creating a poster display or facilitating a discussion. These activities, and many more, may be part of the de facto health-promoting health professional or may equally be part of the work done by skilled health promotion practitioners. Pill and Stott (1990) and Butler et al. (1998) see health promotion work as skilled, but also part of the skills portfolio of primary care health professionals. What defines good practice and how to measure the effectiveness of both process and outcome will matter to the professional as well as to the fund holders who resourced the action or intervention.

Therefore the skills are from many feeder disciplines and this section includes some that are relevant to the general practice context.

COMMUNICATION SKILLS AND ONE-TO-ONE CONSULTATIONS

Communication skills are essential for all healthcare professionals, and health promotion activity within the context of one-to-one consultation builds on those skills.

A number of disciplines inform good practice with regard to health promotion and communication, such as education theory and psychology as well as the 'Stages of change' model (Prochaska and DiClemente, 1986), but also included here are some of the theoretical principles found in counselling. Returning to the earlier definition of health promotion – 'the study of, and the study of the response to, the modifiable determinants of health' – much of the communication work will be to explore what is modifiable in the presenting situation. Pill and Stott (1990) found there was little evidence of a rational approach to personal decision making but that it was more a mix of habit, emotion, impulse, social influences and lack of forward planning. Health, or its absence, was often a consequence of the above mix. Later, their work also suggested that an individual's readiness to change would have to be assessed before advising, if the practitioner is to avoid harm to the doctor–patient relationship, which they argue is paramount. In conclusion, the notion of 'modifiable' is complex and unique, and will only be established through skilled communication work. Accepting and assimilating contested and contradictory information is a demanding task. Most of us, argues DeBono (1971), build on our knowledge base, adding to it in a complex and complementary way. Resistance is often encountered if we have to revisit some basic understanding and reconstruct our knowledge base. A simple example here is that of our construct about a suntan being a sign of health rather than being an indicator of skin damage.

The counselling arena offers three approaches to guide us in this exploratory task.

The first is the problem-solving approach advocated by Egan and Woolfe (Egan, 1982), involving three stages:

1. the present scenario,
2. the preferred scenario,
3. getting there.

This requires open and closed questioning, listening and assessing the client's resources and skills, and providing appropriate information and agreeing a goal (Woolfe, 1996).

The second is the person-centred non-directive approach, which aims to help the client become what he or she is capable of becoming, developed initially by Carl Rogers (1980). This involves exploring and listening, allowing a difficulty to be shared but accepting that solutions and actions, expert advice and information may not be relevant.

The third is the psychoanalytical approach, from Freud originally, which assumes the current crisis and problems are related to unresolved earlier problems or conflicts.

Applying one of these three approaches can guide the way in which a professional establishes what is modifiable and what response could be indicated.

COMMUNICATING WITH CLIENTS WHO SPEAK LITTLE OR NO ENGLISH

Textbooks and research publications remain relatively quiet about this situation, and understandably so. The most important need in a clinical context is to ensure that communication about health care is as effective as possible. There are organizational and funding concerns about contracting professional interpreters and there would never be comprehensive cover of all languages encountered in the UK. 'Language Line' is an option for many practices, but its use is usually confined to health care. However, the non-verbal codes that we use in communication are often universal, such as being welcoming. It is probable that some health promotion specialists have looked more closely at addressing this gap in local communities. Audiotapes and videotapes addressing broad health promotion issues have been developed but they are of limited use in the one-to-one clinical setting, where health care, rather than health promotion, is the usual priority.

COMMUNICATION SKILLS AND GROUP WORK

Group facilitation has been the mainstay of community health promotion practice and, for general practice, antenatal groups, smoking cessation courses and weight management classes have been and continue to be provided. Other group work, such as parenting and stress management courses, has also been popular. Community nurses and people in professions allied to medicine (PAMs) as well as practice nurses usually co-ordinate these groups.

The aims and objectives are very important to set because there are two conflicting theoretical frameworks that can be used and clarity is needed at the outset. First, following the theories of adult education and group learning, the experiences of the group and the knowledge of the facilitator are shared; the aims are to increase knowledge and skill and to modify/review attitudes. In the second framework, following the therapeutic models drawn from the disciplines of psychology and counselling, the aims are those of healing or recovery, facilitated by the therapists. Increased knowledge, new skills and modified attitudes may be the outcome, but success is intrinsically linked to reduced morbidity and modified behaviour. The 'Stages of change' model is frequently seen as therapeutic in essence.

COMMUNICATION AND THE MEDIA

It will be no surprise that many National Health Service (NHS) organizations have official spokespersons and dislike or disapprove of the professional who speaks 'off-message'. The power of the media to misinterpret, mislead or cause confusion is legendary, although it is not always the press that initiates the controversy. However, the media can also be an influential ally for the health promoter. Most health promoters will work closely with the press, radio and local television, carefully choreographing what, when and how information is disseminated and then following up the impact. This is evident when major national and international issues are raised, such as World AIDS Day in December and Breast Cancer Awareness in October each year. Here, the local news is compatible with the national news in a co-ordinated campaign strategy. General practice should ideally be central to this activity, as one consequence is that increased awareness leads to increased requests for consultations! There is also an opportunity for those in general practice to consolidate the message.

The innovations in health promotion that have emanated from local general practices need to be shared too, and one Berkshire example was that of *Healthy Walks*, developed and launched by Dr William Bird, a GP at the Sonning Common Practice near Reading, in August 1995. He used local radio, television and the press. By 1999, the initiative was reported in *Bandolier*, by which time there were more than 200 *Walking the Way to Health* initiatives in the UK and an RCT in place to evaluate them, funded by the British Heart Foundation and the Countryside Agency.

In this instance, the media played a vital role in promoting the scheme (*Bandolier*, 1999).

LEAFLETS AND HEALTH PROMOTION

Leaflets represent the single largest resource associated with health promotion and no more so than in the general practice setting. However, the value of the leaflets is related to the skills of health professionals who produce them, how they are accessed or displayed and how they are used. What defines quality and what factors indicate a good leaflet are more than just how it looks, as we see below.

Practical Exercise

Critiquing leaflets – some key questions

❑ Check the date of production and identity of the producer – is this acceptable in your practice?

❑ What advertising is implicit, if any, and how might that impact on the credibility of the leaflet and your practice?

❑ Is the information accurate and reliable and, if the 'message' is contested, how evident is that on the leaflet?

❑ How realistic is the 'message'?

❑ What are the key messages? Are there too many? Are they clear? Are they plausible?

❑ Who is the leaflet intended for and is it relevant for your practice population?

❑ What additional information is available and is it reliable? For example, if contact telephone numbers or help lines are given, have you tried them and are they 24 hour? Are they free? Are they pre-recorded messages?

❑ Is the leaflet likely to offend? For example, is it based on shock tactics? Is there racist or sexist language or pictures?

❑ How large is the print size? (Point 12 is minimum.)

❑ How well is it laid out and how appealing is it?

❑ If it is mainly visual, does it convey the message?

❑ Is the leaflet produced in the most common languages of the practice area and, if it is produced in a language you can't read, how will you critique it?

Essentially, we ask what are the aims and objectives of the leaflet and how should it be used to good effect. However, two aspects of the text will now be discussed in further detail.

Readability

Readability is one of the most important aspects of writing a leaflet. It often has to involve taking complex and contested issues and shaping them into a 'one size fits all' short summary. The common goal of many leaflets is to provide information about an issue, with a view to them contributing to the notion of informed decision making. Formulae used for testing readability are based on the adult population in the UK having a reading age of about 12 years. The formula adapted by the Plain English Campaign is the FOG (Frequency of Gobbledegook). The test considers the number of sentences in a 100-word sample, the number of words in a sentence and other factors such as number of words with more than one syllable. The score is a percentage; the higher the percentage, the lower the readability. A good percentage to aim for when producing or critiquing a leaflet for mass usage would be 24–29 per cent, similar to tabloid newspapers and 10 per cent less than most broadsheet newspapers (Ewles and Simnett, 1999).

Translations

Readability tests for leaflets produced for English language users cannot be applied to leaflets produced in other languages. Here the issue of quality is more related to semantics, and there are no major published studies, although many in health promotion have learnt from the experience of working with local and national organizations and interpreters. Most of my professional practice within health promotion has been in the Berkshire area, a multicultural and diverse county. Health visitors in the early 1990s became frustrated about the lack of suitable material for their diverse client groups, which included those with limited literacy skills as well as those for whom English was a second language. Many of their clients were well educated, but their ability to read English was often limited. Some women from Asian backgrounds could speak some English but could not read in any language.

The Department of Health and the HEA contracted my Health Promotion Unit to look at ways of producing health-promotion-related information for multicultural communities. Summarized in Figure 11.7 is the process we adopted.

We worked closely with the adult education groups and quickly found that the information from English could easily be distorted.

- Words could not always translate and alternatives would have to be used.
- One of the most enlightening experiences was that of the increase in formality in the written word used for some Asian languages.
- The Reading Commission for Racial Equality (RCRE) noticed that Urdu and Punjabi took up more space than English.

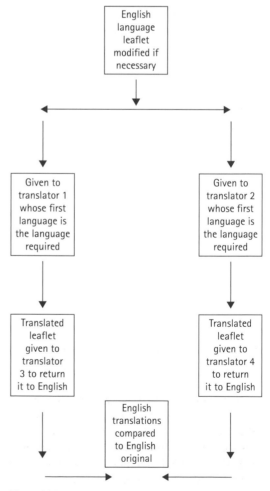

Figure 11.7 Translating health promotion leaflets: a process.

- We found that the translated written word was often similar to the quality of writing in a broadsheet newspaper or, as one community interpreter suggested, 'it was like using a Shakespearean style' that would be inaccessible to many readers and speakers.
- We found in some of the translated leaflets a more direct approach was apparent compared to the original English version. There were sometimes warnings of poor outcome if there was non-compliance with the directive, a type of shock tactic. A typical example was 'Your baby could die if you don't get her vaccinated'. It was in the contested areas that it was most difficult to balance the tone of the leaflet.
- We also found omissions, especially in material about coronary heart disease. For example, smoking and smoking cessation would be given less space in the translated leaflet.
- There was some misleading information. One example concerned the use of fats in cooking. Ghee is a saturated fat used extensively in Indian cooking, but the translated leaflets avoided mentioning this specifically and referred to cooking oils, implying that cooking oils need to be used sparingly, but no such restriction on the favoured ghee. Another concern was related to exercise. Often, the recommendation for women was reworked to imply that exercise was relevant for young women only.

With regard to immunization, many families had seen this as a benefit, and translators who had worked with communities merely used the health beliefs notion – children should be immunized against every disease possible to ward off the risk of death.

It proved difficult to present risk factor advice. Culturally, the changes being suggested to diet (and for some men, smoking) would be 'impossible' and disruptive, and not in line with social norms. What was modifiable for the target communities had to be re-assessed. We were advised that some lifestyle changes could not be even considered, and the leaflet, with its various recommendations, would have no credibility with the intended community. There was also some concern about the notion of premature death in a group of women who felt that, if their husbands died at about 70, that was a good age; why make changes to live longer! However, some of the men from another community had been keen to know more about smoking and coronary heart disease. The leaflets did not explain to them why there was a connection. They accepted smoking carried risks for lung disease, but their understanding of coronary heart disease in their communities was linked to those who drank excessive quantities of alcohol in binge drinking sessions.

It became clear that the cost of producing leaflets in different languages with different alphabets would be high and, if we were to produce them, we must be sure they would be user friendly. This work led to better quality with regard to translated leaflets and the ability to produce local material for the specific communities based on their expressed needs. Many health professionals working in the community became more confident about the information and its reliability but also more realistic about the limitations of leaflets.

Using leaflets

When a leaflet is recommended or given directly to a patient, it is incumbent on the health professional at the very least to have read the leaflet, but preferably to be familiar with it and be confident of its appropriateness.

No matter how good a leaflet is, it is how it is used that matters. The help-yourself option from public areas is appropriate for leaflets with innocuous messages, but would you put leaflets about sensitive sexual information on public display? The chances are that no one will select them unless they are put out especially for a specific clinic such as a family planning clinic. These leaflets may offend some patients and may be the source of amusement for others. Some leaflets are better if used in the clinical context and tailored, if possible, for the user, for example writing on the leaflet personal details or modified goals. Underlining a section or simply explaining in more detail can be helpful.

Generic leaflets can have an important role in health promotion, but this can be enhanced if they are part of a planned intervention and made relevant to the clients' needs. If you are promoting exercise, for example swimming, add some local details, however basic, or have to hand some local information about swimming facilities. Finally, know what the leaflet is about. If it is not ideal for your patient, don't use it; it could mislead or even be harmful!

Practical Exercise

Look at the health promotion leaflets in your practice.
❑ Where are they? Are they well displayed?
❑ What is the range of topics? Are they themed?
❑ Is there a supply of local relevant information?
❑ Have you ever asked or been asked about the usefulness of a health promotion leaflet?
Select one leaflet and do a critique. Does it use active rather than passive tense? If it has a telephone help line, test it out.

POSTERS AND HEALTH PROMOTION

The quality indicators for the health-promoting poster are more subjective than those for leaflets and move into the arena of mass advertising rather than just written language. That said, by returning to the aims and objectives of the intervention, there are some simple indicators to reflect on.

Practical Exercise

Try to visualize the two hypothetical posters in Figure 11.8. Which would you use in a general practice? Would you use both, and, if so, why?

PLANNING FOR HEALTH PROMOTION

It may seem an oxymoron to discuss planned health promotion in the same situation as opportunistic health promotion, but it is and should be possible. The process of planning for health promotion is usually modelled on processes used in the field of education and pedagogy, pedagogy in this instance referring to the science and technology of teaching. These also facilitate evaluation in health promotion. Planning is in itself a skilful activity.

The planning process advocated by Ewles and Simnett (1999) is described in the flowchart in Figure 11.9.

In the one-to-one, opportunistic situation, needs may be identified or expressed by skilful and active listening. The setting of aims leads to a statement of intent about the nature of response to these needs. The objectives are measurable steps that will be taken to reach these aims. Achieving these objectives is dependent on the methods used (such as advice

---

Poster 1 Reduce your risks of skin cancer

This poster could be produced by an authoritative body to be used in a national/European campaign and a batch sent to all NHS sites, together with accompanying leaflets.

The poster lists some risk factors and gives statistics, it informs the reader of the mortality risks and then advises prevention – with a list of 'don'ts' and a small list of 'dos' which includes 'see your doctor if you have a worrying mole similar to the one pictured'. There is a density of written information but the poster is A1 size so large print has been used and the colour is well balanced.

Poster 2 Safety in the sun – three tips!

This poster could be produced by a major commercial organization, which produces skin care products. It would be freely available to the public but also sent to all their retail outlets, local authorities for use in public areas, leisure facilities, day centres, schools and playgroups, childminders, nurseries and youth groups. Large supplies have been sent to health promotion units and the poster is the same as the advertising posters on billboards and buses during May, June and July. The brightly coloured poster has three active tense short sentences:

• Stay in the shade when the sun is at its hottest in the middle of the day
• Wear protective clothing to reduce risk of sunburn
• Use high factor sun block on exposed skin

Each statement has a simple picture to enhance the message.

Figure 11.8 Critiquing health promotion posters.

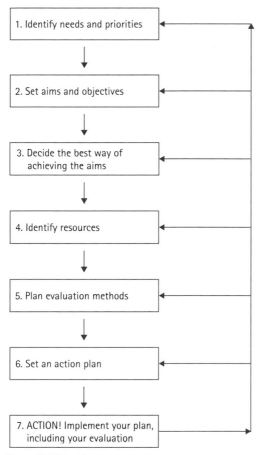

1. Identify needs and priorities

2. Set aims and objectives

3. Decide the best way of achieving the aims

4. Identify resources

5. Plan evaluation methods

6. Set an action plan

7. ACTION! Implement your plan, including your evaluation

Figure 11.9 Flowchart for planning and evaluating health promotion (Ewles and Simnett, 1999).

giving, discussion, demonstration etc.) and the resources needed.

You can evaluate by simply asking the patient or client to summarize or demonstrate, for example. The final aspect of the planning is to set out a realistic, achievable action plan.

Practical Exercise

Your next patient is a middle-aged man recently diagnosed with diabetes who is overweight but not obese. How will you plan the consultation if it is to be health promotion in essence?

Practical Exercise

It is probable that the man has made few changes to his life and diet so far. You will therefore need to explore his feelings about the situation and what he knows about the diagnosis. Your objectives could be to identify his knowledge base about diabetes, to explore his fears, to discuss his current and recent dietary patterns and to negotiate changes that are achievable. The resources may include leaflets, telephone numbers of local support groups or information about the nurse's clinic times. You may see this as a good consultation, patient centred, leading to concordance rather than specifically health promotion. It is, of course, both, but the issue about it being health promotion is related to its planning and its evaluation with regard to a response to modifiable determinants of health.

AIMS AND OBJECTIVES FUNDAMENTAL TO PRACTICE

This planning process, however, is relevant for nearly all health promotion work, including leaflet development, strategic planning, video production and usage, resource packs, media campaigns and facilitating group work. Yet, simple as it may look, writing aims and objectives can be daunting.

Aims need to be realistic statements of intent. They may be informed by public health or government targets, but will usually need refinement for health promotion activity. Let us take physical activity for example. The aims within your practice population could be to increase the access and availability of exercise opportunities for those with disability. The aims may be in line with national targets and local agreements.

So what can the practice do? It could refine the aims to provide information about local facilities to all patients and specifically to explore physical activity with patients who are registered disabled. This would then need to have measurable objectives, such as:

■ to prepare a poster display in the public waiting areas relating to local support and activities and stating where to access add-itional information;

■ to make available a series of specific leaflets both in public areas and for use in all treatment/consultation rooms;
■ to brief the practice team about the project;
■ to do an audit of patients with disability;
■ to liaise with local disability support groups about barriers to physical activity and how to overcome them.

With each of these objectives there is a fur-ther set of skills needed. What becomes clear is that this planned intervention may lead to increased physical activity, but it may not. It will, however, increase knowledge about local facilities and their shortcomings and increase awareness about the needs of people with dis-abilities with regard to physical activities. Planning is therefore an essential and skilful aspect of health promotion work.

If we return to the first objective, poster dis-plays and what needs to be considered, it is back to aims and objectives again. Exactly what is the poster going to convey? Who is it for? Where will it be displayed and is it comple-menting or contradicting other information? Some simple points to consider when develop-ing and using posters include the following.

■ Keep the message clear and simple.
■ Is it appealing to the intended audience?
■ Is it offensive?
■ Will it be legible and visible from the display areas to the viewing areas?
■ Was the cost of the poster affordable or is it free?
■ Does it have a date and the details of its source?
■ Is it free of advertising or sponsorship?

A cluttered poster may have no memorable piece of information; it may offend if the lan-guage is inappropriate; the pictures may be inappropriate; or it targets the wrong age or client group. It may also be lost amongst other posters if not specifically and skilfully dis-played. A simple way of assessing the value of a poster display in general practice is to ask the patients if they noticed it. Did it cause them any concern? What did they think of it and the messages?

In summary, the skills associated with the prac-tice of health promotion in general practice relate to communication skills in the broadest sense, encompassing one-to-one consultations, group work, media activity and the use of leaflets and posters. Evaluation is also skilful and aided by a coherent planning process.

Strategic planning, designing and implement-ing health promotion interventions and commu-nity development will increasingly involve key people from general practice in the UK. It is beyond the scope of this chapter to explore fur-ther the associated skills for such work, but included in the recommended further reading are useful texts such as that by Naidoo and Wills. The skills described in this section could, however, be useful guides to indicators of good practice.

GOOD PRACTICE – ASSESSING AND CONTRIBUTING TO THE EVIDENCE BASE

The systematic review of service provision and activities within general practice is regularly undertaken with a view to assessing if good or best practice is happening and, if not, what changes or training are needed to improve it. These reviews or audits are also related to effect-iveness and efficiency and the accountability of public funds. Audits in general practice may focus on specific areas, often related to clinical practice such as prescribing. However, if an audit of health promotion activity in general practice is being undertaken, the key questions could be as follows.

■ Is the activity defined as health promotion planned, theoretically informed and related to modifiable determinants of health and an informed intervention?
■ Do the activities result in health gain, empowerment and health enhancement and are they undertaken by skilful practitioners, drawing on evidence evaluated and accept-able to all involved?

What counts as evidence-based practice and evidence-based teaching in the field of health promotion is fraught with difficulties, especially with regard to health promotion in the context of general practice.

THE PROBLEMS

The biomedical 'gold standards' of research and evidence are associated with RCTs, which are rigorous and usually large scale. As we have seen, much of health promotion theory and practice is not strictly scientific, but is associated with the social sciences and humanities, where research paradigms differ. Research issues in humanities address reason and rationality, observation and comparison, assessment and review. They may include problem defining, behavioural and theory development research, experimental and action research and dissemination research (Nutbeam, 1996). The research could be linked to identifying determinants and whether they are modifiable or linked to interventions. Most of the research is not generalizable and consists of small-scale studies providing 'greyer' evidence. Interventions are strategic and multi-faceted, with each component being evaluated as appropriate for the practitioners and research funding. This can mean that some interventions have only the most basic of evaluation and no in-depth research aspect.

Health promotion evidence is frequently related to sound argument, judicial approaches and a 'best practice' approach. Not only are some of the research paradigms incompatible with RCTs, but also the results of interventions may be long term and, given the range of variables that cannot be accounted for, it would be unwise to suggest cause and effect. It has taken 40 years in the UK to reduce the smoking prevalence and it is probable that no single approach could be defined as effective (Moore, 2002).

Some argue that the best way to accrue evidence is to fund external research rather than to rely on health professionals having to be practitioner, reflective practitioner and researcher. Many of the problems associated with health promotion evidence relate to intervention evidence. Meanwhile, the research and evidence related to our understanding of determinants and, in particular modifiable determinants, have improved.

THE POSSIBLE SOLUTIONS

Two bulletins, *Bandolier* and *Effective Health Care*, frequently publish reviews of studies related to health promotion, mainly about determinants in the former and interventions in the latter. These publications are now on-line (www.ebandolier.com and www1.york.ac.uk/inst/crd/ehcb.htm) and are easy to read.

The Health Development Agency (HDA) is government funded and has been given the brief to identify the evidence of what works to improve people's health and to reduce health inequalities. In addition, it will provide advice and support. However, it is also able to be realistic about the limitations of evidence in this field, reviewing the intervention's aims and objectives and having informed expectations about proximal and distal outcomes. The HDA's work is helping to further our understanding of important indicators for good practice.

For example, smoking cessation interventions may demonstrate that 12–20 per cent of smokers ceased smoking for 1 week following an intense programme. We would need to see how many people that refers to, how those leaving the programme early are accounted for, and what external factors may have been influencing the behaviour of the group and the individuals. Success needs also to relate to the aims of the programme and the specific objectives, which could have been to raise awareness of smoking cessation support, nicotine replacement treatments and help lines, for example. Realistic expectations for both the health promoter and the smoker influence the evidence base and good practice. Knowing that success rates for smoking cessation can be around 12–20 per cent would enable those involved to consider cost effectiveness and cost benefits before embarking on setting up the intervention. Long-term data on smoking cessation interventions are surprisingly sparse, but this is partially explained by the impact of complex social variables. It would be difficult to claim that a patient who is a non-smoker 12 months after participating in a cessation programme has sustained this non-smoking status as a direct result of the programme.

Interventions may seem to focus on individual behaviour change for success, but if a smoking policy is being introduced for safety reasons in an office block, smoking cessation courses may need to be provided to give smokers the coping skills to be compliant during the working day. Success now is related to compliance with the policy, but none of the smokers needs to become a non-smoker.

In summary, evidence for health promotion practice within general practice is problematic, whether trying to assess evidence or to contribute to the evidence base. Clarity about the nature of the evidence and its application is needed to contribute to good health promotion practice and, increasingly, reliable evidence sources are available on-line. However, the multi-faceted nature of health promotion will result in evidence that is often inconclusive about cause and effect, but can contribute to best practice with regard to interventions and understanding the impact of interventions.

HEALTH PROMOTION AND ETHICAL ISSUES

Health promotion work and values may be seen as a prima facie good activity for the benefit of patients or populations. Yet we have already raised the issue of the potential for harm within the context of health promotion in general practice. The four well-known principles of healthcare ethics (beneficence, non-maleficence, autonomy and justice) together with the Seedhouse Grid (Seedhouse, 1988) are the familiar approaches to ethical issues within health promotion practice. However, much of what is classified as health promotion activity can be potentially harmful.

Screening, for example, is dependent on a critical mass of the target group taking up the screening option. This requires dissemination of the screening provision and encouragement. But screening is about pre-symptomatic disease detection. The possibility of false positives or false negatives may cause distress or foster anxieties. Is early detection always beneficial to both the patient and the health professional? Immunization can hold similar concerns. The need is to have high levels of compliance in the population, so the public are encouraged or advised to be immunized, but what are the individual's risk of getting the disease and/or of a full, uneventful recovery from this disease? Are the public misled about the limitations of immunization and how can we know that individuals have made an informed choice when the evidence is contested or inconclusive?

Working with behavioural change models could result in a challenge to autonomy, victim blaming and coercion, but justified because of duty, a sense of justice and a patient's right to receive expert information or advice.

The public purse is also part of the ethical debate for health promotion: is it just in a democracy to fund interventions that curb people's freedom of choice? Equally, if funds are lacking, what level of sponsorship can be sought, who decides and what impact will that have on the credibility of the interventions?

What are the parameters of health promotion per se and within general practice? As inequalities and social issues are established as determinants of health and disease, what is reasonable and applicable for health promotion activities in general practice needs to be addressed.

We return to Doll and Hill's work in 1964: should a GP raise the issues of smoking with a patient who has come for an unrelated reason? According to the Wanless Report (2001), the health service should be concerned and responsive to disease prevention and reduction. But how does that authorize health professionals to raise lifestyle issues with patients and what harm might that do to the doctor–patient relationship if the patient is unlikely to be able to modify the situation (McLellan, 2002)?

Finally to the notion of being informed and informed consent: how has the information been modified, edited and presented? Are shock tactics acceptable? Is the issue contested and has this lead to empowerment or confusion, apathy or discredit?

Cribb argues that health promotion is inherently contentious and, as such, ethical dilemmas are the norm (Cribb, 2002). The ethical issues may differ or even conflict with those related to health care in general practice, but they should be confronted. As a consequence, activity defined as health promotion may be unacceptable and inappropriate in some instances, while in other situations what was planned may need to be modified.

HEALTH PROMOTION BEYOND THE MEDICAL ARENA

This chapter has already drawn the reader's attention to the work of health promotion beyond the medical arena. This section briefly summarizes the range of issues and settings that are integral to health promotion work.

The issues that have come to be central to most health promotion activity are related to health inequalities at the local level, at a national level, at a European level and globally. In terms of health-related issues, this translates into:

■ nutrition, dietary habits and food safety,
■ violence, crime, drugs and relationships,
■ sexual and reproductive health,
■ accident prevention/risk reduction,
■ mobility,
■ tobacco usage.

This list could easily expand, and all of these issues fall within the remit of many other professionals but within the context of health promotion work, they have come to be part of the mainstay. The definition I have used for health promotion – 'the study of, and the study of the response to, the modifiable determinants of health' – enables health promotion activity to focus on addressing specific issues and to develop aims.

The settings that dominate are schools, workplaces, local communities and neighbourhoods, as well as the healthcare sector. In all these settings, addressing inequalities is central to the activity. It is probable that for those in general practice and primary care, the community setting will be of most interest. In the community or neighbourhood setting, concepts such as social capital have been seen as determinants of health, with social capital being linked to social cohesion, social networks and active involvement. Indeed, the lack of social capital is arguably a factor in crime and fear of crime, according to Wilkinson (1996; Acheson, 1998). Many initiatives are now part of the generic remit of health promotion activity in the community, including addressing crime and safety, the physical environment such as traffic and green space, the social environment and the provision of services.

Finally, I would like to mention the need to be global when thinking about health promotion. The local issues are, of course, central to most of our work, but we need to see where these are in the context of the bigger picture. We need to work with initiatives that complement the WHO policies such as *Health Cities* programmes and *Agenda 21*, and to be aware of the global challenges associated with drug trafficking and the needs of vulnerable mobile populations such as refugees. We also need to be aware of the WHO priorities for health promotion, which include human immunodeficiency virus/acquired immunodeficiency syndrome (HIV/AIDS), tobacco, maternal health, food safety and mental health. The WHO also sees health promotion activity as relevant to the global challenge of certain diseases, their prevention and reduction, diseases such as malaria, tuberculosis, cancer, coronary heart disease and diabetes, the focus predominantly being on reducing inequalities and increasing social capital. Worthy aspirations indeed, but the task is to take them from rhetoric to meaningful reality.

SUMMARY POINTS

To conclude, the most important messages in this chapter are:

■ health promotion is an integral part of general practice work;
■ health promotion is difficult to define, is eclectic and contested, as well as political in nature;
■ a number of theories and models are used to guide practice and identify relevant skills for practice;
■ within the context of general practice, health professionals can be health promoting in their practice and can engage specifically in planned health promotion interventions;
■ the planning of health promotion activity facilitates evaluation, thereby contributing to the growing evidence base that is related to interventions rather than determinants;
■ evidence is from qualitative and quantitative paradigms;
■ ethical issues need to be identified and considered;
■ health promotion seeks to address health inequalities at local, national and international levels, through collaborative working, mainly outside the medical arena, endorsing WHO charters and declarations.

REFERENCES

Acheson, D. 1998: *Independent inquiry into inequalities in health: a report.* London: Stationery Office.

Ashton, J. and Seymour, H. 1988: *The new public health.* Basingstoke: Open University Press.

Bandolier 1999: Exercising the way to better cardiac health. Oxford University, September, 3–5. Also available online at: www.jr2.ox.ac.uk/bandolier

Beattie, A., Gott, M., Jones, L. and Sidell, M. 1993: *Health and wellbeing: a reader.* Basingstoke: Macmillan.

Butler, C.C., Pill, R. and Stott, N. 1998: Qualitative study of patients' perceptions of doctors' advice to quit smoking: implications for opportunistic health promotion. *British Medical Journal* 316(7148), 1878–81.

Cribb, A. 2002: Ethics: from health care to public policy. In: Jones, L. Sidell, M. and Douglas, J. (eds) *The challenge of promoting health*, 2nd edn. Basingstoke: Macmillan, 261–73.

DeBono, E. 1971: *Mechanisms of the mind.* London: Penguin.

Department of Health 1992: *The health of the nation: a strategy for health in England.* London: HMSO.

Doll, R. and Hill, A.B. 1964: Mortality in relation to smoking: ten years' observations on male British doctors (completion part). *British Medical Journal* 5396, 1460–7.

Downie, R.S., Fyfe, C. and Tannahill, A. 1993: *Health promotion models and values.* Oxford: Oxford University Press.

Duncan, P. and Cribb, A. 1996: Helping people change – an ethical approach? *Health Education Research* 11(3), 339–48.

Egan, G. 1982: *The skilful helper.* Brooks/Cole.

Ewles, L. and Simnett, I. 1999: *Promoting health: a practical guide*, 4th edn. London: Baillière Tindall.

Fisher, B. 1994: The Well's Park Health Project. In: Heritage, Z. (ed.) *Community participation in primary care.* Occasional Paper 64. London: Royal College of General Practitioners.

Graham, H. 1988: Women and smoking in the United Kingdom: implications for health promotion. *Health Promotion* 3(4), 371–82.

Graham, H. 1993: *Hardship and health in women's lives.* London: Wheatsheaf.

Health Education Authority 1993: *Helping people change: training course for primary care professionals.* (Pamphlet.) National Unit for Health Promotion in Primary Care. Oxford: Health Education Authority.

Hilton, S., Doherty, S., Kendrick, T., Kerry, S., Rink, E. and Steptoe, A. 1999: Promotion of healthy behaviour among adults at increased risk of coronary heart disease in general practice: methodology and baseline data from the Change of Heart study. *Health Education Journal* 58(1), 3–16.

Illich, I. 1976: *Limits to medicine.* London: Marion Boyers.

Jones, L. and Douglas, J. 2000: The rise of health promotion. In: Katz, J., Peberdy, A. and Douglas, J. (eds) *Promoting health: knowledge and practice*, 2nd edn. Basingstoke: Macmillan, 58–79.

Lalonde, M. 1974: *A new perspective on the health of Canadians.* Ottawa: Ministry of Supply and Services.

McLellan, A. 2002: Public health: has its time come at last – again? *Health Service Journal*, 28th November, p. 17.

Moore, A. 2002: Through a glass darkly. *Health Service Journal*, 7th November, pp. 14–15.

Naidoo, J. and Wills, J. 2000: *Health promotion: foundations for practice*, 2nd edn. London: Baillière Tindall.

Nordenfelt, L. 1995: *On the nature of health: an action theoretic approach*, 2nd edn. Dordrecht: Kluwer Academic.

Nordenfelt, L. 1998: On medicine and health enhancement – towards a conceptual framework. *Medicine, Health Care and Philosophy* 1, 5–12.

Nutbeam, D. 1996: Achieving 'best practice' in health promotion: improving the fit between research and practice. *Health Education Research* 11(3), 317–26.

Pill, R. and Stott, N.C.H. 1990: *Making changes: a study of working class mothers and the changes made in their health-related behaviour over five years.* Cardiff: University of Wales College of Medicine.

Prochaska, J.O. and DiClemente, C.O. 1986: Towards a comprehensive model of change. In: Millen, W.R. and Heathen, N. (eds) *Treating addictive behaviors: process and change.* New York: Plenum Press, 3–27.

Rawson, D. 1992: The growth of health promotion theory and its rational construction: lessons from the philosophy of science. In: Bunton, R. and Macdonald, G. (eds) *Health promotion: disciplines and diversity.* London: Routledge, 202–24.

Rogers, C.R. 1980: *A way of being.* Boston: Houghton Mifflin Co.

Rowntree Foundation 1995: *Rowntree report on income and wealth.* York: Joseph Rowntree Foundation.

Seedhouse, D. 1988: *Ethics: the heart of health care.* Chichester: Wiley.

Seedhouse, D. 1997: *Health promotion: philosophy, prejudice and practice.* Chichester: Wiley.

Tones, K. 1991: Reflections on health promotion and education. *Health Education Research* 6, 1–3.

Townsend, P. and Davidson, N. 1982: *Inequalities in health: the Black Report.* London: Penguin.

Wanless, D. 2001: *Securing our future health: taking a long-term view: interim report.* London: HM Treasury.

Wilkinson, R. 1996: *Unhealthy societies: the afflictions of inequalities.* London: Routledge.

Woolfe, R. 1996: Becoming a counsellor. In: Hales, G. (ed.) *Beyond disability.* London: Sage.

World Health Organization 1986: *Ottawa Charter for Health Promotion.* Geneva: World Health Organization.

World Health Organization 1997: The Jakarta Declaration on Leading Health Promotion into the 21st Century. *International Journal of Health Education* 35(4), 133–4.

Wylie, A. 2002: Health promotion in medical undergraduate curricula: a question of definition. The 10th Ottawa Conference on Medical Education, Ottawa.

FURTHER READING

Jones, L., Sidell, M. and Douglas, J. (eds) 2002: *The challenge of health promotion,* 2nd edn. Basingstoke: Macmillan (Open University).

This is a text book used by level 3 students on the K301 Health Promotion course at the Open University.

Katz, J., Peberdy, A. and Douglas, J. (eds) 2000: *Promoting health: knowledge and practice,* 2nd edn. Palgrave/Open University.

This is both a stand-alone book and one used by level 3 students on the K301 Health Promotion course at the Open University, preparing for the award of honours degree. It is comprehensive, well referenced and provides the reader with questions and exercises to develop critical thinking and practical application of concepts.

Naidoo, J. and Wills, J. 2000: *Health promotion: foundations for practice,* 2nd edn. London: Baillière Tindall.

This text is seen as standard reading for both health promotion practitioners and students regardless of level. It is pragmatic, covers theoretical and practical issues and provides good background information.

Seedhouse, D. 1997: *Health promotion: philosophy, prejudice and practice*. Chichester: Wiley.

This textbook raises issues about values and ethics, provides the reader with a framework for critical thinking about the health promotion in our society and considers some parameters for practice.

Tones, B.K. and Tilford, S. 2001: *Health promotion: effectiveness, efficiency and equity*, 3rd edn. London: Stanley Thornes, Chapman Hall.

This textbook is standard reading for those doing higher degrees in the field of health promotion, but is also valuable for those who plan at strategic level and want critically to evaluate health promotion activity.

12

HEALTHCARE ETHICS AND LAW

Broader questions about what is best for patients or staff, what it is right to do, or whether we are acting within the law commonly arise in practice for anyone who reflects on their work. This chapter suggests ways of approaching these issues and reaching conclusions that are satisfactory for all concerned.

LEARNING OBJECTIVES

By the end of the chapter, you will be able to:

- identify where moral and legal questions may arise in your work;
- understand how the law, professional regulation and medical ethics may ask different things of the practising doctor;
- confront the complexity of these requirements by thinking about potential duties and possible consequences in practice;
- understand the contribution of thinking in terms of a balance of principles, giving weight to important values, and exploring the different perspectives of all involved to creating the best outcome possible in each situation.

CONFLICT AND COMPROMISE

Becoming a doctor may seem a very complicated process. There is a great deal to find out about and a lot of new skills to develop. Creating order from so many different intellectual sources is hard. General practice may seem even more confusing, as the focus of each new consultation, or the focus within each consultation, moves from topic to topic. It is possible to feel like a cork in a strong current, bobbing about from pool to pool, losing your sense of direction, and with it your view of what properly should be done. In order to make good sense of what you are doing, and to end the day feeling you have done things right (on balance), at least you have to *start* with a clear idea of what it is best to do and what sort of person you should be. If this is challenged by events, you should have some way of sorting out the conflicts that seem to present themselves.

Ethics and law help with this process. Consider this situation.

CASE STUDY 12.1

The patient was 35, and had just been discharged from hospital after treatment for his first grand mal fit. Further investigations were in progress, but the specialist thought it wise for him to be on anti-epileptic drugs for the moment. The patient tells his GP that he is very pleased to get out of hospital and they treated him well.

His wife has recently been made redundant after she was injured by a hit-and-run driver. They have four young children, one of whom may need to go to a special school. The patient is self-employed, and needs the money. He wants to get back to work. He drives a taxi.

There are lots of further details the GP might want to know. The diagnosis is not completely certain yet. The balance of the patient's drugs needs care. He can't remember what happened to him, so he is not unduly worried. But the regulations, enshrined in law in the UK, are clear. After a fit like this he is not allowed to drive for the moment, certainly not a public service vehicle.

On the other hand, the doctor knows all too well, because she also looks after the wife and family, how desperate things are at home: the welfare of the whole family depends on the patient. The doctor has several other patients who she thinks should work but don't. This man wants to work, and can't see why he shouldn't. Without his income, this family is going to be in trouble financially, and so possibly in other ways. The fit may never happen again. If all goes well, no one will know.

The doctor is under enormous pressure from different sources. She has to resolve this in the consultation quickly. But she has to get it right. If he does have another fit, at the wheel of his taxi, many people, including himself and his passenger, may get hurt. There are problems posed by the illness, the treatment, the family, the man's attitude and issues of communication. But most of all, the doctor has to decide what is right.

When you are not sure what to do, there is a temptation to gather more and more information, to amass more details. Surely something extra we can find out may help? This is certainly true in the sense that the investigations may find a cause of the fit. But they won't tell the doctor what it is best to do. She has to know the law and the regulations about driving. She has to convince the patient. She also has to think through her attitudes to the various harms that could come from each action, or lack of action (for even doing nothing is in this case a kind of action with consequences). In her head, or with colleagues, she will have an ethical discussion.

Discussion in ethics is concerned about right and wrong. Factual evidence may be important, but values are even more so. It is less about 'what' than about 'why' or 'how'. The origins of ethics are in custom and behaviour, in questions that are often called normative. In order to know what could be wrong, and what is best (or better) in the circumstances we find ourselves in, we shall need to be able to look at both (or all) sides of a question, and to balance the arguments for and against on each side. We shall need to know something about what are good and what are bad arguments, and what are good processes for reaching an outcome when people disagree.

Although a kind and caring doctor may have been put on the spot by the taxi driver's determination to return to work, to someone who has not yet taken over clinical care of patients there seems to be a right answer waiting somewhere. Similarly, for you as a student about to sit in on a consultation with a teaching GP, there may be a series of quite obvious, but nevertheless important, questions to ask. How are you going to spend your time together: sorting out the patient's problems or helping you to learn medicine? Is the patient happy to have someone sitting in on the consultation and hearing what is said? Has the patient been warned, and has he or she the option of asking the student to leave or of seeing another professional without a student? Conventionally, these last questions bring together the two issues of *confidentiality* and *consent*. However, other issues may be lurking in the wings that may creep up unawares, as it were. You may be keen to learn, but have to get away to prepare for another class. The doctor may have to sort out an employment problem in the practice or squeeze other activities between the surgery and her afternoon visits. In the rush, you may find yourself watching or even being asked to do something that does not feel to you to be the *best practice*. Have you done all you could, or even the best you could in the circumstances? Have all the patient's concerns been properly addressed? You and your teacher may be involved in a *conflict of roles*. The satisfaction of the patient is set against the demands for preparation for the student, or one properly sorted medical presentation against the needs of the practice or another patient. There are trade-offs and compromises to be made to get through a working day, and sometimes these leave us with a lurking dissatisfaction or guilt – or even, perversely, a sense of pride in coping which our best selves know is only waiting for a fall.

Luckily, however, as humans we are used to these sorts of conflicts. We are equipped both to detect them and to make decisions about them. We have what has been called a moral sense, which helps us to think about what is best or right, and helps us to decide when things are going wrong. It has links with all sorts of functions in our body and mind. It links with our emotions as well as our memories, our hopes and our plans. Its activation often seems to be a thing called conscience, and its guidance depends on what we believe in and value. Although religion may have a lot of say about what we should do, the approach to thinking about how we should live, whatever our beliefs, is called ethics or morality. Although different groups of people may end up with slightly different ways of looking at things, it is clear that humankind is at one in needing to make ethical judgements. These judgements, when groups of people agree, may be represented in different cultures and contexts as moral rules or as laws.

Some things that ethics may help with include:

- deciding when there is a moral question to be addressed,
- naming or describing that question,
- giving us the language to address the question,
- helping us to understand the concepts in that language,
- enabling us to look at the arguments for different approaches,
- deciding what are good and what are bad arguments,
- coming to a conclusion so that we know what to do,
- enabling us to express clearly the justifications for that choice.

MEDICAL ETHICS AND LAW

If ethics and law tell us about right and wrong, is there any reason why we need a specific knowledge of medical ethics? Is medicine any different from other things that people do? Can doctors make reasonable claims to be exempt from everyday rules? We are all citizens or members of a social group even when we are doctors. We are bound, as everyone else in society, by laws or traditions of conduct. We know that in moments of calm reflection, but it is very easy to forget it in the heat of the moment, if as clinicians we get too enthusiastic about or exhausted by the demands of medical practice. Responding to sick people and saving lives seem sometimes to have an imperative that overrides other considerations. What has been clear to doctors and patients for hundreds of years now is that, although doctors are bound by society's rules or laws, something *extra* is required in medical relationships and in the organization of health care. A trainee on a supermarket checkout would not have to ask the customer before watching the process. What the customer bought would not have to be secret. Centuries ago, doctors in ancient Greece thought about medical practice and decided that the doctor was in a strongly privileged but also a vulnerable position. To practise medicine properly, he (doctors were men in those days) would have to behave in a certain way, and promise solemnly to do so under all circumstances. Most of the oath attributed to a man called Hippocrates rings true today, even though our lives have changed so much. (It did not cover everything: some challenges, like whether to tell patients the truth about their condition, were never mentioned in the original oath.) Doctors need to have a particular view of their own conduct or character in order to maintain the trust of the society in which they work.

The Hippocratic Oath is traditionally linked with a doctor who lived in Greece in the ninth century BC, though who wrote the original oath is uncertain. Kenneth Boyd, in the *New dictionary of medical ethics*, sums up the oath as:

A solemn promise: a) of solidarity with teachers and other physicians; b) of beneficence and non-maleficence towards patients; c) not to assist suicide or abortion; d) to leave surgery to surgeons; e) not to harm, especially not to seduce patients; f) to maintain confidentiality and never gossip.

Most medical schools these days do not ask qualifying doctors to swear an oath, but all who practise in the UK must work to the rules laid down by the General Medical Council (GMC). This body publishes clear guidelines, which have recently become even more explicit in the UK after pressure from government and society in the wake of recent medical scandals. Most other countries have the same or similar arrangements, some directly following the lead of the GMC. Doctors could act completely within the law of the country they work in and still find themselves in trouble with their regulating authority. These rules, guidelines or statements act like a sort of evolving 'oath in progress'. We may not think about them all the time, or even at all, and may not be able to quote them, but they exist to form and frame the world we work in. Some of this helps to make it clear when we might fall foul of the law, were we not doctors, and some of it helps to clarify legal requirements.

Sometimes, however, it appears more complicated than that.

THE LAW AND PROFESSIONAL REGULATION IN PRACTICE

The frameworks of legal and professional regulation on occasion appear to differ greatly in what they demand or offer to doctors and patients. This is strange, because both are derived from what a society considers it right to do. As the emphasis or balance of thinking in any society may change, so may laws and professional regulations. As an aside, we should also be aware that there might be important differences between different countries from time to time. Any health professionals going to practise in another country would be foolish not to check out the approaches in that country; some countries might require them to take a special course or pass a new exam, and would probably want them to join a new local regulatory body. How and why do the approaches of these different regulating forces differ?

It is easier to answer this question in terms of how each responds when things go wrong. The law often says little specific about things that matter a lot in medical practice. For example, until recently, the law in England and Wales on medical confidentiality was very sparse. Doctors are seen in law as having to do things that other people usually do not do, hence the need for examinations, regular appraisal and a special registration. The law expects doctors to get on with being doctors without being told what to do. It is only likely to become involved if something criminal happens. It may not, of course, be absolutely obvious what would constitute a crime; in the words of one English lawyer, 'the law doesn't tell you what to do, it only tells you after you've done it whether it was lawful or not'. This may sound alarming, but in most countries courts and judges know all too well how difficult it is to make good judgements in the heat of the moment and so are reluctant to criticize doctors. What is more, they are likely to be cautious about making a legal decision that would have the consequence of depriving patients of medical care because doctors would be unable or too nervous to act. Most judgements will therefore follow, rather than lead, major changes in public opinion. This is certainly important in countries where the law is based on the English legal system, which relies to a great extent on cases and precedent. In this system, judges base their own legal opinions and advice to juries on the foundations of the thinking about previous similar cases. From time to time, the government may intervene and pass new laws. These new laws will then have to be applied to specific cases, which may need further legal deliberation. Doctors, too, learn how to make judgements in specific cases based on an amalgam of science and practice. So the major protection from falling foul of the law (or any supervisory body for that matter) will always be to think clearly about the options. We should think *why* we have made a particular choice, and then, whenever possible, we should *write down our reasons* as well as just the decision. If we can be seen to be acting intelligently and rationally in our proper professional capacity and not just on a whim, even if others subsequently disagree, we can feel at peace with ourselves. We did what we thought was right at the time based on good reasons and clear thinking.

Things do not always turn out the way we hoped and intended they would, however, so there remains another anxiety about the law. Even if we act within the law, if something goes wrong, will we be sued for damages? This concerns a different part of the law, and is too complex to be dealt with here, but again we are protected by good professional conduct. If we asked for consent to a procedure, for instance if we explained what we were going to do, introduced the other options and warned a patient properly about possible harms, and then we did in the procedure what we said we would do, if things eventually do go wrong, we may be upset but we need not feel to blame or personally at fault. All doctors must have insurance, at all stages of their professional lives, to cover this sort of eventuality, which protects the patients as well as the doctor against sheer bad luck.

So if we are good citizens, the likelihood of falling foul of the criminal law is remote, and we

are protected, provided we act properly, if patients sue us when things go wrong. What then is the role of bodies like the GMC? Here, the focus is more specifically medical and the concerns and penalties are different. Medical processes as well as outcomes are important. Standards rise all the time, in practice as well as in the application of science. These changes will be reflected much more rapidly in what the GMC expects of us than they might be in the law. What is expected, in turn, will usually be clearly expressed in written form, and may be much more prescriptive. We should read what is written in all GMC documents carefully, and take careful notice of how the views of that body change.

There will be a further level, where patients may complain locally within the health service, either to the general practice itself or to one of the local regulatory bodies linked to the current structure. Managed well, such complaints can often have a positive effect: with the guidance of a disinterested party, misunderstandings can be corrected, apologies made and the relationship repaired. Sometimes, as professionals, we can actually improve our approach or raise the standards of the service by reflecting on these complaints. Another approach would be to use a potential mistake or 'near miss' as a critical incident to challenge and improve practice. It is hard to see it this way sometimes, because we feel upset when people complain about us, but mistakes remain a potent source of education all our working lives.

GOOD PRACTICE AND THE MORAL STRANGER

If falling foul of the law or the GMC happens only to the careless or unfortunate few, and many patient complaints can be used (whilst apologizing) to improve our practice and set things straight, nevertheless it would be a narrow, sad or neurotic doctor whose sole or even main aim was just to keep out of trouble. If we want to be good doctors and deliver the best practice, every single contact between one person and another has the potential for improving things, or the reverse, and so has a moral component. It is almost as if each consultation has its own little textbook of medical ethics waiting to be written about it. But even if half the medical profession were employed by regulating authorities to write about how the other half were doing it, this could (thank goodness!) never cover all the eventualities. The chart may be there, as it were, but *we* need to do the navigation. One of the earliest writers on ethics or how people should live, a Greek philosopher called Aristotle, regularly used two analogies to illustrate his thinking – the work of a ship's captain and the profession of being a doctor. For the captain, there is the tide, the wind, the type and condition of the boat: even with the latest computer, anyone who ventures to sea has to use all their knowledge, skill, professional experience and intuition to get the best out of the voyage and return safely to land.

So it is in the consultation. What is uncharted here may also be very extensive, especially in general practice. We see elsewhere in this book the many different things patients may bring to their GPs. It is likely they, too, will be wondering what sort of doctor they are going to meet and what his or her approach will be. Even if patient and professional know each other well, the tide and weather of anxiety, exhaustion, depression or excitement may overwhelm the usual responses on either side. One of the fascinations of medicine (and law) is that when the lid is taken off individual lives, what happens in private is often very different from what the outside world might expect. The bouncer who listens to Mozart, the social work manager who goes on gambling holidays, the vicar who beats up her husband, the doctor who seems the model medic but is struggling to keep up: life is full of surprises. Pluralistic modern society raises further problems. It might be possible in very settled societies to be clear about what the 'rules' are, or how each family would 'play it', but in a modern urban society, even these direction signs are few and far between, or may even point in the wrong direction at times of crisis. People of different generations and with different experiences may make choices for themselves outside their ethnic, religious or family tradition. So each patient comes to us as what the American ethicist Tristan Engelhart has called a 'moral stranger'. We do not know how they will approach a particular

problem before we see them. As doctors, we certainly have to get to know our patients' medical problems, but we also have to get to know their way of thinking and the choices they intend to make – their moral responses. We have, as it were, to make a *value diagnosis* as well as a medical one; and we need to do it swiftly and surely and without compromising our own values or moral position – assuming, that is, that we can identify and have thought through the issue we find ourselves facing.

MORAL ANTENNAE: WHAT ARE THE ISSUES?

At the beginning of the chapter it was suggested that some moral issues we meet in the consultation might, in theory, be absolutely obvious: just by sitting in with a GP, a student raises a set of questions about the patient agreeing to have a third person in the consultation. However, in practice, it may not be quite so easy to see all that could go wrong, even if we have that agreement. A sensitive student, paying attention, may see that the patient is looking uneasy or trying to talk about something that the doctor, because of his or her interest in the physical symptoms or in teaching, has not noticed. A question from the clinician may catch the patient off guard, and the patient may start to unburden himself about something deeply personal; it may be clearly inappropriate for the student to be involved and the student may feel the need to withdraw. All of these observations may be part of the skill that some have in abundance, but others may need to develop: of being sensitive to moral and psychological issues and responding appropriately. It may not always be easy to name precisely all of these issues. What we may have is a *feeling* that we cannot immediately put into words, or one that may not be adequately expressed by the words available. However, the importance of noting that something is going wrong or that there is a hidden problem that needs addressing cannot be overstated. Our natural moral antennae link to our emotional awareness, and it is this as much as anything else which helps us to find our way on the moral chart. Unnoticed or unaddressed, the issue may act as a trap for all involved, and the emotional feeling, instead of being a signal for reflection or for going carefully, may burst out. Someone may get angry or become upset. Responses may be inappropriate; the treatment may be poorly directed or key issues may be held back and missed. A patient may complain or leave the list, a doctor may go home dispirited or go off to do some other type of work. So one of the important things to notice in medical work is a change in the emotional climate, within oneself, in the patient, or in the interaction. It signals, usually, a moral problem – one that is unidentified or unaddressed, but desperately needs attention.

ROLES, RULES AND DUTIES

One thing that commonly causes a consultation to stall is confusion about what is being done, the task in hand, as we have seen in the teaching situation. With the best will in the world, clinicians may find themselves changing what they are doing or being asked to do without realizing fully what is happening. Staying with the teaching situation, a fellow GP from another room suddenly lights on an unusual physical sign, and breaks into the teaching consultation to ask the student to come and see something. The student, delighted, goes out into a room where a patient is unprepared for teaching. The patient demonstrates the sign (or, worse, becomes 'teaching material') and the second doctor teaches the student extensively; then the student leaves and the patient is bundled out of the room. It would be very funny if it weren't so destructive, or if it were more unusual.

We saw above a role conflict for a doctor between duty to an individual patient and to running the service as a whole, but even within one consultation, roles may suddenly change. A patient may reveal something that may challenge the doctor as a fellow citizen – such as a crime or major misdemeanour. Either party may start a conversation that owes more to friendship or more intense feelings than to a professional relationship. Other conflicts of role may simply be built in, and there all the time. A country doctor may have to look after his staff's medical

problems, or his own family's. The counsel of perfection would be to avoid these conflicts, but if that is not possible, at least to be aware of them, even if they are not made explicit.

One of the main reasons to keep a close check on the task in hand is that each role may carry its own rules, separate from those of clinical practice: a teacher may be bound by one set of regulations, a researcher by another; a citizen may feel bound to act, or a neighbour be inhibited from doing so. These rules may seem to get in the way, designed to trip us up, but in reality they are to protect us from making these sorts of mistakes. They look ahead, as it were, to the job to be done and say: 'If you are to do this sort of job or to be in this sort of position, you must be prepared to be the kind of person who acts in this sort of way'.

In order that other people who are to be involved know what they are going to be involved in, you make *promises* about what you are going to do and how you are going to do it, and these promises become part of broader *duties* that we undertake. Without them, people could not know what to expect, and how to trust us in difficult situations. Without them, we as professionals would not know how to resist other desires or outside forces that come to frustrate these promised actions. We are only human, and get tired, bored, fascinated by something else. Our shift is over, we get a phone call or a text message and our concentration goes elsewhere. Our promise in practice keeps us at the task until we have completed it. Our duties define what else we could or could not do in the course of our work.

ABSOLUTE DUTY?

Duty is a word with rather a heavy feel to it. It is something we owe, because we said we would. People then have a claim on us to deliver. They have a *right* to expect something from us. But we must be consistent as well as reasonable. We cannot pick and choose, say, to tell the truth on Fridays but not on Mondays or on our own in outpatients but not when we are put on the spot in a ward round. Because that consistency is so basic to our lives, such duties (and, reciprocally, other people's rights) are often thought of as

HEALTHCARE ETHICS AND LAW

absolute. To go back to the issue of confidentiality, patients would not be as open as they should be to doctors when discussing some conditions if they did not know that what they describe or relate will be kept in confidence between them and the doctor. The patient asks, 'Is this absolutely confidential?'; it forms the basis of trust between the two parties. This is why a student who joins a teacher comes under that banner, enters with that promise. Were that not so, medicine and teaching medicine as we know it now would not be possible. Any discussion of that consultation elsewhere, after the patient has left, is bound by the same duty. To ensure this, notes in the practice must be kept secure. Anything a student writes and takes away must be completely anonymized.

But an uneasy feeling is creeping in already. This does not feel like *absolute* confidentiality. A third person has come into the interaction. The patient gave his consent to the student being there; but was it also given to the discussion afterwards, and the taking away of anonymous notes? The consent for these could be considered, by extension, to be implied. But what if the student shares this information with a teaching group? What if the doctor needs to write a letter to a specialist and so has to put the letter on a tape to be typed by a secretary? What about a receptionist making a phone call about the patient, or the doctor consulting a colleague about the best form of referral? From inside the system, we can see that any of these situations may be necessary for effective care and proper teamwork, so all these people – student, group teacher, secretary, receptionist, professional colleague – are still bound by the same duty of confidentiality, and that this formed a *cordon* around this group of people. It is a shock to find in researching such an area that the general public does not understand it this way (Carmen and Britten, 1995), so there is probably some informing of the public to be done. But could the idea and ideal of absolute confidentiality be stretched to apply to a group? Some may feel that the phrase has now lost its meaning.

However, the idea of absolute confidentiality may be challenged in another way. It is not difficult to envisage a situation in which a clinical secret kept within a group committed to the duty becomes completely impossible to keep. Someone is being abused, or someone is in danger. In these circumstances, duty suddenly stands on its head. There now seems to be another duty we have signed up to, whether as doctor or citizen; in this case, to protect vulnerable people in danger. Society expects us to deal with medical harms, but we may also feel we have to deal with some harms unearthed in the consultation that go beyond the strictly medical. Confidentiality is not 'absolutely absolute', after all. How can we negotiate these new and difficult waters and decide what to do?

HANDLING DUTIES AND CONSEQUENCES

When we make a promise, we may not have foreseen all the possible situations that may arise which may challenge that promise. For instance, it is unlikely that two people who promise to love and look after each other would at the beginning think through what this would mean if there were a war and one of them was called away to wartime duty. But in medicine, we should know enough at least about the possibility of conflicting demands and so should think ahead. For example, if we think there is even the outside chance that we might have to break confidentiality, say in a case of child abuse (which the GMC and most legal authorities would think there is), we should not make an absolute promise: we should be adding the rider 'under normal circumstances' at the very least, and be prepared to indicate where we thought normal circumstances would end. Perhaps it would be when there was another (and potentially overriding or trumping) claim on us. Although some might say this was too meticulous, at some level or other the public needs to know, and perhaps even be reassured, that we, too, accept the force of the other claims that society would feel had overriding importance.

However, duties do not only face competition from other duties. Medicine judges itself in scientific terms or in terms of evidence assessed largely by *outcomes*. Is this treatment better than that? What should we do in order to improve lives or reduce suffering? In some situations, where one outcome would clearly be the best

('best' in the limited sense of best for the immediate people we are concerned with), duties prevent us from overstepping the mark. A single daughter of 60 faces retirement looking after a completely demented mother who has previously said she would rather die than be a burden to other people. The better *consequences* here may be in clear opposition to the duties set by medicine (to maintain life) and certainly by the law (not to kill). Clearly, we should look for other options – an old people's home, extensive day care services or whatever would enable both mother and daughter to live reasonable lives in their different ways. But sometimes the balance may seem more difficult. Before the 90-year-old mother developed her dementia, a routine blood test demonstrated that she had some leukaemic cells in her white cell series. These were mildly aggressive, and certainly not likely to threaten her life more than other things: the specialist advice was to do nothing. But when she asked whether her blood test was all right, what should we have said? Telling her that she had leukaemia but that we were going to do nothing about it would probably raise unnecessary anxiety which we would have no chance of settling, and which might even cause her to lose faith in her doctor. There may be many ways round this, but at this stage, this pits a clear *duty* that the doctor has – to tell the truth to the patient about issues which concern her health – against a *consequence* – telling her about something that might cause major anxiety, and possibly blight the rest of her life.

This is one of the many situations in which we find ourselves trying to balance things that not only are not similar, but that are not even measured on the same scale. These are incommensurable, and we just have to accept that. We are left to make a moral balance. Outside bodies are unlikely to have the answer. It is just that professionals tend to act in one way, while perhaps our intuitions or conscience may point in another, and so we may be left confused. The culture of our society may be in transition, or people may differ. We need a way of assessing the options and coming to a decision.

At least three different ways have been advanced to help us try to bring incommensurable things to a balance. In the first, we can try to analyse what *principles* underlie different arguments and bring them together to create a way forward. As another way of thinking, we can focus not so much on what to do as on what sort of person we should be, and try to act in that way by looking at *virtues* and *values*. Finally, we could examine the different *perspectives* of the actors in each drama and combine them into a type of story, turning our responses into a narrative, and try to 'tell our way' through the problem.

In the paragraphs that follow, we look at each of these approaches. One may be more appealing than the others; one may fit the circumstances better than others. There may be yet other ways of looking at things that may be important for individuals, or may help particular branches of the healthcare professions. Probably, however, the best (or better) option requires us to use at least all three of these approaches as part of the 'ethical circuit' of thinking (Fig. 12.1).

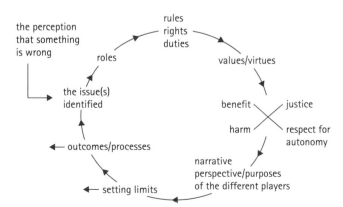

Figure 12.1 The 'ethical circuit' of thinking.

FOUR PRINCIPLES AND SCOPE

The elderly woman with her abnormal blood count brings us to the quite obvious idea that at work we are trying to help or benefit people, and certainly to reduce things that may be or are threatening to be harmful to them. The first, the principle of doing good for people – often called in medicine a duty of care – is known as *benefi-cence.* The contrast with commerce may be too simplistic, but however ethical a company, the bottom line in business is profit for shareholders, not benefit or care for customers. However, even in business, a company might get into trouble if it caused harm to its customers, and in medicine the imperative to minimize or avoid harming people is even stronger. The principle of reducing harm is called *non-maleficence*: it has defined our decision that we might break confidence if a consultation revealed abuse. Sometimes even more important is the idea that in order to help people we actually have to do things that, outside medicine, would be considered as harms: the surgeon has to cut; the medicine has side effects. So doctors usually cannot avoid the possibility of harm, but have to reduce it as much as possible and set it against the good to be achieved. Thus we have to balance, in our work or life, benefits and harms, just as politicians or economists balance these ideas.

However, for the last 40 years or so in Western medicine, another idea has become important. Even if the doctor can see what is best done to help a patient, what about that patient's own view of what should be done? More and more, we have realized recently that even if the doctor knows best in general, second guessing a patient's own personal choices or preferences is not the right way to work. People should be able to choose what happens to their own bodies and lives. Overriding their decisions, with the best of motives, is likely to lead to a poor outcome or may actually disable the individual into being a 'permanent patient'. It may simply be illegal. Helping people to achieve their own goals increasingly seems like a great benefit. Doing something that seems like the best medicine at the time but which the patient does not want is a major harm.

These sorts of ideas lie behind keeping medical secrets and getting people's permission before we do anything that affects them directly. This thinking about individual choice grew out of the political arena in Europe and America over the last 400 years (the earlier part of which is sometimes called 'the Enlightenment' because it opposed the traditional but unscientific approaches of mediaeval times). So the words used were similar to those used in political discussion about countries wishing to rule themselves. Each individual was seen as his or her own sovereign in matters of personal choice. It was considered important to recognize that each person should be treated as an autonomous individual. *Autonomy* means ruling or providing the laws for oneself. That could be interpreted as each person doing what he or she liked, but that freedom is, of course, constrained by other people's freedom, so some of the boundaries are clearly set. As one Enlightenment thinker, Jeremy Bentham, said, 'your freedom to swing your stick ends where my nose begins'. Every person should acknowledge the importance of the choices individuals make about their own lives: we should *respect their autonomy* in being able to think, desire and actually do what they wish whenever we can if that is not in conflict with the autonomy of other people.

That freedom to make choices about things that concern our own personal lives has been translated from the grand political scene into that of personal politics in some sectors of modern life in the West. Between consenting adults in private, for instance, their sexual preferences are their business and theirs alone, much as choice of clothes, music or flowers to put in a window box are theirs (in our ideal world!) and no-one else's. Where there are clashes, in home or at the workplace, we prefer shared or negotiated decisions to someone simply being told what to do. We believe that people should achieve their potential and should, wherever possible as adults, be empowered to make their own decisions and choices.

However, in health care this has seemed less easy to achieve. One of the reasons why individual choice is difficult to apply is that people often cannot easily make medical judgements about themselves. Patients cannot easily examine parts of their own bodies. If they can, they may not know what that examination means or what to do about it because they lack the medical knowledge. That drugs are dangerous poisons as well as potential cures means that most important ones are available only on a doctor's prescription. So, until the middle of the last century, most medical (and healthcare) practice was largely *paternalistic* in style: doctor or nurse knew best; the patient's duty was to obey orders. Whether there are still situations in which that still applies is under debate, but even with improving self-diagnostic aids, more access to medical knowledge for lay people, and over-the-counter medicines, it is still clear that patients are often not able to express their choices properly. They may be disabled by anxiety, too ill to think straight, or actually unconscious. If the healthcare worker is to act properly, the autonomy of the patient has to be *respected* even if it cannot be expressed. This may be done by acting as the person would choose to act, or we know did choose to act before they became ill, by working to get patients into a situation in which they can really make their own choices again, or by avoiding going beyond certain sorts of boundaries in decision making – unless there are overwhelming reasons to do so, defined by obvious benefits or harms. This is important whether the concerns are major or the decisions are everyday ones. (Emergencies carry their own special duties: no one who suddenly collapsed in the waiting room would expect the staff not to attempt a resuscitation just because they hadn't had a chance to get permission for it.) However, the terminally ill patient who has thought things through and wants no further treatment of the current type should have his or her choice respected, even if clinicians are disappointed with this choice. The same sort of thinking defines the approach to time off work for a nasty but self-limiting illness like 'flu, the approach to understandable depression, or choosing alternative medicine. By not listening to the patients' decisions or choices, healthcare workers can treat them like children. This is not only wrong in itself, but sometimes delays recovery.

Thus three important principles contribute to resolving a conflict – doing good, avoiding harm, and respecting autonomy. However, our choices may be limited not only by what we know or can comprehend, but also by what can be afforded. A practitioner in Somalia may have a different range of options from one in Southwark or Saskatchewan. We may regret that, but it is reality. Equally, in different countries the healthcare system may have made different decisions about what type of care takes priority for funding, or how one chooses between two people with the same condition when only one can be treated. These are issues of *justice*.

We are all brought up in our families to have a view of what is fair, and how to address the situation when something is unfair. Most political movements are driven by similar thoughts writ large. These ideas of what is fair or just permeate health care too, whether it be to deal with a problem when someone has overstepped the mark and done something really wrong (*retributive* justice), or in circumstances in which there is not enough of something to go round (*distributive* justice). Some people think that there is a natural ceiling for healthcare demand, when everyone has enough for their needs.

The National Health Service (NHS) in the UK was planned with that in mind: it was assumed that as people got healthier, calls on the service would be reduced. For whatever reasons, however, most people now do not think it works that way. It seems as if however much is put into any healthcare system, it will be inadequate for everyone's wants and for improvements in health care. Distributive justice in this view will always be with us. This approach not only sees a problem of how to distribute resources such as curative drugs or doctors' time, but also (whether funding comes from the state or some commercial system) detects a general shortage of what is needed to satisfy the needs of the population overall. If the majority are right, or if the political will to correct an overall deficiency is not found, people working in health care will always have to make awkward decisions about how to allocate resources, not only on the expanding edge of bioscience but also in the centre of routine medical work. We saw at the beginning of the chapter the dilemma that might have faced the student and the busy teaching GP concerning how to make sure each patient's needs were properly addressed and that some of the other calls on the student's and doctor's time were attended to. Good communication and time management skills may have helped, but something more was needed: choices had to be made.

Some progress may be made by looking at the *scope* or *limits* of the issue under discussion. A patient may present a problem, such as a dispute with a neighbour, which is quite properly not in the doctor's province. Someone else may want to talk so extensively about a psychological problem or have such a complex complaint that specialist help is needed. Perhaps the student should have prepared for his afternoon session the night before, or the doctor not allowed the management demands of the practice to impinge on her afternoon visits. Drawing lines in anticipation may be common sense but also may need clear thinking, and the time given to thinking things through has limits too. Decisions have to be made.

VALUES AND VIRTUES

One of our own built-in shortcuts, which modern developmental psychologists might say is 'wired in' to human thinking, is that we live life with pre-existing preferences, and do not have to work things out from scratch each time. Where these ideas are not available for reasoning or reflection, they might be called prejudices, but even if we would like to challenge and discuss complex beliefs, we each have casts of character that are quite obvious to our friends and family if not to us. We may be good timekeepers or decision makers, excellent at listening to people, open and honest about our opinions, and so on. These we conventionally call *virtues*, and we prize them. They may make us effective in certain circumstances, and prone to make certain sorts of choices. Some of these choices will lead us into certain types of job, or in medicine, into particular branches of care. Neurosurgery and community psychiatry may share many things, but the virtues required of doctors and nurses in each area are likely to be very different. This in turn is in part because the jobs are different (the outcomes expected and the processes used are dissimilar), but also

because the values of each area, though they may overlap, extend across a different range. The house officer who tolerated the bizarre behaviour of someone with a rapidly increasing brain haemorrhage or the psychiatrist who insisted on opening up patients' skulls are probably stories from the past (we hope). In these two areas of work, the balance is struck differently between tolerance and active inquisitiveness or intervention. (Perhaps this is in part due to the different dangers that each area of work poses for its patients.) The moral challenge may thus be not so much about what a doctor should *do*, but about what sort of person (or professional) he or she should *be*. To the degree that we change this – and we can probably all change our professional practice a lot more than we might think – we have to identify the important attributes to develop in a certain area of work or to display in a certain situation. Thus a particular approach may prevent problems arising (or the reverse!). The doctor facing the elderly patient with an incidental and probably irrelevant blood test abnormality may simply not have a problem if he or she is always open and honest with patients. They have grown to trust their doctor and respect her truthfulness and judgement.

What applies to individuals can, to a degree, apply to groups. In this context we usually talk about a deliberate choice of *values*. A particular service, say an oncology department or a group practice, may make a conscious decision to take a particular approach for the benefit of patients, or to reduce or stop their commitment elsewhere in order to give their work a particular focus. There may be local factors that are decisive. A group practice in a poor inner-city area with a high morbidity from alcohol or opiate drug use may decide to tolerate a fair measure of chaos in order to keep open the contact with people with disorganized lifestyles, and may encourage doctors to follow their instincts when it comes to calling time on a prolonged consultation. There are likely to be trade-offs here, too, though. The same practice might find it difficult when patients from a part of the locality that has gone 'upmarket' come in with Internet printouts and complain about being kept waiting past appointment times. So both values and virtues are on a spectrum: the tolerance the above practice develops will be a menace for a busy executive superwoman who just wants her pills and to get home to take over from the au pair. Someone appearing to be brave in one situation may in another appear simply foolhardy. If we value choice, we also need to value choice of values, and each of us may have made particular choices of our values because of experiences we have had, or new goals we now need to achieve.

PERSPECTIVE AND NARRATIVE

The proposal was made early in the chapter that each encounter with a new person could be not only a meeting between strangers but also a meeting between moral strangers. Understanding one person's relevant aims and goals may be quite a task, but understanding the culture of a group or family, and how one individual blends with or differs from that group, gives a special extra dimension to family practice that makes decision making, when there is dissonance, a real skill. Respecting the patient's choice may be supported by the law, regulating bodies and principles, and is unlikely to be far from the value set of most modern practitioners or service groups. However, within families these concepts may begin to unpeel like an onion, as illness or distress upsets a previously established and artificial harmony between different people's expectations, needs and experiences. Choice implies that there is also something that is not chosen, and the path not taken, the unvalued expectation, an unmet need or a negative experience may need to be addressed before progress is made. So each person who has a stake in a difficult moral decision ideally should have the opportunity to offer his or her own perspective where it is appropriate to do so. This is (partly) the theory behind case conferences. However, in practice this is all much more difficult. Whereas professionals may be expected to present coherent options and the justifications for and against a particular approach, most people are more concrete thinkers, and express their preferences in ways that may not appear so neatly logical.

Some of this concrete thinking is expressed in our desire to tell and hear stories. While most of us respond well to people telling interesting stories, the imperative in modern medicine to look for scientific evidence in treatment evaluation has led to some clinicians insisting that such things are 'mere anecdotes'. This seems not only to misrepresent at least what some patients are doing when they are telling stories, but also to misunderstand what such stories may hold at their heart. We are probably used to the idea that a religious leader may use a narrative to illustrate a moral point or clarify a particular belief, but modern novelists or soap opera directors are often doing the same. Though writers usually have several ideas they want to get across, the point is the same: telling about events is usually the vehicle for presenting the clash between ideas. When this happens in the consultation, there is seldom *not* a purpose to the story told, and this purpose is usually to help define, in the circumstances, what sort of person is consulting and how the patient can help the doctor make sense of what has and is happening to him or her, separately or together.

Those who find this idea far-fetched or impractical may prefer to stick to the concept of perspectives. Understanding where each person in an interaction 'is coming from' is not the only aim of modern ethical practice – we still have to put each point of view together and reach a reasoned and reasonable conclusion – but it is certainly a good starting point.

PUTTING IT ALL TOGETHER

Much professional medical ethics derives from philosophical thinking down the ages, and law is made by judges and juries deliberating at length. No one would want to make a virtue out of work pressure, but the passage of time means something different in medicine. For the clinician, the patient is there in front of him or her and is likely to remain so unless some sort of decision is made. Other problems clamour for attention in the waiting room. Medical practice worldwide would grind to a halt if clinicians took time out to think deeply and extensively through each dilemma that came their way.

Equally, even the most strident political advocate of patient choice would not expect clinician to act like a dispensing machine, simply waiting for their buttons to be pressed. The practice of medicine is complex, but many of the difficult decisions have already been made. These decisions may be made by the people who set up the service, or by the GMC or the government. They may be based on the choices that patients or relatives have made before they arrive. They may be affected by the place in which the encounter occurs, or by the way two people interact. But two things at least stand out. One is that patients spend quite a lot of time afterwards ruminating about what happened, and that doctors do too. This is the moment to bring together the sort of thinking processes we have looked at here, so that in follow-up, or the next time something similar happens, our thinking may be clearer and our responses more coherent. As one ancient Greek doctor said, 'If treatment is good, treatment after thought must be better'.

The other marker we need to lay down is that we should try our best not to be pressed into doing something that we know, in our heart of hearts, is wrong. This is even more so if the pressure is simply of routine or workload. Medical ethics and law are often annoyingly short on prescriptions, and we may not find it easy to know what we should do, but it is extraordinarily obvious, in most cases, what we should not do.

Thinking in medical ethics and law can be exciting or challenging, and can take us to some unusual places. However, the 'bottom line' is that it helps us to practise well and stay out of trouble.

Learning through case studies

The following elements should be considered when preparing a response to case studies in medical ethics and law.

1. Summarize the case study.
2. State the moral dilemma(s).
3. State the assumptions being made/needing to be made.
4. Analyse the dilemma(s) in terms of general ethical principles.
5. Analyse the dilemmas(s) in terms of outcomes.
6. Spell out possible solutions or ways forward, giving reasons for accepting or rejecting each one.
7. Note any legal implications.
8. Come to a conclusion about what to do.
9. Consider how practice could be improved/changed in the light of this particular case study.

SUMMARY POINTS

To conclude, the most important messages of this chapter are:

■ you should be clear what laws and regulations govern your work before you start to practise medicine, especially in primary care, which can be either very supportive or isolating, depending on *your* approach to your work;

■ you should keep alive your own sense of right and wrong in all aspects of your work, and particularly be alert to unusual or unexpected emotions that may arise, as these may indicate that there is a moral problem for you to think about;

■ emotional reactions are not enough, however, and your moral intuitions need to be subjected to scrutiny through some or all of the approaches suggested here to keep your health care in good shape;

■ doing that thinking or discussion and coming to conclusions that you feel are justified, respecting the wishes and needs of people you work with and protecting them from harm, will enable you to feel good about your work and sleep in peace at the end of the day;

■ having conversations with other colleagues within the cordon of professional confidentiality can be very helpful, so it is important to find careful and responsive colleagues who can help you to think through difficult issues that may arise wherever you work.

REFERENCES

Boyd, K.M., Higgs, R. and Pinching, A.J. 1997: *The new dictionary of medical ethics*. London: BMJ Publishing Group.

Carmen, D. and Britten, N. 1995: Confidentiality of medical records. *British Journal of General Practice* 45, 485–8.

FURTHER READING

The General Medical Council (www.gmc-uk.org) publishes booklets on good medical practice, consent, confidentiality, doctors in management, and other issues of importance that arise. These are required reading for all doctors who intend to practise within UK or related jurisdictions.

The *Journal of Medical Ethics* (www.jmedethics.com) is the leading journal that discusses ethical issues, and this site provides a list of classified websites, articles from the journal and abstracts of many articles published in the last decade.

Her Majesty's Stationery Office (www.legislation.hmso.gov.uk) provides publications detailing UK statutes.

Blackburn, S. 2001: *Ethics: a very short introduction*. Oxford: Oxford University Press.

As it says, very short, but extremely readable introduction to modern ethical thinking and writing.

Brazier, M. 1992: *Medicine, patients and the law*. London: Penguin.

Campbell, A.V. and Higgs, R. 1982: *In that case: medical ethics in everyday practice*. London: Darton, Longman and Todd.

Gillon, R. 1986: *Philosophical medical ethics*. Chichester: John Wiley and Sons.

Glover, J. 1977: *Causing death and saving lives*. London: Penguin.

This is the classical study of this area, which has never been surpassed.

Harris, J. 1985: *The value of life: an introduction to medical ethics*. London: Routledge.

This is an exciting and challenging book about many of the issues at the expanding frontiers of medical science.

Hope, T., Savulescu, J. and Hendrick, J. 2003: *Medical ethics and law: the core curriculum*. Edinburgh: Churchill Livingstone.

Kuhse, H. and Singer, P. 2001: *A companion to bioethics*. Oxford: Blackwell.

This and its companion volume *A companion to ethics* are very useful gateways to the range of modern writing.

Parker, M. and Dickenson, D. 2001: *The Cambridge medical ethics workbook*. Cambridge: Cambridge University Press.

A very wide-ranging explanation of approaches to bioethics that is designed to be used in a similar way to this book.

CHAPTER
13
CLINICAL AUDIT IN GENERAL PRACTICE

Medical knowledge and technology change at a seemingly ever-increasing rate. Government and patient pressure for improved quality of care and best value makes the efficient use of resources vital. Ensuring that new and effective treatments become available to patients requires good managerial strategies and clinical skills. This chapter examines the ways professionals cope with rapid change and develop their clinical skills.

LEARNING OBJECTIVES

By the end of this chapter, you will be able to:

- understand the key elements of four commonly used research methods and the sorts of data they can provide;
- understand why effective linkage between research evidence and improvements in patient care is often over-estimated;
- have a detailed understanding of how clinical audit, by combining research technologies with a potentially effective change mechanism, can overcome these difficulties;
- be in a position, by following the discussion points and practical exercises throughout the detailed explanation of the audit cycle, to plan effective changes in care where change is appropriate.

FROM RESEARCH EVIDENCE TO QUALITY IMPROVEMENTS IN PATIENT CARE

This chapter is about the management of change in primary care and uses a number of examples in ischaemic heart disease to illustrate the complex relationship between research evidence and subsequent changes to clinical practice. It starts by exploring the nature of research evidence and outlines four commonly used approaches to generate evidence for primary care. It then moves on to describe the processes and systems that have been developed to try to ensure that research evidence is applied to everyday clinical

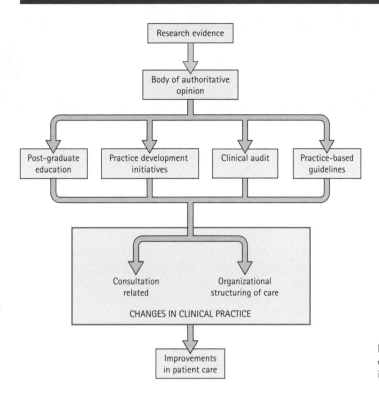

Figure 13.1 A flow diagram linking evidence to changes in clinical practice in primary care.

practice and discusses the new quality improvement agenda within clinical governance. It also briefly describes the change management processes that have been incorporated into the proposed new general practitioner (GP) contract. Finally, it provides a detailed explanation and guide to clinical audit, the change management process that the authors consider to be the most effective for primary care.

Figure 13.1 shows a somewhat idealized model of how research evidence leads to improvements in clinical practice. The crucial link is through the quality improvement methods that have been given new impetus within the clinical governance framework. For the purposes of this chapter, clinical governance is best seen as a bringing together of a range of already existing quality improvement tools rather than as introducing any new methods. There are obviously other quality improvement methods that are not shown here; we have focused on the most common.

The various sections in what follows will take you through the model shown in Figure 13.1, giving illustrations and prompting thought concerning change.

Thinking and Discussion Point

What is clinical governance?

Clinical governance is a system through which NHS organisations are accountable for continuously improving the quality of their services and safeguarding high standards of care by creating an environment in which excellence in clinical care will flourish.

(Scally and Donaldson, 1998)

For a detailed discussion of clinical governance in primary care, see Zwanenberg and Harrison (2000).

RESEARCH EVIDENCE

Research, by itself, rarely leads to any change in professional practice. Indeed, we know that some of what we currently accept as standard clinical practice has been refuted by research findings and that much of the work we do has little or no basis in scientific research at all. Research has also shown wide variations in the processes and outcomes of care from different National Health Service (NHS) services treating similar conditions. The flow diagram linking clinical evidence to changes in practice (see Fig. 13.1) is clearly an idealized model. It is, however, a model that the NHS has determined to move towards, and very real progress is now being made in a variety of projects, large and small, up and down the country. For example, the NHS has an extensive established research and development programme which has injected fresh impetus and resources into health services research. The National Institute for Clinical Excellence (NICE) has been established since 1999 to disseminate the results of scientific research into effective health care through its evidence-based guidelines and health technology appraisals. The Cochrane Collaboration (Chalmers et al., 1992) has been expanding its work in collating and disseminating the results of randomized controlled trials (RCTs). Research networks such as the South Thames Area Research Network (STARNET) have been established in primary care settings to research, monitor and implement proven effective healthcare programmes; and healthcare professionals and managers at regional, district and local levels are increasingly becoming involved in research, audit and evaluation. The impetus for much of this interest in research has come from governmental pressure to set priorities for NHS spending and get best value from increased NHS resources. Coupled with this has been the Government's declared aim of moving towards a primary-care-led NHS (NHS Executive, 1994). The establishment of primary care trusts, primary-care-led commissioning and purchasing and the increasing emphasis on health care in the community have put primary care right in the middle of this need for research evidence. Much of the health service's research that will take place in the next decade will be undertaken within primary care.

So what is research and how can it help inform us when making changes to the way we work? For the purposes of this chapter, research is defined as 'an attempt to find out what we should be doing'. In effect, research is a form of enquiry that aims to gather evidence. As a form of enquiry, research is distinguished by its 'scientific' or rigorously systematic processes and, in healthcare settings, research has typically been of one of four types.

1. *Experimental research*, principally using RCTs, tests the effect of an intervention.
2. *Survey research*, using either questionnaire or interview studies, measures the frequency or distribution of something within populations such as patients' or GPs' views of a particular service.
3. *Evaluation research* evaluates the process, outcomes and sometimes the cost effectiveness and acceptability of a new service.
4. *Needs assessment research* is used to measure the health needs of patient populations. Health authorities and primary care trusts have become interested in using needs assessment so that they can commission the quantity and quality of service actually required by their patients.

Of course, these are not the only sorts of research going on in primary care, and the list could be almost endless. However, these are the areas that the student of primary care needs to be broadly familiar with. Nor do these types of research projects necessarily employ distinct methods. For example, many evaluations of a service incorporate a RCT with a survey. Equally, needs assessment studies frequently draw on survey methods to identify patients' needs. There is, in fact, a huge variety of research taking place, and many research projects will be based on more than one particular method.

EXPERIMENTAL RESEARCH: THE RANDOMIZED CONTROLLED TRIAL

Experimental research often takes the form of a RCT, and much of the search for new clinical evidence has focused on the collection of results from these sorts of studies. The great value of controlled trials to primary care is that they allow the researcher to draw conclusions about the relative benefits of one treatment or therapy compared with another.

CASE STUDY 13.1

In the Scandinavian Simvastatin Survival Study (1994), the authors set out to test the effect of prescribing the cholesterol-lowering drug simvastatin on mortality and morbidity in patients with coronary heart disease. A large sample of patients (4444) with a history of heart disease and high cholesterol levels was randomly assigned equally to an intervention group, prescribed simvastatin, and to a control group, prescribed a placebo. The study was designed as a 'double-blind trial', which simply means neither the patients nor their doctors knew which individuals were receiving the real drug and which the placebo. This method ensures that the doctors interact with control and intervention group patients in the same way, and thus the possibility of bias is reduced.

The patients were followed up over an average of 5 years, and the authors reported 189 coronary deaths in the placebo group but only 111 in the simvastatin group. In the control group, 622 patients (28 per cent) had one or more major coronary events, compared with 431 (19 per cent) in the intervention group. Total cholesterol levels in the intervention group were reduced by an average of 25 per cent.

It is obvious from these results, which were confirmed by statistical analysis, that the patients in the intervention group gained tremendous benefit from the use of simvastatin. The authors were able to conclude: 'This study shows that long-term treatment with simvastatin is safe and improves survival in CHD [coronary heart disease] patients.'

In Case study 13.1 (above), the Scandinavian Simvastatin Survival Study compared the effect of prescribing a cholesterol-lowering drug with a placebo in patients with coronary heart disease, and clearly demonstrates the long-term benefits of using the drug. The advantage of this sort of study, which in this case has used a large sample over a long period, lies in the robustness and reliability of the results. The research has demonstrated, beyond any reasonable doubt, the benefits derived from this particular therapy and has formed a vital part of clinical evidence about the best management of patients with coronary heart disease.

The key methodological issue in a RCT is ensuring that the memberships of the control and intervention groups are similar, so that at the end of the study the researchers can be sure that they are comparing like with like. The example study would have been worthless if all the most poorly people had been in the control group or all those least likely to be compliant were in the intervention group. The problem for researchers is that no two humans are the same, and nor will their physiological, psychological or behavioural responses to disease and treatments be the same. The only solution for researchers is to ensure that patients have an equal chance of being assigned to either the control or intervention group, and this is achieved by selecting membership of each group at random. Probability theory assures us that, providing the sample is large enough, the variability within the sample will be equally distributed between the two groups. This randomization procedure can be achieved by the simple tossing of a coin, but, normally speaking, more sophisticated methods, involving the use of randomly generated numbers, are used.

There is a major ethical consideration that affects the RCT. The patients who were assigned to the control group, purely by chance, in the example study were given a placebo and, as a result of the research process, denied what became clearly for many people a life-saving drug. Researchers must, of course, obtain patients' consent for all forms of research, but the dilemma of withholding new and possibly life-saving treatments from patients as a result of the research process remains.

SURVEY RESEARCH

... surveys are essentially a research tool by which facts can be ascertained, theories confirmed or refuted, ideas explored and values identified and illuminated. So the sorts of questions with which surveys are concerned relate to the distribution and association of facts and attitudes.

(Cartwright, 1983, p.1,
cited in Ong, 1993, p.21)

Cartwright's widely accepted definition of survey research notes that surveys are really about the frequency and distribution of facts and attitudes. Survey methods have been widely used in healthcare settings, and Ong (1993) neatly summarizes Cartwright's review of subjects in healthcare contexts where survey methods have been applied:

> These include the use of general measures of health and sickness to make comparisons over time, understanding the nature of disease by, for example, uncovering causality or identifying syndromes, assessing health and health care needs of populations, evaluating the use of services, examining the effects and side effects of care and studying the acceptability of services or investigating the organisation of care.
>
> *(Ong, 1993, p.23)*

Survey method normally involves the use of a questionnaire or interview schedule to collect the attitudes or facts being reviewed. The key methodological issue in survey research is one of bias, which is a particular problem at two stages of the research process. First, bias can inadvertently be built into the questionnaire or interview schedule during the design stage. Researchers have to take great care in the formulation and wording of questions so that they do not encourage particular answers. Second, bias can creep into survey research during the sampling process. Survey samples should be chosen strategically rather than for convenience, and target only the population for whom the facts or attitudes being surveyed are relevant. There would be little point in a GP sending a questionnaire enquiring about his or her patients' views of the practice's maternity care to a randomly chosen sample of all the practice's patients. Most of the patients will not have had any contact with the practice's maternity services, nor will they be likely to. It is also important that the sample size is large enough to be representative of the population as a whole. In Case study 13.2 (below) of GPs' perceptions of current treatments for angina pectoris, the researchers were able to include the whole population (of GPs with access to the regional cardiology centre at Southampton) in their study group because there were only 217 in the entire population. Often in surveys, the population is too large to interview or for a questionnaire to be posted to everybody and so representative samples need to be drawn. The exact size of the sample required will depend on the size of the population and the nature of the questions and research design. There are statistical procedures that help researchers to determine sample sizes.

In Case study 13.2, the researchers' aim was to assess GPs' perceptions of current treatment for angina. They collected facts about the GPs' referral practice to hospital units and about the beliefs and attitudes the GPs held about current treatments. The researchers can be sure that these attitudes and referral patterns are representative of the population of GPs with access to the regional cardiology unit, because they asked them all and because so many of the GPs (79 per cent) replied. Assuming that the rest of the study design was equally unbiased, this piece of research gives powerful evidence to healthcare planners about the nature of GPs' referral patterns to the cardiology unit and about their understanding of current treatments for angina. Healthcare planners will be able to reorganize services and plan educational and information initiatives as a result of the research.

CASE STUDY 13.2

'This survey set out to assess GPs' perceptions of current investigation and treatment for angina pectoris' (Ghandi et al., 1995). The authors of this survey, who were based at Southampton University, set out their aims and posted a questionnaire to 217 GPs who had access to a regional cardiac centre. One hundred and seventy-one GPs returned the questionnaire, making a very good response rate of 79 per cent. The authors reported that these GPs appeared to hold 'divergent and contradictory opinions about exercise testing and the scientific evidence for the benefits of coronary angioplasty and coronary artery bypass surgery' (Ghandi et al., 1995).

In brief, the main results of the survey were that:

■ 80 per cent of GPs reported referring 10 per cent or fewer of patients with angina to the regional centre;

- 72 per cent of GPs reported referring 25 per cent or fewer of patients with angina to a hospital physician;
- 77 per cent of GPs considered exercise testing useful for diagnosing angina;
- 47 per cent of GPs were uncertain about the prognostic value of exercise tests;
- 79 per cent of GPs were not confident about interpreting the results of an exercise test;
- 79 per cent of GPs believed there was scientific evidence to show that coronary angioplasty relieves symptoms;
- 21 per cent of GPs believed that coronary angioplasty prolongs survival;
- 96 per cent of GPs believed that coronary artery bypass grafting relieves symptoms;
- 62 per cent of GPs believed that coronary artery bypass grafting prolongs survival.

Clearly, the authors were able to show that GPs held divergent opinions about the benefits of current treatment for angina pectoris. They recommended that access to cardiology investigation should be easier and that more information about the value of exercise testing and survival benefits from coronary intervention should be made available.

This particular survey was chosen as an example because it fits into our theme throughout the chapter of coronary heart disease, for its simplicity and because the subject matter highlights the need for clinical professionals (GPs in this case) to be in a continuous process of learning, developing skills and changes to their practice. Any one of hundreds of surveys that are published in medical and healthcare journals every week might have been chosen. We might have taken examples from a survey of patient satisfaction, or a health status survey that had employed one of the widely used health questionnaires such as the Nottingham Health Profile (Hunt et al., 1986), or we might have chosen an interview study that explored, in depth, patients' experiences of living with an illness. The point is that whichever the example, the type and form of the data and evidence that arose from the project would essentially be the same. Surveys, provided that they are properly carried out, provide robust and reliable evidence of how things are and what people think.

EVALUATION RESEARCH

This type of research forms an important piece in the jigsaw of gathering evidence. Evaluation normally involves the systematic measurement of the process, outcome and impact of a new healthcare service, and to do this evaluation, researchers draw on a variety of research methods, including survey research, sometimes RCTs and sometimes cost effectiveness and cost–benefit analysis. In practice, evaluation research in healthcare settings tends to take one or a combination of two forms: evaluation of processes and evaluation of outcomes. The study described in Case study 13.3 combines a process and outcome evaluation. Process evaluation is concerned with describing the structures, organization and activities of a healthcare service, whilst outcome evaluation is concerned with measuring the extent to which the service being evaluated meets its own stated objectives.

The first and foremost methodological issue in evaluation research is in setting objectives. Objectives need to be set for the evaluation itself (i.e. what is to be evaluated, what will be measured) and also for the healthcare service being evaluated. It is usually most helpful if these are all set at the same time. It is vitally important that objectives are set at realistic levels and that the objectives of the evaluation tie in with the objectives of the healthcare service being evaluated. This is often a complex procedure because different stakeholders in any given service are likely to have differing views of its main purpose and will be likely to want to measure different processes and outcomes. Furthermore, it is often difficult to break down long-term aims and goals (such as the reduction of mortality due to coronary heart disease) that might have driven the establishment of a new service in the first place into shorter-term, measurable objectives (such as the reduction of cholesterol down to target level in patients post myocardial infarction). It is vital that these objectives are all set and agreed upon at the outset of an evaluation, simply because it is against these objectives that the service will be evaluated. If set objectives are too ambitious or ill-defined or the objectives of the evaluation do not match those of the service being evaluated, it is inevitable that the evaluation will produce negative feedback regardless of the success or otherwise of the service in practice.

CASE STUDY 13.3

In this study (Schellevis et al., 1994), the researchers set out to evaluate the process and outcome of the formulation and implementation of guidelines for follow-up care in patients with hypertension, diabetes, chronic ischaemic heart disease and osteoarthritis. Fifteen GPs were involved in the project and took part in the development of the guidelines, set out to implement them in their practice and contributed the patients to the study.

Over 21 months, the researchers measured the performance of the doctors and the disease status of the patients using disease status indicators. The researchers reported that even though during the study the GPs did tend to work to the guidelines, especially in routine matters, there were no statistically significant changes to the patients' disease status over time.

There could have been any number of reasons for the findings of this study. The objectives may have been too ambitious to measure in the time period. The health status indicators may have been too insensitive to incremental change. The samples may have been too small or the guidelines themselves may conceivably have been poor. Nevertheless, the example reveals the sort of evidence that can be gained from doing an evaluation. Processes and outcomes can be described and measured to show whether a service meets its own objectives. This sort of evidence is particularly useful for healthcare planners who wish to monitor the effects of their interventions.

NEEDS ASSESSMENT RESEARCH

The assessment of patients' needs in the NHS has become more common since the Government's 1989 White Paper 'Working for Patients' (Department of Health, 1989). This recommended needs assessment to inform the new purchasing and commissioning arrangements following the split between purchasers and providers in the government's health service reforms. However, as with evaluations, there is little agreement about methodologies, or even about the definition of 'needs'. Needs assessment studies therefore tend to employ a wide range of research methods, including surveys, secondary analysis, in-depth interview studies and reviews of routinely collected information. In the main, however, needs assessments studies have adopted the following definition of healthcare needs.

> The need for health care is ... dependent on the availability or potential availability of health care and prevention services to respond to the disease or risk factors – and to secure an improvement in health, i.e. the ability to benefit from effective health care or prevention services.
> *(National Health Service Management Executive, 1991, p. 4)*

By matching healthcare 'need' to the 'ability to benefit from effective healthcare intervention', this definition underscores the distinction between healthcare 'need' and 'demand'. Demand in this context refers to patients actively seeking and asking for services. This distinction is important because sometimes patients ask for health care that is inappropriate to their needs. For example, GPs are often asked by their patients for antibiotics to treat a common cold. On the other hand, we know that some patients who might benefit do not demand a healthcare intervention, either because they do not know that they might benefit or simply because they do not want to have any form of treatment. Amongst these patients we can identify 'unmet needs'. Unmet need is also apparent for those patients who have demanded a service but who remain on waiting lists.

The purpose of a needs assessment study therefore is to quantify and describe patients' needs from a given population and for a given effective form of health care and to identify, quantify and describe where current service provision is meeting needs (effectively) and where patients' needs remain unmet. With this information to hand, healthcare professionals can plan the development and implementation of services that are designed to meet patients' needs fully in the most effective way possible.

CASE STUDY 13.4

A group of GPs has become aware of the benefits that patients with a history of coronary heart disease might gain from attending a rehabilitation service following a cardiac event. Their knowledge of these benefits was gained from their reading of a range of research papers that showed a reduction in mortality following exercise programmes (see, for example, Oldridge et al., 1988). At a meeting, the GPs decide to commission a needs assessment study of their patients' needs for cardiac rehabilitation.

The aims of the needs assessment study will be to quantify the need for this service, to examine where these needs are already being met and where they are not, and to identify the level of service required to meet identified need.

The following tasks face the researchers.

- To calculate the incidence and prevalence of coronary heart disease in these GPs' patients. This could be achieved by examining patients' records, by reviewing disease registers or from records held at the local hospital cardiology unit. This will tell the researchers the total number of patients who might benefit from cardiac rehabilitation.
- To carry out a lifestyle survey of the patients with coronary heart disease to identify those who are presently taking very little exercise and who therefore would benefit most from being invited to take part in an organized and structured exercise programme.
- To identify where patients' needs for cardiac rehabilitation are presently unmet. This can be achieved by an activity survey of hospital and primary care workers to see what and how much, if any, cardiac rehabilitation services are being provided. What are the aims and objectives of current services and how many patients are receiving them?

Having collected the information outlined above, the GPs will be in a position to know exactly how many of their patients might benefit from this particular intervention and therefore have a 'need' for cardiac rehabilitation. This will allow them to calculate the resources required to establish a rehabilitation service for their patients.

In the needs assessment study proposed in Case study 13.4, a group of GPs wishes to employ a cardiac rehabilitation nurse to develop exercise programmes for their patients. However, they are unsure about how much need there is for the service and so are unable to decide how many nursing staff to employ. By commissioning a needs assessment survey such as that described above, the GPs will be furnished with clear and reliable evidence of the numbers of patients who will benefit from the proposed service and will be able to calculate exactly the level of service required to meet their patients' needs.

Thinking and Discussion Point

Find a copy of the latest edition of the *British Medical Journal* and read the 'Original Papers'.

- ❏ How much new knowledge does each of the papers add and how much do they contribute to a growing body of opinion?
- ❏ Which of the papers report the findings of RCTs and which use other approaches?
- ❏ Consider how the findings of the papers might be implemented in general practice to improve patient care. What could be done to ensure that this happened?

LINKING RESEARCH TO CHANGES IN CLINICAL PRACTICE

WHAT HAPPENS TO RESEARCH EVIDENCE?

In practice, what often happens (and this can clearly be seen in our example of coronary heart disease) is that the body of evidence steadily grows in weight, and bodies of authoritative opinion tend to coalesce around it. These bodies of opinion are further informed by collaborative overviews of research findings, which seek to combine the results of individual research studies to bring about more convincing and definitive evidence. Such reviews are a common feature within medical journals.

CASE STUDY 13.5

The aim of this study (Antiplatelet Trialists' Collaboration, 1994) was 'to determine the effects of "prolonged" antiplatelet therapy (that is, given for one month or more) on "vascular events" (non-fatal myocardial infarctions, non-fatal strokes or vascular deaths) in various categories of patients'.

The study was based on the secondary analysis of research results published by March 1990. By combining the results of 174 RCTs, the researchers were able to present convincing evidence concerning the benefits of antiplatelet therapy, especially to 'high-risk' patients. The authors concluded:

> Taking all high risk patients together showed reductions of about one third in non fatal myocardial infarction, about one third in non fatal stroke and about one third in vascular deaths.

The importance of the review described in the example above to the movement towards implementing change in working practices lies primarily in its size and the enormity of the improvements shown. Evidence based on the outcomes of 174 RCTs is particularly powerful.

Unfortunately, from the researcher's perspective, the results of research projects often seem to sit on library shelves gathering dust and there can be lengthy delays between the publication of results and the implementation of new ways of working. There are many reasons for this, including the following.

- There are only limited change mechanisms in place that can be utilized to bring about new ways of working in response to research evidence. Some of these, such as postgraduate education and development initiatives, are discussed below.
- Some research results are so at variance with established ways of thinking and working that people will not respond to them until the results have been re-tested and re-proved several times.
- Many research topics are derived from the particular interests of the researcher rather than from the information needs of policy makers and service providers, and it is often only once these interests and needs overlap that the speedy implementation of research results is seen.
- Often, research studies, for practical and resource reasons, are limited in their scope.

It is rare for any one research paper to provide the definitive answer to a question or problem.

It is in part for these reasons that NICE was formed as part of the NHS on 1 April 1999. NICE aims to provide the NHS and its patients with current, relevant and reliable evidence of 'best practice'. It does this by setting up expert review panels that review the relevant research findings and produce evidence-based guidelines that *must* be implemented by NHS trusts. In the longer term, this process will have the effect of helping to speed up the process of linking research findings to clinical practice.

The Department of Health has also taken an active interest in speeding up the implementation of research evidence by producing a number of National Service Frameworks (NSFs). The purposes of the NSFs are to provide guidance and a set of standards for clinical practice and the organization of healthcare in key areas. At the time of writing, the Department of Health has produced NSFs in *coronary heart disease* (2000), for *older people* (2001) and *mental health* (1999). Further NSFs are imminent in *diabetes* and in *children's services*. One aspect of the NSF for heart disease, for example, states that all appropriate patients should receive antiplatelet therapy – aspirin.

However, even though these new initiatives are compulsory – that is, all NHS trusts must implement the guidance within prescribed timescales – change management tools and strategies are still required to make this happen. It is not sufficient simply to produce research evidence, publish, synthesize, and put it in a framework for professionals to change their practice automatically. An approach to implementing clinical evidence is required that is as rigorous and systematic as that used for collecting the evidence in the first place.

In the following pages we discuss some of the key approaches currently used for implementing change and concentrate on the most effective of these, clinical audit.

CONTINUING PROFESSIONAL DEVELOPMENT

In historical terms, GPs have relied heavily on local postgraduate education groups for their continuing professional development. Such groups commonly have a format of clinical seminars, perhaps presented by a local consultant, at which an academic discussion takes place around best practice. Other educational activities might include attendance on particular courses, for example those run by the Royal College of General Practitioners. Currently the Postgraduate Education Allowance Scheme exists, whereby GPs are remunerated for gaining sufficient points from course attendance over a 3-year period. Points have to be gained in the areas of health promotion, service management and disease prevention. Clinical assistant schemes are again becoming more common in which a practitioner works within the secondary care setting to gain expertise in a particular area. Hospital outreach clinics are a feature in some practices where consultants attend the practice to see patients. One objective of these is to increase the knowledge and clinical skills of general practice as well as to improve the specialists' understanding of the primary care role.

The role of pharmaceutical companies in the education of practitioners has always been somewhat controversial. There is little doubt, however, that such companies continue to play a major role in education through extensive medical research, sponsoring educational events and producing educational material. (Whether we feel this is desirable or not continues to be a matter for heated debate.) Since the formation of primary care trusts, general practice clinical staff have been engaged in schemes for critical appraisal and have been supported to develop their own professional development plans. In this way, clinicians are encouraged to engage in lifelong learning.

In recent years, the role of primary care within the overall strategy of the health service has been enhanced. Much work has resulted to facilitate the development of primary care services. In our own district, this has been spearheaded by funding of projects by the local health authority and the involvement of academic departments of primary care situated at our district medical schools. Such projects seek, through facilitation, to provide training for practice professionals in their clinical and managerial skills. In addition, useful development tools are created for areas such as health promotion, practice management and clinical audit, to be used by the practices.

IMPLEMENTING CLINICAL EFFECTIVENESS

Increasingly, healthcare professionals are involved in defining more clearly their clinical practice through the development and use of clinical guidelines. Research suggests that guidelines can play an important part in improving clinical care provided certain conditions are met. In primary care it seems that guidelines are more likely to be adopted if they have been developed or adapted at a local level and the process of their development seeks to involve a wide group of professionals. Such guidelines need to be relevant to primary care while retaining a basis of good research evidence as much as possible. Their implementation can be enhanced when they are supported by clinical audit.

There now seems to be a whole industry of 'guideline development' at national and local level, the most obvious being the guidelines produced by NICE and the NSFs. It is still too early to assess the impact of NICE guidance and the NSFs on primary care, although there is some evidence that where these guidelines have been supported with change management action plans, the impact can be significant.

CLINICAL AUDIT

The term 'medical audit' was first described as being an expected part of the professional duties of all doctors in the Government White Paper *Working for patients*, published in 1989. (Department of Health, 1989). Since that time, the term 'clinical audit' has taken its place and reflects the fact that audit is now a multi-professional activity involving many clinical professionals and managers within their respective teams (Fig. 13.2). Two definitions of medical audit can be found overleaf.

The idea of receiving appropriate feedback concerning our performance is an integral part of human learning behaviour. It is familiar to all students in a variety of forms whether from peers, tutors or through examinations. Our need for feedback remains an essential part of postgraduate professional development and yet the

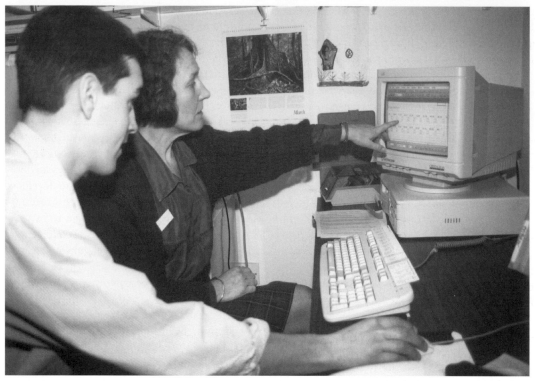

Figure 13.2 Practice computing: patient monitoring.

> **Definitions of medical audit**
>
> The systematic, critical analysis of the quality of medical care, including the procedures used for diagnosis and treatment, the use of resources, and the resulting outcome and quality of life for the patient.
>
> Clinical audit involves: ...looking at what you do in a way that allows you to see how you might do things better, making appropriate changes and then looking again to assess improvement in clinical practice.
>
> *(Department of Health, 1989)*

> **Difference between clinical audit and research**
>
> Research is an attempt to find out what we should be doing, whereas in clinical audit, we know what we should be doing but are trying to determine how well we are doing it.

opportunities for it can be limited. Clinical audit can provide such feedback, allowing us to assess our clinical practice and its impact on patient care against our expectations and those of our profession. It is not surprising, therefore, that clinical audit activity has expanded greatly and

that resources have been channelled to support it. In recent years, the basis of clinical audit has developed to be much more focused on the agreement and subsequent implementation of realistic plans to improve patient care. Such change plans, rather than being in the form of vague recommendations, can take on the rigour of plans familiar to the business community and can be informed by a variety of professionals, managers and, increasingly, the patients themselves.

Clearly, there is a fundamental difference, summarized in the box above, between the aims and objectives of clinical audit and those of research, even though they may borrow aspects of methodology from each other.

THE AUDIT CYCLE – THE STANDARD MODEL FOR CLINICAL AUDIT

The basis of audit is that incorporated within the audit cycle, an example of which is shown in Figure 13.3. This shows a simple model for undertaking audit. However, within it lies a variety of complexities if professionals are to respond to an audit by being willing to make changes to their clinical practice.

CRITERIA AND STANDARDS

An audit consists of a group of criteria, measurable statements about the clinical topic, and an agreed standard for each aspect of care under review. Criteria are arrived at by discussions within the team and may be informed by external information such as research evidence, local or national guidelines, and other audits performed or designed elsewhere. Each criterion is agreed by the practice team and represents an important measurable aspect of care that can be influenced within an appropriate time scale by the practice team. Criteria are constructed specifically to allow them to be judged as present or absent when data are collected.

In practice, criteria can be devised to look at clinical care from a range of perspectives. A convenient classification for criteria would be to divide them into structure, process and outcome. Examples of criteria classified in this way, for an audit of patients with known ischaemic heart disease, are shown in Case study 13.6 (below). Structural criteria look at the structures needed to be in place for care to occur effectively. Process criteria look at actual events in clinical practice that have or have not taken place. Outcome criteria look at whether those events have resulted in a positive effect on the health of the patient.

CASE STUDY 13.6

■ Structure.
  – A register of all patients with ischaemic heart disease exists/does not exist within the practice.
  – A recall system is/is not in place to review all patients with known ischaemic heart disease at least annually.
  – The practice has/does not have agreed guidelines for risk factor management in patients with ischaemic heart disease.
■ Process.
  – The records show that patients eligible for aspirin therapy have/have not been prescribed aspirin.

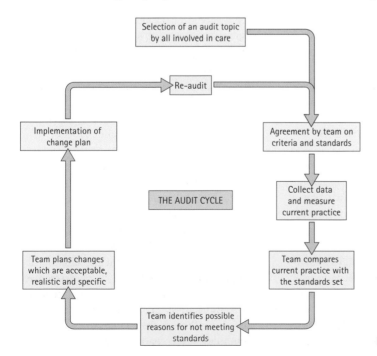

Figure 13.3 The audit cycle.

- The records show that a serum lipid result is/is not present.
- The records show that for patients with abnormal serum lipids dietary advice has/has not been given.
- The records show that a patient's blood pressure has/has not been measured in the last year.

■ Intermediate outcome.
- The records show that patients with abnormal lipids prior to 1 year ago now have/do not have a lipid measurement within the target range agreed.
- The records show that the last blood pressure reading for patients with hypertension diagnosed prior to 1 year ago was/was not below 90 mmHg diastolic.

■ Long-term outcome (not usually appropriate within audit – see text).
- The mortality rate of patients with known ischaemic heart disease.
- The incidence of strokes in patients with known ischaemic heart disease.

OUTCOME CRITERIA

In recent years we have seen a greater emphasis on trying to define outcome criteria for our patients. However, within general practice, any use of long-term outcome measures is severely hampered. Let us consider a major goal in clinical care, to reduce the mortality rate of certain groups of patients with ischaemic heart disease. The meaningful demonstration of this rate is impossible within a single practice due to the small numbers of patients concerned and the general turnover of patients who change practices. The same would be true for blindness or renal failure in diabetes. However, intermediate outcome measures (or proxy outcome measures) can be used where research evidence has shown that a specific intervention can result in health gains for the individual patient. Research supports the assumption that our patients' health may well gain if we can show that patients with hypertension have their blood pressure controlled.

STANDARDS

The setting of standards is an important step in audit, as, following agreement by the team, this defines what is an appropriate level of performance in delivering clinical care. Standards are used in different ways.

■ Clinical standards: these describe what to expect from a clinical service.
■ Standards for best practice or 'gold' standards: these are idealized standards.
■ Minimum standards: these may be used to identify poor performance.
■ Target-based standards: a percentage goal is attached for each criterion. We recommend that you use these standards wherever possible, as they set realistic goals for performance.

A target-based standard is set specifically for each criterion in the audit. The actual level of standard set can be influenced by a number of factors. It is meant to be a realistic target of the level of care you feel is appropriate at a particular time, given the resources and systems you have in place. It follows that, as a result of audit, these resources and systems may change and so realistic standards may well increase in subsequent audits. Standards can also be informed by external factors such as research evidence, other audits and recommendations from organizations such as the British Diabetic Association or the British Hypertension Society.

Examples of standards are shown in Case study 13.7 (below) for an audit of patients with known ischaemic heart disease. (The particular percentages given here are arbitrary).

CASE STUDY 13.7

■ Structure.
- A register of all patients with ischaemic heart disease *should exist* within the practice.
- A recall system *should be* in place to review all patients with known ischaemic heart disease at least annually.
- The practice *should have* agreed guidelines for risk factor management in patients with ischaemic heart disease.
■ Process.
- Eighty per cent of patients eligible for aspirin therapy should have been prescribed aspirin.
- A serum lipid investigation should have been carried out in 80 per cent of patients with ischaemic heart disease.

- Seventy percent of patients with abnormal serum lipids should have been given dietary advice.
- Eighty per cent of patients should have had a blood pressure recording in the last year.
■ Intermediate outcome.
- Sixty per cent of patients with abnormal lipids prior to 1 year ago should have a lipid measurement within the target range agreed.
- Eighty per cent of patients with hypertension diagnosed prior to 1 year ago should have a blood pressure reading below 90 mmHg diastolic.

PLANNING AN AUDIT

The first aspect to consider when planning an audit is the primary care environment in which it takes place. The time available for staff to undertake the audit has to be balanced against many other priorities. Individual audits need to be kept simple and be quick to complete if a number of audit topics are to be covered systematically, giving a wide review of clinical practice. Criteria need to be designed to prompt appropriate change and not just present 'interesting' data for discussion. The cost of audit (usually in terms of time doing and implementing it) must be realistic compared with the resources available, and the benefits of carrying it out need to be clear from the start.

Thinking and Discussion Point

Most of the examples in this chapter are based on evidence supporting interventions in patient care for ischaemic heart disease. You may wish to use the following topic for your audit design or choose something else you have experience of in general practice.

Audit aim: to assess the level of care aimed at reducing coronary risk factors of patients with ischaemic heart disease in the practice.

Remind yourself at this stage of some of the research evidence mentioned in this chapter that supports risk factor management in ischaemic heart disease. You may want to search for other research evidence to support your clinical practice.

Choosing a topic for audit

While choosing a topic for audit may seem simple, a number of pitfalls arise, even at this stage, that need to be avoided. Examples abound of one professional choosing an audit topic that is a high priority for him or her or is an area he or she sees as being dealt with deficiently by other members of the practice. There are other examples of topics being chosen, an audit designed, and data collected and presented to other professionals without gaining their involvement at all. The chance of successful audit in such cases (i.e. a team of professionals identifying and implementing improvements in the quality of care) is very limited. For this reason, topics for audit need to be reached by consensus. A group of professionals involved in an area of care need to define the audit structure and method together in a way that they feel comfortable with. They also need to feel able to take an active part in planning changes. Audit is most effective when all those on whom changes may impact are involved in the process from the start.

Change analysis

Thinking and Discussion Point

Clinical audit of necessity frequently involves making changes to our clinical behaviour. The factors involved in successfully changing our behaviour, or indeed the behaviour of others, are not straightforward. Factors such as motivation, costs versus benefits and having change easily blocked all contribute. Think about the last time you changed some aspect of your social lifestyle, e.g. joined a club, started exercise.
❑ What motivated you to change?
❑ What did you need to enable you to make the change?
❑ In what way did you gain from the change?
❑ What were the costs for you or others?
❑ What did you need to maintain the change?
You may wish to discuss aspects of your thoughts with other students. It is hoped that you will have been reminded of some of the important factors that influence changes in our behaviour.

Even at the early stages of an audit, you should be able to develop some idea in broad terms of what changes might be needed. It is important at this stage to spend time on this, as it will greatly influence how you go about setting up the audit from the beginning. Considering our audit topic, try to answer some of the following questions.

- On whom are these changes likely to impact and therefore who should be involved and when?
- Do people want to change things related to this topic or not? (Are they likely to want to change once they know more about it?)
- What do people need in place to bring about change? (Consider motivational factors such as their role being supported and valued, as well as actual resources, for example time. Are there ways of re-prioritizing rather than expecting everyone to 'work harder'?)
- Is it likely that the necessary resources in time and possibly finance can be found? If the motivation to change and the necessary resources cannot be found, go no further! Audits in these circumstances rarely help matters.

It is hoped, having performed this change analysis, that you are now much more in tune with the potential requirements for a successful audit. You should be able to identify the consequences for you and the members of the primary healthcare team of implementing the planned changes that result.

Defining and identifying the audit population

You are now in a position to plan the audit method and content more specifically. The first step in your audit will be to find a group of patients with certain characteristics who make up your audit population. You may feel that just defining your audit population as all those with ischaemic heart disease may be the answer; but how are you going to find these patients? Practices have only fairly recently had morbidity registers for conditions such as ischaemic heart disease and this has resulted from local implementation of the coronary heart disease NSF.

How were these registers formed? Even with a computer, patients often did not have a definitive diagnosis entered: a range of diagnoses may have been entered on the computer by different health professionals for the same basic condition. Examples might be ischaemic heart disease, myocardial infarction, angina, coronary artery disease or coronary artery bypass graft. All of these might fall into the group you are trying to identify. The quality of information in general practice increases greatly in the area of prescribing and so many registers were initially constructed by finding all patients prescribed nitrates. Even without computerized prescribing, those patients currently on nitrates could be found over a period of time as they present for repeat prescriptions. The actual quality of the register is an issue and, for a topic such as ischaemic heart disease, a range of methods of identifying patients might need to be combined, such as those on the current register, patients identified from nitrate prescriptions, and morbidity searches on computer systems if they are available, in order to be comprehensive. Even then, there will be one or two patients who escape the net. One of the consequences of this audit may well be better recording of diagnosis as the patients present in future.

Defining criteria and standards (see 'The audit cycle', pp. 237–9)

Successful audits are often simple and therefore not as costly in time. Try to keep your audit to, say, fewer than six criteria. You may want to include both process and intermediate outcome criteria. Discussion and agreement of

Thinking and Discussion Point

Discuss within your group how you are going to define your audit population. You may need to talk to staff at a practice to determine a satisfactory way of actually finding the patients who fit your definition. Write down the final definition you have chosen.

Define some criteria and standards for your audit. (See 'The audit cycle', pp. 237–9, for help.) Try to keep it to, say, fewer than six criteria and include some process and outcome criteria for your audit. Ensure that you word the criteria in such a way that a definite answer can be determined 'present' or 'absent' when you are collecting data.

target-based standards is an important step at this stage, as it defines what you expect as a team.

Collecting data

Once the population for investigation has been defined, there needs to be a collection of the relevant data. A variety of methods exist, as shown below. The choice of method will be determined by the type of information you need to collect.

Examples of audit methods commonly used in general practice

Prospective analysis The clinical details of patients are audited as the patient is encountered, for example auditing the next 30 patients who attend for blood pressure readings to see whether or not their blood pressure is controlled. Such information may be recorded on a specially designed encounter form to simplify data collection.

Retrospective case analysis The medical records of a defined group of patients are examined to see if particular events occurred or to identify if particular clinical outcomes have taken place (e.g. the last recorded blood pressure is below 90 mmHg diastolic). Again, this process is speeded up by designing specific data collection forms.

Patient questionnaires/interviews Questionnaires may be used where various aspects of patient satisfaction are being audited. They have also been used to quantify patient symptoms and educational knowledge of patients.

Telephone surveys These are an alternative to patient questionnaires.

Critical event analysis The notes of patients in whom a defined event has occurred are reviewed, sometimes against standards or guidelines. A meeting is then held with a wide range of staff, at which any lessons to be learnt are discussed and decisions made as to how to change the system in order to prevent recurrence. An example in practice might be to analyse the notes of all patients admitted with asthma, to see whether there is anything that can be done to reduce the likelihood of re-admission.

Peer review Various forms of this exist. One example might be the use of video or observers to analyse consultation techniques against defined criteria. Primary care trusts now undertake to engage all general practice staff in appraisals and encourage staff to have a practice development plan. It is also likely that this method will form a major part of the revalidation process for GPs currently being developed.

Random case analysis A selection of cases seen for a particular condition is chosen randomly for discussion in a peer group.

Multi-practice audits Frequently, groups of practices get together to audit particular topics and to compare results anonymously (benchmarking). Many multi-practice audit programmes are in existence nationally for conditions such as diabetes and asthma.

Having decided on a method of data collection, it is often easier to design and use a form specifically to record information as it is encountered. An example data collection form for an audit in ischaemic heart disease is shown in Case study 13.8 (below). The form allows the person collecting data to enter 'Yes' or 'No' in each of four columns as they examine the patients' medical records, depending on whether or not the criteria are met. There is a row at the foot of the form for totals, i.e. the number of times 'Yes' was entered, to be summed.

CASE STUDY 13.8

Criterion: the records show that within the last year all coronary heart disease patients are taking aspirin unless contra-indications or side effects preclude it.

The following data should be collected (Table 13.1).

■ The records within the last year show that the patient is taking aspirin.

■ The records show that the patient has stopped aspirin due to side effects.

■ The records show that aspirin is no longer being taken, reason unknown.

■ The records show that aspirin was considered but not recommended due to contra-indications.

The patients in column C of Table 13.1 had no recorded legitimate reason for stopping, and therefore are not included in the calculation.

Table 13.1 Data collection form: aspirin and ischaemic heart disease

Patient identification	A. Patient currently taking aspirin	B. Aspirin not being taken because of side effects	C. Aspirin stopped, reason unknown	D. Aspirin considered but contra-indicated
Patient 1	Yes	No	No	No
Patient 2	No	Yes	No	No
Patient 3	No	No	No	Yes
Patient 4				
...				
Total 'Yes'	56	3	5	5

Audit population = 108.

Criterion level of performance = total A/[audit population − (total B + total D)].

Criterion level of performance = 56/(108 − 8) = **56 per cent**.

Thinking and Discussion Point

For your audit, design a simple data collection form. Check that you will collect all the information you need to calculate the level of performance for each of your criteria.

Sampling techniques in audit

The benefits of audit are to some extent reduced by the time and effort required to collect, analyse and present the audit data. For this reason, many of the most profitable audits are simple and require little time. Auditing the total target population for, say, diabetes may involve in some practices examining 200 sets of medical records, a task requiring a considerable investment in time. For this reason, a practice may choose to take a sample of the population. In practical terms, this can be either a random sample, by assigning a number to each record and then choosing the records using random number tables, or a systematic sample, by choosing every third (or tenth) set of notes until the required sample is gained. (You should ensure that notes are extracted from the full range of the population, as the records are not ordered randomly.) The size of the sample you take is determined by the error you will find acceptable within the audit. The exact calculation of the sample size is beyond the scope of

this text and will be dealt with within your statistics teaching. Suffice it to say that for 200 sets of records, only 100 of them might need to be looked at to have 95 per cent confidence that the result will be within 5 per cent of the value of your total population. As a result, your workload will be greatly reduced.

How to deal with audit results in practice (Fig. 13.4)

Thinking and Discussion Point

For your audit, sketch out how you will present the audit results to the group.

The analysis and presentation of results need to take account of how the results will be used by the team in their development planning. Is the team likely to study them in detail or is the plan for the results to be presented at a meeting? On the whole, simple graphical or tabular formats are sufficient, provided that care is taken to ensure that the participants easily understand the mode of presentation. This can be achieved with very little in the way of technical requirements, although excellent presentations can be prepared very quickly if spreadsheet technology is used (e.g. Microsoft Excel, Lotus 123 etc.). The presenter needs to be fully conversant with the specific wording of

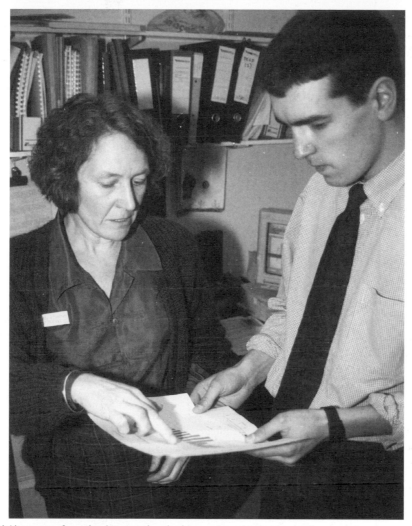

Figure 13.4 Making sense of practice data: a serious business.

the criteria and standards. Part of the discussion needs to consider what errors may occur within the results so that spurious claims for improvement are not made. For example, if a sample has been taken, a 5 per cent error may arise simply by taking a sample. A 5 per cent error may or may not be important for the audit.

An example of the presentation of audit results is shown in Figure 13.5.

Planning relevant changes and alterations to working practices

Earlier in the chapter you were encouraged to do a change analysis before you undertook to do the audit. This will ensure that all the people on whom the audit impacts are involved in it and that they will be ready to plan changes together that are realistic and can then make the necessary changes to their own working practices. It is probably true to say that if audits fail to achieve their purpose, it is usually at this stage. Thinking about what is needed for change early on in the audit process helps to reduce the risk of the audit not meeting its potential.

So, once people decide to meet to plan change, what happens? All those involved need the opportunity to voice their ideas without

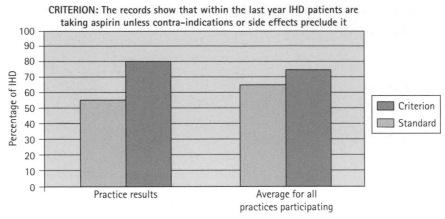

Figure 13.5 Audit results for a simple audit of aspirin use in ischaemic heart disease (IHD).

planning meetings being dominated by one or two individuals (often the doctors) if a team approach is to be supported. One technique that can be used for this is *brainstorming*.

- Each member of the team is asked in turn to suggest in a sentence possible ways in which improvements might be made and these ideas are recorded for everyone to see. Ideas are expressed without elaboration or comment from other members. The ideas are not meant to be well-thought-out structures at this stage. The main purpose is to gain as wide a view of the topic as possible so that change plans do not focus only on a narrow aspect.

- Examine the ideas from your brainstorming in the light of available resources. Planning of this nature does not necessarily mean doing more, and it is important to ask 'Can we do some things less?' Unless this occurs, professionals will quickly feel overburdened and will not be able to make the changes necessary. Good management needs priorities to be set that take account of the limitations of resources, for example people's time and expertise.

- Formulate a consensus agreement of changes that are possible as well as of how such changes are to be implemented. It is important to document the steps involved in your action plan and include time scales as well as who will do what.

- Document how the implementation will be monitored, e.g. re-audit, practice review.
- Set up an early review of the plan and implementation to identify practical blocks to change and to find ways round this. If things do not happen, there is usually a practical reason – avoid a 'we must try harder' mentality, as this invariably misses the real reasons for things not happening. Either such blocks can be overcome or the plan can be re-formulated. The most important thing is not to lose the momentum generated by the team's involvement in the process by ignoring difficulties.

Thinking and Discussion Point

For your audit, assuming that your criteria were below the standards you set, identify changes that could happen.
- ❑ Who is involved in these changes?
- ❑ What do they need to change?

Identify possible practical blocks to change at this stage (e.g. are your plans realistic given the setting/resources?). Try writing down your plan, including time scales and who will fulfil each part of it. Resolve how you are going to check whether your planned changes have been implemented.

CLINICAL AUDIT: CURRENT AND FUTURE DEVELOPMENTS

SYSTEMATIC AUDIT USING COMPUTER DATABASES

Practices are increasingly turning to audit to look at a range of clinical areas. By using their computers more effectively, a larger range of audits becomes possible in the time available. As a result, practices are able to move towards a more systematic approach where repeating audits at regular intervals becomes a part of their practice systems.

ELECTRONIC AUDIT

Increasingly, audits are written to query the computer patient record. The results can then be collated electronically to formulate audit reports. This does demand that record keeping is in good order for a particular condition. To aid this, many practices are increasingly using disease templates to prompt good record keeping.

Developing electronic audit is vital if we are to progress towards an extensive integrative quality system in practice.

INTERFACE AUDIT

Many aspects of clinical care involve the transition of patients between primary and secondary care, or areas of joint responsibility such as diabetic care. Audit is becoming more popular as a tool to try to improve the communication between these two groups and for professionals to understand more clearly the differing roles of primary and secondary care professionals. These audits can be complex and need to involve professionals across the interface in planning changes if they are to succeed in improving patient care.

CONTRACTING AND AUDIT

It is common practice in secondary care for audit activity within certain clinical topics to be a part of the contract between a trust and the local health authority. While the specific audit results remain confidential, the trust is required to show in what ways changes have been planned to services and then implemented. In primary care, audit is required as an activity if remuneration is given in the care of diabetes and asthma and, more recently, in practice incentive schemes, where practices are asked to prioritize their efforts towards a particular clinical topic.

PATIENT INVOLVEMENT IN AUDIT

Practices are increasingly aware that involving patients in planning their services can be extremely helpful. The most common involvement is in the form of a patient satisfaction questionnaire. However, more important work is beginning in the area of involving patients in defining clinical outcomes; these can then be the basis for audit. An example of this might be in considering morbidity and prognosis after myocardial infarction. Clinicians would tend to measure satisfactory outcome in terms of increased survival, myocardial infarction recurrence rates, re-admissions to hospital and perhaps changes in measured exercise or even anxiety rating scores. From the patient's perspective, however, things might be measured very differently. Our patients' perspectives on outcome relate more to their particular health beliefs and expectations and how their condition affects their ability to function in the context of their family, social and work environments. What constitutes a reasonable outcome for one patient might be intolerable to another. An example of this might be two patients who have no residual ischaemia after angioplasty. One patient may be delighted to be able to take up sport once again, while another is unable to return to normal sexual relations with his partner because of both their fears about further heart attacks. Both might represent good outcomes on the clinician's scale, but clearly things are not always so good from the patient's point of view. By learning more about how patients see outcomes, we will improve our clinical decisions and, in audit terms, be closer to assessing improvements in the quality of life of our patients. (See the definitions of audit on p. 236.)

SUMMARY POINTS

To conclude, the following are the most important messages of this chapter.

- Effective linkage between research evidence and improvements in patient care is often over-estimated and this remains a continuing source of concern for those involved in the health service.
- There are problems and lengthy delays in implementing even well-founded evidence, because research methods largely do not embody any form of change mechanism.

   The example of ischaemic heart disease we have used throughout this chapter is a case in point. Aspirin usage in patients with ischaemic heart disease has been the subject of research, review, clinical guidelines and, more recently, audit. This process has taken of the order of 20 years. Only with the use of audit has the patient group in particular general practices who need aspirin therapy been fully quantified, allowing them to be actively sought and their 'need' met.

- The Department of Health is attempting to resolve these issues by setting up clinical governance structures, NICE and NSFs.
- Clinical audit, by combining research technologies with a potentially effective change mechanism, can overcome these difficulties.
- By following the explanation of the audit cycle within this chapter, you should be in a position to take part, with others, in audit activities and begin to plan effective changes in care where change is seen as appropriate.

REFERENCES

Antiplatelet Trialists' Collaboration 1994: Collaborative overview of randomised trials of antiplatelet therapy. 1. Prevention of death, myocardial infarction, and stroke by prolonged antiplatelet therapy in various categories of patients. *British Medical Journal* 11(308), 81–106.

Cartwright, A. 1983: *Health surveys in practice and potential.* London: King Edward's Hospital Fund for London.

Chalmers, I., Dickersin, K. and Chalmers, T.C. 1992: Getting to grips with Archie Cochrane's agenda. *British Medical Journal* 305, 786–8.

Department of Health 1989: *Working for patients.* London: HMSO.

Department of Health 1993a: *Research for health.* London: HMSO.

Department of Health 1993b: *Improving clinical effectiveness.* London: HMSO.

Department of Health 1999: *National Service Framework for mental health: modern standards & service models.* London: HMSO.

Department of Health 2000: *Coronary heart disease: National Service Framework for coronary heart disease: modern standards and service models.* London: HMSO.

Department of Health 2001: *National Service Framework for older people.* London: HMSO.

Department of Health 2003: *Research and development programme.* Available online at: http://www.doh.gov.uk/research/index.htm

Ghandi, M.M., Lampe, F.C. and Wood, D.A. 1995: Management of angina pectoris in general practice: a questionnaire survey of general practitioners. *British Journal of General Practice* 45(395), 328–9.

Hunt, S., McKenna, S. and McEwan, J. 1986: *Measuring health status.* London: Croom Helm.

National Health Service Management Executive 1991: *Assessing health care needs.* DHA Project Paper. London: Department of Health.

NHS Executive 1994: *Developing NHS purchasing and GP fundholding: towards a primary care led NHS.* EL(94)79. Leeds: NHS Executive.

Oldridge, N.B., Guyatt, G.H., Fischer, M.E. and Rimm, A.A. 1988: Cardiac rehabilitation after myocardial infarction. *Journal of the American Medical Association* 260, 945–50.

Ong, B. 1993: *The practice of health services research.* London: Chapman & Hall.

Scally, G. and Donaldson, L. 1998: Looking forward: clinical governance and the drive for quality improvement in the new NHS in England. *British Medical Journal* 317, 61–5.

Schellevis, F.G., van Eijk, J.T., van den Lisdonk, E.H., van den Veldon, J. and van Weel, C. 1994: Implementing guidelines in general practice. Evaluation of process and outcome of care in chronic diseases. *International Journal of Quality in Health Care* 6(3), 257–66.

Simvastatin Study Group 1994: Randomised trial of cholesterol lowering in 4444 patients with coronary heart disease: the Scandinavian Simvastatin Survival Study. *Lancet* 344, 1383–9.

Van Zwanenberg, T. and Harrison, J. (eds) 2000: *Clinical governance in primary care.* Abingdon: Radcliffe Medical Press.

FURTHER READING

Belsey, J. and Snell, T. What is evidence based medicine? Available online at: www.evidence-based-medicine.co.uk

Cartwright, A. 1983: *Health surveys in practice and potential.* London: King Edward's Hospital Fund for London.
This remains a key text for health services research.

Department of Health 2000: *Building a safer NHS for patients.* Available online at: www.doh.gov.uk/buildsafenhs/index.htm

Department of Health 2000: *The NHS Plan.* London: HMSO.

Irvine, D. 1991: *Making sense of audit.* Abingdon: Radcliffe Medical Press.

Irvine, D. and Irvine, S. 1996: *The practice of quality.* Abingdon: Radcliffe Medical Press.
Irvine's *Making sense of audit* will be found on the bookshelves of just about everybody who has ever had any interest in clinical audit, and *The practice of quality* is an ideal companion text.

Ong, B. 1993: *The practice of health services research.* London: Chapman & Hall.
This book is especially useful for the chapters on qualitative, evaluation and multi-method research methodologies.

National Institute for Clinical Excellence 2002: *Principles for best practice in clinical audit.* Abingdon: Radcliffe Medical Press.

Pringle, M. 1991: *Making change in primary care.* Abingdon: Radcliffe Medical Press.
In this book, Pringle tackles head-on the thorny issue of developing change.

Roberts, G. 2002: *Risk management in healthcare,* 2nd edn. London: Witherby.
This book provides a detailed account of risk management.

Robson, C. 1993: *Real world research.* Oxford: Blackwell.
A really down-to-earth, practical approach, which is still, nevertheless, packed with theory.

Van Zwanenberg, T. and Harrison, J. (eds) 2000: *Clinical governance in primary care.* Abingdon: Radcliffe Medical Press.
This book gives a detailed account of clinical governance.

APPENDIX: EXAMPLE OF CHANGE ANALYSIS FOR AN AUDIT TO ASSESS THE QUALITY OF CARE AIMED AT REDUCING THE RISK FACTORS OF PATIENTS WITH ISCHAEMIC HEART DISEASE IN THE PRACTICE

CONSIDERING OUR AUDIT TOPIC, WHAT BROAD AREAS WHERE CHANGE MIGHT BE NEEDED CAN YOU IDENTIFY?

Possible areas for change

- Increased use of opportunistic contact with patients to give education, appropriate monitoring and treatment of risk factors might be needed.
- A system to record regular reviews of patients with ischaemic heart disease might be needed.
- A recall system for inviting patients who have not been reviewed opportunistically might be required.
- Training of staff will need to be considered, e.g. doctors, nurses and clerical staff, in recording clinical reviews and running the recall system.
- Re-prioritizing time for the practice nurse and some doctors may be required, e.g. spending more time on reviews for this group and less on monitoring controlled hypertension.
- Practice nurse time might need to be increased by employing a nurse for more hours.
- More money might be needed to fund increased nurse time.
- The health visitor is interested in ischaemic heart disease and would consider contacting and supporting patients post myocardial infarction, but would need the practice to identify patients and tell her about them.
- The district nurse is currently undergoing training in offering cardiac rehabilitation for post myocardial infarction patients in conjunction with the hospital cardiac rehabilitation services. Any service she offers needs to be understood and co-ordinated with the other practice initiatives.

WHO ARE THESE CHANGES LIKELY TO IMPACT ON?

- All doctors.
- Practice nurses.
- Practice clerical staff.
- Health visitors, district nurse.

WHAT DO PEOPLE NEED TO MAKE SUCH CHANGES?

Motivational factors

These have a major impact on whether realistic changes are planned, implemented and, most importantly, maintained. A team approach to care is often linked to high-quality services. The team approach relies on each professional seeing him/herself as a valued member of the team whose role and work are understood by the team's other members.

The following are often prerequisites for successful change.

- All those who might need to change their working practice need to be involved in the audit process.
- Each professional involved needs recognition of his or her time limitations, current contribution and work priorities.
- Team members often need to see change in behaviour by others; they may need continued feedback on performance in a non-threatening environment.
- The team needs to demonstrate success for individuals and as a whole in planning and implementing improvements in the quality of care if a focus is to be maintained.

Resources

- All those potentially involved need to spend time meeting together to plan the audit, discuss the results and consider what changes are realistic.
- These plans might need to look at re-prioritizing people's workloads and determining how key people might free up time for this area by doing less of something else.
- A further audit cycle might be needed fairly soon to give people direct feedback on whether their implementation was successful.
- Leaflets and other educational material may need to be ordered and their re-ordering included within the practice stock-taking systems.
- There might be financial implications based on the extra use of stationery, phone calls etc., as well as staff time to run recall systems.

CHAPTER 14

THE MANAGEMENT OF GENERAL PRACTICE

For general practices everywhere to deliver high-quality health care to patients, a team of health-care professionals and support staff is needed. The job of a practice manager is to create an environment in which members of this team can work together successfully to achieve the best possible service to their patients, the greatest possible job satisfaction for themselves, and financial viability for the practice.

LEARNING OBJECTIVES

By the end of this chapter, you will be able to:

- understand why general practices need management;
- grasp the basic principles of management;
- appreciate general practice's place in a National Health Service;
- understand the function of a management team;
- identify the different aspects of a practice manager's job.

WHY DO WE NEED MANAGEMENT IN GENERAL PRACTICE?

When you go into a general practice today, you are likely to find that it has a practice manager. It may even have a management team consisting of a practice manager, an assistant practice manager and perhaps a finance manager or a development manager. Why?

General practices are businesses. In Great Britain, since the 1990 General Practice Contract (National Health Service, General Medical and Pharmaceutical Services, Regulations 1974 as amended 1990), a more business-like ethos has entered general practice. General practitioners (GPs) are expected to serve their community, to treat patients and to act as a gateway to hospital and specialist care. But they also have to run their practice profitably, to market their services and to think of their patients as customers.

Most general practices are now also complex organizations. They are group practices with several GP partners, employing practice nurses and other professionals, supported by clerical and reception staff. Usually they are housed in purpose-built or adapted practice premises. A wide and varied range of services is offered to patients/users by general practices. On their part, patients rightly expect a high quality of care from their doctors, and general practices have to be organized to provide this. In addition, within a health service climate of limited resources, government health initiatives, clinical governance and the need to be profitable, all demands for services have to be weighed and balanced carefully against each other and against available staff, time and finance.

Such complex businesses, within a constantly changing health service environment, need specialist management. For high-quality, appropriate patient care to be provided in a financially viable way, high-quality management by managers who are equipped for the task is vital. All aspects of the service need to be managed. General practitioners need managers with whom financial management, strategic planning, decision making, the management of change and day-to-day operational responsibilities can be shared. They cannot manage today's general practices on their own, without taking quantities of time out from their clinical roles. It is practice managers who take the lead, in consultation with the practice GP partners, in planning, organizing and working with the whole primary healthcare team. They manage the practice, sometimes on their own with the GP partners, but more often with a management team, which also contains any other team members who perform a management role, for example the senior practice nurse.

Practical Exercise

Make a list of all the members of the primary healthcare team in your practice, clinical and non-clinical.

❑ Is there a practice manager?
❑ Is there an assistant manager?
❑ Is there an identifiable management team?
❑ How long has the practice had a manager?
❑ Was the manager appointed to make the practice more businesslike?
❑ Have the services offered by the practice (e.g. clinics, minor surgery) increased?

Ask the practice manager.

WHAT IS MANAGEMENT?

Management is getting things done through people and systems. A manager has to conduct an orchestra of people and systems through the steps of 'what to do', 'how to do it', 'who to do it', 'doing it' and then checking if it has been done as well as possible.

To put it more formally, managers have to:

■ establish objectives,
■ research background,
■ define roles, policies, procedures,
■ determine priorities,
■ decide on resources – people, finance, systems,
■ negotiate the plan,
■ lead and motivate the team,
■ review performance and progress,
■ modify and change – according to experience and outside factors.

Figure 14.1 shows the cycle of management.

In order to do all the above, managers have to use different skills:

■ interpersonal skills: team building, negotiating and persuading, leading, liaising and communicating;
■ information gathering and analysis skills: auditing, analysing, communicating results;
■ decision-making skills.

PRACTICE MANAGEMENT

In order to manage in general practice, a manager has to do all these things and use these skills. The basics of management are the same in every organization, but general practice

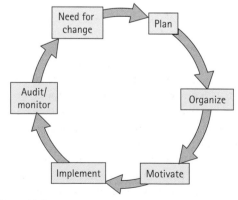

Figure 14.1 The management cycle.

management has some different aspects. Most managers work in a specific function within a large organization. They may be working in personnel, finance, marketing or other areas. Hospital managers are like this; they work in a single department of the hospital and manage that section alone. Next time you are in the hospital, ask to look at a management chart and see how many managers there are. The general practice manager works in a relatively small organization, with perhaps 10–40 staff, but has a much wider range of responsibilities: patient/user relations, staff, finance, office procedures, audit, planning of services, service delivery, marketing, interface with other medical services, building maintenance, clinical governance, health and safety, and more.

Practical Exercise

Ask the practice manager in your practice to give you examples of his or her responsibilities under the following headings:
- ❏ human resources,
- ❏ finance,
- ❏ customer relations,
- ❏ marketing.

GENERAL PRACTICE'S PLACE IN THE NATIONAL HEALTH SERVICE

A general practice is usually an independent small business owned by a GP partnership and independently managed by a management team of GPs and practice manager or managers. However, it does not genuinely stand alone. In Britain it is part of a large public sector organization, the National Health Service (NHS). To a large extent, it is funded and resourced by the NHS, but practice management teams can make decisions about how their resources can be used and which services they will offer, within the constraints of either the General Medical Services (GMS) contract or the Personal Medical Services (PMS) contract. These two kinds of contract lay down the rules under which GPs work.

PERSONAL MEDICAL SERVICES AND GENERAL MEDICAL SERVICES CONTRACTS

In Britain since 1997, GPs have been able to choose to work under two distinct contract frameworks. The GMS contract is the standard national contract to which all GPs worked until 1997. The contract specifies set terms of service that govern what core services GPs must provide, how they must provide them and what they must not provide.

In a PMS arrangement, a GP practice contracts with the local primary care trust (PCT) for the services it will provide. General practitioners remain independent contractors. The PMS is an alternative contract framework that offers a new, more flexible way of delivering services. It covers exactly the same core services for patients as GMS, but has the flexibility to extend to cover a much wider range of services than GMS. PMS practices can offer services aimed specifically at local needs. The PMS also offers flexibility in how services are organized. This includes the options of employing salaried GPs and the use of nurse practitioners instead of GPs. PMS practices are funded differently from GMS practices (see below).

At the time of writing, the GMS contract is soon to be replaced by a new GMS contract under which GP practices will contract with their local PCT. This will still be a national contract, but will offer practices greater flexibility to determine the level of service they wish to provide.

PRIMARY CARE TRUSTS

General practices provide what is called primary care. They are contract managed by their local PCT, the NHS organization that is responsible for ensuring the provision of primary and community care to the whole population of the area that it covers. PCTs are therefore responsible for supporting and developing primary care within either GMS or PMS contractual arrangements. They are general practice's link to the wider NHS. The PCT managers offer support to practices; they allocate funding for service development and they performance manage their practices.

PRACTICE INCOME

Most general practice income is received from the NHS. Only a small element can be privately earned. Much of the NHS income can be varied according to the number of patients a practice has, the amount of work it does and the type of services it offers.

General Medical Services GPs are paid under a prescribed funding mechanism known as the 'red book' (the statement of fees and allowances). Their income mainly consists of:

■ capitation fees (based on numbers of registered patients),
■ deprivation payments (for patients living in areas of high deprivation),
■ item of service fees (for which the practice has to submit claims),
■ targets and health-promotion payments.

The rest of the NHS income is made up of subsidies from the NHS to enable the GPs to do their job of carrying out their contract. These subsidies are:

■ rent and rate reimbursement (all rent and rates are paid),
■ basic practice allowance,
■ staff reimbursement (a large proportion of practice staff salaries and National Insurance and pension contributions is funded by the NHS).

Personal Medical Services GPs agree an annual fixed contract sum with the PCT, which they receive in monthly instalments. This sum is based on what is agreed as an equitable payment for the services they provide. It is based in the first instance on their previous GMS income and can be altered up or down as practice circumstances (for example numbers of patients registered) change. All the subsidies described above are included in PMS contract payments.

Under the new GMS contract framework (see above), it is intended that practices will be paid a global sum of money for the work that they do, with the opportunity of further payments for quality and additional services.

Although the GP is subsidized, the practice can still affect its income substantially. Within the constraints of the GMS or PMS contracts, it can decide how many patients it wishes to serve and how to offer services to those patients.

PCTs will allocate funding to practices to enable them to provide additional services if they judge a practice to be working efficiently and effectively and to be providing a high quality of service.

THE MANAGEMENT TEAM

General practitioner partners and practice managers ensure that practices run smoothly and profitably by working together in a general practice management team. Each member of the team plays an important part in the management of the practice. The management team provides leadership for the practice and decides (often in consultation with the whole primary healthcare team) on the 'vision' it wants for the practice and the ethos or culture of the practice. Having decided these things, the team members have to act as role models in the practice and build towards their vision. They need to have asked themselves the following questions.

■ What are we doing?
■ What is special about us?
■ What can we do?
■ Where do we want to go?

Then they can all move forward together. They can develop a practice development plan and use it as a basis for all planning and assessment of training needs and to monitor progress.

Both the GP partners and the practice manager lead the practice, but it is the practice manager who has the executive function of making the development plan happen, bringing forward issues for discussion and following through decisions made whilst monitoring new items for consideration. The practice manager is in an unusual position as a vital team member, but, because the GPs are the owners of the organization, the practice manager is an employee. There are now examples of practice managers becoming partners in general practices, but this is not widespread.

The practice manager has to advise the partners on policy and planning and has to manage them as well as the employed staff. He or she has to forge agreements on practice policy, procedures and new health initiatives (such as National Service Frameworks), and ensure that these are followed by all the primary healthcare team, including the GPs. Everyone has to be involved if the practice is to run well and provide high-quality care to patients.

Practical Exercise

Does your practice have a management team? Do its members meet regularly for management meetings? Ask if you can attend one such meeting. Watch how the practice manager functions in the meeting. Write a short description of the meeting, describing the role of each participant. (Remember that if confidential staff or financial matters are to be discussed, you will probably be asked to leave.)

WHAT DOES THE PRACTICE MANAGER DO?

Practice managers' jobs fall into several different areas. They have to juggle their responsibilities and constantly assess their priorities.

PATIENT/CUSTOMER CARE

Good patient care is central to the 'vision' of the practice management team. Patients require a quality service from the practice and the practice manager has constantly to keep this in the forefront of the team's minds. Both doctors and staff will work more happily if they are giving a good service. The income of the practice depends on numbers of patients registered and services provided. Patients must be attracted to the practice and then kept. In the UK it is now extremely simple to change one's GP: patients merely have to ask to be registered at a new practice, and do not need to inform their previous GP. A good practice is one that keeps its patients. The manager has to ensure that this happens in his or her practice. How is this done?

Ask the patients what they want and learn from them

The manager has to check that appropriate services are being provided.

- Are clinic and surgery times acceptable?
- Is the surgery accessible?

- Are telephones manned at the right times?
- Is the practice leaflet helpful and informative?
- Are practice staff helpful and informative?

Once the manager gets answers to these questions, they can be acted upon and changes can be made if necessary. There are various ways that patients can be asked: user groups, questionnaires, focus groups, and quick surveys in the waiting room or over the reception desk.

Practical Exercise

Ask the practice manager at your practice what customer opinion surveys have been carried out. Devise a short survey about an aspect of the practice's service delivery. Show it to your GP tutor and the practice manager and ask if you can question a sample of patients in the waiting room. Analyse the results and present them to the practice management team.

Make sure that systems work and that a good service is always given

Patients want a practice to run efficiently and to have systems which work. It is the practice manager's job to ensure that a good service is given to patients every time. If mistakes do occur, the manager should look into them at once and, if necessary, change the process if a weakness is found. The manager should also check the standard of service being offered through audits and patient surveys and make changes if necessary.

Deal with complaints at once

Inevitably, there will be times when patients feel that they are not getting the service they expect. All practice staff need to know that patients do get angry and frustrated, sometimes with good reason, and they need to be able to handle such situations. Often tact and a listening ear can solve the problem, but frequently complaints have to be dealt with by the practice manager and, in the case of complaints about medical care, the doctor or nurse has to be involved. Practices have procedures for handling complaints. The most important factor is that the complaint is investigated and dealt with speedily and an apology is immediately offered if necessary. It is the responsibility of the manager to see that this is done.

Practical Exercise

Ask to see the practice complaints procedure. Are there different levels of complaint? Ask the practice manager how he/she applies it, and about the last complaint dealt with.

Explain to patients how you do things

If the patients do not understand the system, they will at best be confused and at worst angry. It is important that systems are explained to them. Clear and informative practice leaflets, notices in the waiting room, handouts about specific services, clear signs in the practice building and helpful reception staff all help to inform patients.

Practical Exercise

Ask for a copy of the practice leaflet at your practice. If you were a new patient, would it tell you what you needed to know? Ask the receptionists what they do when new patients ask to register. What information do they give them?

Make sure the practice looks good

The practice manager needs to ensure that the practice image is good. Patients will prefer to come into a surgery that looks attractive and is comfortable. They want to be greeted by friendly, sympathetic staff. Of course the medical care they receive is the most important factor of their contact with the practice, but the reception area is the first thing they see and the receptionist's voice is the first they hear over the telephone. All staff should be aware that it is practice policy to be as helpful as possible to patients and that smiling is important.

The following things should be organized and attractive:

- the waiting room,
- the reception area and layout,
- notice boards and posters,
- practice leaflets,
- practice signs,
- the receptionist's manner and dress,
- telephone answering,
- car parking.

Provide information for patients

The practice is a central point in any community. It has a vital role to play in disseminating information to patients. The manager should ensure that the practice can provide information on:

- health education,
- disease prevention,
- local services, e.g. playgroup, libraries, transport,
- local medical services, e.g. dentists, hospitals, chiropodists,
- local schools,
- welfare rights,
- local organizations, e.g. Women's Institute, National Childbirth Trust.

STAFF MANAGEMENT

A successful general practice is dependent on good staff. A motivated and well-trained workforce is the backbone of a good practice. This means that the manager should invest a lot of time in the staff.

Imagine that you are a patient walking into a practice reception area. Would you prefer to be greeted by:

- a smiling receptionist, wearing a name badge, who answers your query and offers you an appointment; or
- the back view of a receptionist who is gossiping with a colleague and then cannot answer your question or find the relevant appointment page on the computer?

The answer is obvious. Effective recruitment and training of staff, together with ongoing motivation and job satisfaction for them, are the keys to an effective practice.

For the doctors to function well, they need the support of confident reception staff who answer the telephone, make appointments, manage patient records and deal with happy and unhappy patients successfully. For the practice to function well, referrals have to be made, entries have to be made on the computer, new patients have to be registered, supplies have to be ordered, and so on. The entire organization can only be a success story if all members of staff do their work well and with confidence and offer a quality service to the patients.

The manager of a typical practice might have the following employed staff to manage:

- receptionists,
- clerical staff,
- secretaries,
- general practice clinical assistants,
- salaried GP(s),
- practice nurse(s),
- practice counsellor,
- clinical psychologist,
- physiotherapist,
- osteopath,
- cleaning staff,
- maintenance staff.

In addition, there may be the following attached staff, employed by the PCT but managed by the practice manager in relation to the work they do for the practice (the practice manager will manage these staff in consultation with their employers, of course):

- health visitors,
- midwives,
- dietician,
- district nurses,
- special nurse advisors.

You will see at once that some of these staff are clinical and some are not. Practice managers are not involved in the clinical element of the work clinical staff do, but they are accountable to the manager for the way in which their work is done and the type of services that are delivered, e.g. timings of clinics, numbers of patients to be seen, recording of work, and so on. The practice manager is also responsible for planning with them and the management team any changes in their work.

How does the practice manager manage the staff?

Recruitment

First of all, the practice manager has to recruit good staff. The process is as follows.

- Look at the post that needs to be filled and decide with the management team what the practice requirements for the post are.
- Write a job description for the post that needs filling. This should list the purpose of the post and all the tasks the jobholder needs to carry out. It should also include the hours of work and the salary.
- Write a person specification. This describes the type of person you want for the job, detailing skills required, qualifications needed and personal qualities necessary.
- Agree these documents with the management team.
- Advertise the post.
- Provide an application form.
- Shortlist candidates using the job description and person specification.
- Hold selection interviews. Usually the selection panel will consist of the practice manager and two or three other members of the management team.
- Take up references.
- Send a letter of appointment to the successful candidate.
- Agree a contract of employment and fix a start date.

This probably seems a long and time-consuming process in order to appoint a member of staff. However, it is worth it. The wrong person is far less likely to be appointed if careful joint planning goes into the selection process. Good members of staff who fit into their jobs are vital to the health of the practice.

Induction: introduction to the practice

When a new member of staff starts work in the practice, the manager arranges a programme of induction training for him/her. New staff cannot be thrown in at the deep end: they must be made welcome at once; they need to get to know the layout of the practice, the other staff, the GP partners, the services the practice offers and the ethos of the practice. They also need to learn their new job. This may mean in-house training or external training, which the practice manager must organize. This is a very important stage in order to ensure that the new staff member is functioning happily and efficiently in as short a time as possible.

CASE STUDY 14.1

Miss M, the new practice receptionist, was told to come in for her first day at 8.30 a.m. on a Monday. No one in the reception area welcomed her as they were too busy answering the telephone and preparing for morning surgery, which began at 9.00 a.m. The practice manager did not get in until 9.30 a.m. Miss M stood in the reception area, uncertain as to what to do until then. At one point a doctor asked her for some medical notes urgently and snapped at her when she could not produce them. By 9.30 a.m. she was terrified and unhappy.

Thinking and Discussion Point

❑ Is this a good beginning?
❑ What could the practice manager have organized to make Miss M's first day a happier and more productive one?
❑ As a medical student, how did your first day in a general practice feel?

Ongoing training and support

All practice staff continue to need training and updating on changes throughout their careers in order to do their work well and confidently. They also continue to need support and encouragement from their manager. The practice manager needs to have ensured that each member of staff has a personal development plan that sets out their training needs and achievements. Based upon this plan, the manager can arrange in-house training sessions and external courses for them and give them regular support and information through one-to-one interviews and group meetings. General practice is a stressful working environment. Staff members are in constant contact with patients who are anxious, unwell and often demanding. They require a lot of praise and support as they deal with difficult situations.

Appraisal

The practice manager will appraise or organize appraisals for all practice staff. At least once a year, a manager sits down with each member of staff and discusses his or her performance during the year, strengths and weaknesses. Staff members are invited to discuss their aspirations for the future, their feelings about their jobs and the practice. Then, together, the manager and each staff member produce a personal development plan for the future in which any training needs or changes in approach to work by the employee can be set out. Both the manager and the employee will aim to work to that plan until their next meeting. Then they review progress and modify the plan if necessary. This should be an ongoing process and should be as positive and supportive for the staff member as possible, not destructive. Appraisal and personal development planning should help employees perform better.

Discipline

If staff members fail to carry out the duties expected of them, or act in a manner that is contrary to the rules of the practice, the practice manager has to discipline them. In disciplinary matters, general practice in Britain usually abides by the ACAS guidelines (Advisory, Conciliation and Arbitration Service, UK, 1977). These lay down stages to be followed, depending on the gravity of the misconduct. There is an emphasis on counselling and discussion with employees about any problems they may be encountering that might have a bearing on their conduct, for example persistent lateness because of a sick relative. The range of disciplinary stages a manager can use includes:

- informal verbal warning/counselling,
- formal verbal warning/counselling,
- written warning,
- final written warning,
- dismissal with notice,
- dismissal without notice.

Grievances

If a member of staff has a grievance about the way he or she is treated or about the behaviour of a colleague or manager, the practice manager has to deal with this, and should listen to the grievances and take them seriously. Again, there should be an emphasis on counselling and discussion, and again, in Britain the ACAS guidelines for dealing with grievances apply (Advisory, Conciliation and Arbitration Service, UK, 1977).

OPERATIONAL MANAGEMENT

The practice manager is responsible for the organization and day-to-day work of the practice. Procedures, policies and services are all decided upon by the management team, in consultation where necessary with the whole primary healthcare team. However, daily work rotas and daily organizational problems have to be dealt with by the practice manager or assistant practice manager. When staff or doctors phone in sick, new arrangements have to be made; if a violent patient threatens to damage the waiting room, the patient has to be calmed down and, in extreme cases, the police have to be called; if vandals have broken surgery windows overnight, repairs have to be organized. This has been called crisis management, but the nature of general practice with its emphasis on people (staff, patients, the surrounding community) is such that 'crises' do frequently occur. A well-organized manager will have contingency plans and procedures for most eventualities, though inevitably things occur of a totally unforeseen nature, and have to be dealt with: 'the show must go on'. Patients cannot wait as the customers of some organizations can.

A busy doctor does not have time to deal with these day-to-day issues. Doctors rely on their managers to cope; they have employed them to manage.

Practical Exercise

Ask the practice manager in your practice how many on-the-spot decisions he/she has had to take today in reaction to events.

Protocols

Most areas of practice work, including potential 'crises', are best organized through practice protocols and systems. These protocols are worked out by the management team (often as the result of an audit) as the most efficient and effective

way of operating at that time. The practice will run better and staff will feel supported when there is a structure in place. Of course, there has to be flexibility in certain cases, but a good manager will have laid down ground rules for working. Even with such rules, conflicts can occur, but a structure is in place to be referred to.

CASE STUDY 14.2

The practice standard for non-urgent repeat prescriptions to be ready is 48 hours. (This is a reasonable standard which most practices would find workable.) A patient comes to the reception desk and demands a repeat prescription for aqueous cream at once. The receptionist rightly points out the 48-hour rule, and feels justified in doing this. A doctor standing in the reception area overhears and gets the prescription done on the computer there and then. The receptionist feels let down by the doctor and will complain to the practice manager.

CASE STUDY 14.3

There is a practice rule that during surgeries no telephone calls are to be put through to doctors and nurses by reception. The only exception is if a member of their family calls. A receptionist puts through an urgent call from the PCT to a doctor during a consultation. He is justifiably annoyed and complains to the practice manager.

Can you see that both 'guilty' parties in case studies 14.3 and 14.4 could argue that they were being helpful in their actions? Can you also see that it did not help other patients and the overall smooth running of the practice in the long run?

CLINICAL GOVERNANCE

As discussed in Chapter 13, general practices have to deliver high-quality care through clinical effectiveness, risk management and clinical audit. Each practice has a clinical governance lead who will be a senior clinician, but the practice manager has to be fully aware of clinical governance issues in his or her work. Clinical and operational risk management is a high priority and the manager has to ensure that risk assessments are carried out regularly on both practice premises and procedures. Critical incident/significant event reporting is also an area with which the practice manager must be involved, taking a lead in ensuring that full reports are made of any incident and that the primary healthcare team is fully debriefed, with appropriate learning and reflection. The practice manager will also organize any necessary follow-up action or change in procedure.

TEAM MANAGEMENT

We have seen how the manager supports and works with individual staff members. Practice managers also have to work to manage the entire primary healthcare team and the smaller teams within it. You have seen in Chapter 9 how, although doctors and nurses may work alone clinically, effective teamwork is vital in providing good-quality and effective medical care. It is the job of the practice manager to ensure that there is effective teamwork.

Decision making and communication

Effective teams must make good decisions. These must then be communicated to and understood by the whole practice team. Equally, everything that happens which affects the work of the practice needs to be communicated to the entire team. It is the practice manager's responsibility to see that these things happen.

Meetings

These are vital for decision making and team building. The practice manager must ensure that meetings are organized and well run. There are different types of practice meeting, e.g. clinical meeting, management meeting, receptionists meeting etc. The manager must ensure that the meeting includes all relevant team members, that there is an agenda and that the meeting is effectively chaired, that briefing papers are available where necessary, decisions are taken and minutes written and circulated. The manager must also ensure that any decisions taken by any smaller core meetings are communicated as necessary to the whole primary healthcare team. Even when the subject of a meeting is entirely clinical, it is always important for the manager to play a part. The manager needs to be aware of

the implications for the organization of the issue at hand, and frequently has an important contribution to make to the discussion.

CASE STUDY 14.4

The doctors and nurses in a practice decided to reorganize the family planning clinics. They planned to hold clinics in the early morning and the late evening. Neither the practice manager nor the reception manager was present at the planning meeting. They would have been aware of the implications for the staffing of reception at the times chosen, and would have been able to start planning for this change.

Team building and development

As part of the practice manager's responsibility for training the team and implementing the practice development plan, team-building exercises are vital. All team meetings are team-building exercises, as team members learn to work together and take joint decisions; however, managers often organize special 'away days' when the whole team, or one of the smaller practice teams, goes away from the practice and works together in small groups, possibly brainstorming a problem or discussing aims and objectives for themselves and for the practice. This is invaluable training for the team, which has to work as a unit and to get to know other team members' aspirations. Some PCTs are now funding their general practices to close for one afternoon a month to facilitate this type of practice team education and development. Social events and team expeditions are another tool the manager can use in welding the team together.

Practical Exercise

Ask the practice manager at your practice what team-building exercises the primary healthcare team has had in the last year. Ask a team member how he or she benefited from one of these.

STRATEGIC PLANNING

The practice manager will take a lead in strategic planning for the practice. He or she will meet regularly with the management team to look at practice objectives and to plan for new services and expansion as necessary, and will also need to react to changes in government, health authority and local authority policy (such as National Service Frameworks, Health Improvement Plans) which may affect the work of the practice. Every aspect needs to be considered as part of the planning process:

- finance
- staff
- buildings
- systems
- clinical governance
- equipment
- external factors
- patient opinion.

Any research needed has to be put in train by the manager. Audits may have to be carried out before decisions can be taken. Cost has to be considered very carefully. There will almost always be a conflict between demand for services, clinical need and limited resources. The manager and the team have to look at all options and come up with a plan. This planning will be an ongoing process – remember the management cycle (see Fig. 14.1).

FINANCE MANAGEMENT

The practice manager has to run the finances of the practice in such a way that it does not go into the red. As we have seen, the practice is a large and complex organization, employing staff and purchasing supplies and services. It has to be financially viable and provide acceptable incomes for the partners.

Income

It is the responsibility of the manager to ensure that all possible income comes into the practice. The manager of a GMS practice is responsible for overseeing all claims made to the funding authority and has to check that all fees and allowances are paid correctly to the practice. Staff pay reimbursement has to be checked, and rent and rates reimbursement. Obviously, some of this work can be delegated to clerical staff, but the manager has overall responsibility. The PMS manager has to ensure that the monthly cash flow accounts are kept up to date and that

any changes in practice work levels are highlighted so that variations to the PMS contract can be justified.

Practice income can be increased by good financial management – achieving quality standards and efficiently run services to earn the maximum amount of income. When the new GMS contract is introduced, practices will no longer need to make claims for individual items of service, but efficient financial management will still be essential.

Expenditure

The largest element of practice expenditure is staff pay. The manager is responsible for ensuring that the practice staff are paid and must manage this carefully. The manager has to keep any overtime within set limits and endeavour to stay within the staff budget.

The manager also has to manage all other expenditure very carefully, ensuring that the most reasonable suppliers are used and that practice purchases fit in with the cash flow.

Financial planning

This is an important element of all strategic planning for the practice. The practice manager prepares annual and 5-year business plans for the practice, including cash-flow forecasts, and then uses these as a yardstick for progress during the financial year.

Accounts

In most practices, the practice manager has responsibility for preparing the annual accounts for audit by the practice accountant. Each general practice is a business and has to have audited accounts.

INFORMATION TECHNOLOGY

Computers are now integral to the work of general practice. Information can be generated for audit and for planning purposes. Computerized registers and call and recall systems have made the management of health promotion much more effective. The management of chronic disease has been made easier with computer databases. Practices are now linked directly by computer to PCT finance and patient registration departments. Computerized appointment systems make reception work more efficient and help to monitor clinical output in the practice. Hospital appointments can be booked on line by primary care, and pathology results are being returned to practices via computer links. Work has begun on producing an electronic patient record that can be shared between primary, secondary and social care. Many practices are planning to become 'paperless'. This has been a massive change for general practice and all practice staff are having to adjust to it. Practice managers have had to manage this change, planning for it, communicating to staff about it, arranging training and support, negotiating new ways of working and getting agreement.

BUILDINGS

Most general practices work in purpose-built or specially adapted premises. The maintenance of these premises is the responsibility of the practice manager. The manager may delegate the tasks, but is personally responsible. Inevitably, the wear and tear on a practice building is great because of the number of patients who pass through daily, so regular maintenance is vital. It would be unsafe to leave damaged premises or equipment unrepaired. Equally, from the point of view of hygiene, practice premises have to be cleaned at least daily. Equipment has to be regularly serviced and checked. Any building expansion will be managed by the practice manager, as will the allocation of rooms in the building. Often, a complicated rota has to be worked out to accommodate the various clinical staff working in the building.

HEALTH AND SAFETY

As employers and providers of services to patients, the management team is legally responsible for providing and maintaining a safe working environment. All equipment, buildings and methods of working should be safe and free of risk to health. The manager must ensure that there are practice policies and protocols to make sure that health and safety laws are adhered to, must check regularly that the protocols are being followed, and must organize regular risk assessment procedures.

SUMMARY POINTS

To conclude, the most important messages of this chapter are:

- general practices are complex and ever-changing organizations and need specialist management;
- good-quality patient care needs good-quality management;
- management is getting things done through people and systems;
- general practices are independent businesses in the UK but very much a part of any health service;
- management in general practice is best done by a practice management team led by a practice manager;
- the conflict between rising demand and the need to provide quality service in line with government and local policy and limited resources in general practice means there is a need for strategic planning by the manager;
- a general practice manager has many different areas of responsibility: patients, staff, operational management, clinical governance, team management, strategic planning, management of change, finance, information technology, buildings, health and safety.

REFERENCES

Advisory, Conciliation and Arbitration Service, UK 1977: *Code of practice on disciplinary rules and procedures in employment*. London: HMSO.

National Health Service Act 1977, General Medical and Pharmaceutical Services Regulations 1974 as amended 1990: *The terms and conditions of service for general practitioners*. London: DHSS.

National Health Service (Primary Care) Act 1997, UK (General Medical and Pharmaceutical Services) 1997: *The statement of fees and allowances (The red book)*. London: DHSS.

 The practice manager of the general practice to which you are attached will have copies of these or their equivalent.

FURTHER READING

Dean, J. 2000: *Making sense of practice finance*, 3rd edn. Abingdon: Radcliffe Medical Press.

 A good general text for students interested in the financial management of general practice.

Drury, M. and Hobden-Clarke, L. (eds) 1995: *The practice manager*, 4th edn. Abingdon: Radcliffe Medical Press.

 A very comprehensive volume of chapters on all aspects of practice management, written for practice managers and senior receptionists.

Huntington, J. 1995: *Managing the practice: whose business?* Abingdon: Radcliffe Medical Press.

 An excellent and down-to-earth approach to management in general practice, written by a well-known guru.

Haman, H. and Irvine, S. 2001: *Good people, good practice*. Abingdon: Radcliffe Medical Press.

 A useful book about managing and employing staff.

PREPARING TO PRACTISE

A placement in general practice offers opportunities for learning that are relevant to your development as a practising clinician whatever your final career choice. The variety inherent in the cases you will deal with should encourage you to look beyond the immediate case to the common elements; the thinking and learning processes you employ will be generally applicable to all types of medical practice. This chapter considers some of the practical ways in which you can use these opportunities.

LEARNING OBJECTIVES

This chapter is based around nine selected learning objectives, and springs from experience gained designing and running a course for senior undergraduates, Eight Weeks in General Practice and Community, at Guy's, King's and St Thomas' School of Medicine, King's College, London.

By the end of this chapter, you will be able to:

- select and apply relevant methods of clinical reasoning;
- demonstrate good written communication skills;
- demonstrate good working relationships with members of a primary healthcare team and other agencies;
- show evidence of good timekeeping and organizational skills;
- implement strategies for managing uncertainty;
- demonstrate an awareness of your own limitations and an understanding of when and where to seek help;
- accept and utilize constructive criticism, be willing to reflect on your own strengths and weaknesses, and act upon them;
- maintain sound professional conduct;
- adopt strategies for lifelong learning.

INTRODUCTION

These nine learning objectives, one of which heads each section, consider aspects of your learning that are all achievable in the general practice setting, and are designed to be as relevant to those who will *not* eventually specialize in general practice as to those who will.

The sections can be considered separately, but they do interrelate, and there are cross-references. Much of the activity which leads to the achievement of these learning objectives is based in clinical practice, i.e. seeing and consulting with patients yourself, ideally in a separate room from your tutor but in close proximity, and with supervision and sanctioning of your decisions by your tutor. Reflection on what you have been doing in those consultations will yield interesting and useful information, so we encourage you to keep log diaries of some of your clinical sessions. Looking through the sections of the chapter, especially the thinking and discussion points and practical exercises, will give you an idea of the sort of information you could record in your log diaries.

Log diaries can be updated between consultations with patients or by reviewing the notes at the end of a clinical session. Sometimes it is useful to use different techniques, because, for instance, recording immediately after a consultation will be more influenced by the emotional impact of the individual consultation (an important factor that has to be considered in its own right), whereas recording at the end may illuminate how one consultation affected others in the same session.

Take opportunities to discuss more than individual cases with your tutor; consider also how your performance is changing, evolving or getting stuck. Make sure you think about the big picture as well as individual cases; take opportunities to see the common ground, the similarities between cases or between management strategies, as well as the differences – these will enable you to generate ideas within a consultation even when the case itself is one you have not seen before, because you have something similar to draw upon.

You will already have developed or be developing your own personal style; an aspect of this individuality is that we do not respond in the same way to patients, and some consideration of the impact different patients have on us as individuals is necessary so that we understand how this can influence our decision making. Discussions of these aspects of your development are good areas for tutorial work in one-to-one sessions with your tutor, and sometimes in group sessions with your peers.

In group sessions, everyone is a source of information, expertise and views, and all contribute; you are all responsible jointly for each other's learning. The function of these sessions may include:

- sharing individual experiences, learning vicariously about unusual cases,
- sharing ideas of expected levels of competence,
- providing support for each other,
- debating difficult or sensitive issues in a protected environment,
- practising peer review and receiving constructive criticism,
- working collaboratively on a particular topic,
- practising skills through role plays and group discussion,
- recruiting expert support in certain shared areas of learning need.

The ideas and concepts discussed in each section may overlap with those of other sections; experiential learning involves elements of different learning objectives in varying proportions. The reinforcement this provides is one of the strengths of this kind of learning, and is why clinical students enjoy and appreciate learning in the clinical environment. Reflection on the activities and experiences of your clinical time will further enhance and consolidate your learning.

SELECT AND APPLY RELEVANT METHODS OF CLINICAL REASONING

WHAT IS CLINICAL REASONING?

Many students coming into general practice from a hospital environment are struck by the apparently very different consultation technique, and the speed at which the consultations occur.

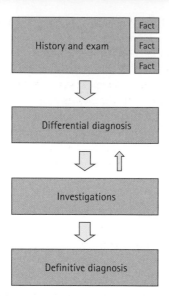

Figure 15.1 Inductive reasoning.

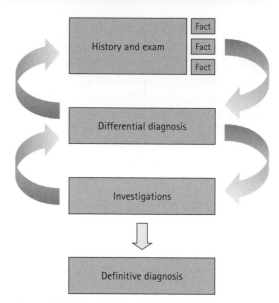

Figure 15.2 Hypothetico-deductive reasoning.

Naturally, they ask how they can perform consultations the same way. First, it is important to put aside speed as an independent goal – it is easier to learn to do the job well and then speed up than to learn to do it quickly and then get better. The second point to consider is: is this technique really as different as it seems?

Some words about clinical reasoning may shed some light on this. Undergraduate medical students are taught to take a history, perform a physical examination and write up case notes with the differential diagnosis at the end, as though it could only 'appear' at that point. This linear model of thinking is known as *inductive* reasoning, which can be described as the completion of a comprehensive information-gathering programme before thinking begins (Fig. 15.1).

Most experienced clinicians actually use a different model, *hypothetico-deductive* reasoning, which involves the postulation of an hypothesis during the consultation and the gathering of supporting or refuting evidence – sometimes known as 'guess and test' (Fig. 15.2).

A necessary part of this kind of thinking is pattern recognition, which depends on experience and which, at one extreme, may occasionally telescope the whole reasoning process (Fig. 15.3).

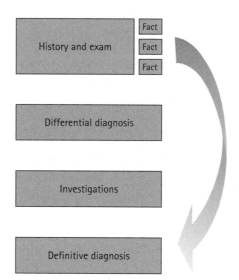

Figure 15.3 Pattern recognition.

Clinicians are able to use all of these models interchangeably, shifting the emphasis according to the situation (Fig. 15.4).

During training, most doctors use the inductive method, as it is thorough and tends to avoid error; experience makes it easier to use hypothetico-deductive reasoning. Different tasks may also influence the type of reasoning used: the specialist must explore possibility, reduce

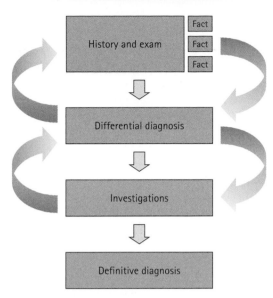

Figure 15.4 A synthesis of clinical reasoning.

uncertainty and marginalize error, so may make more use of inductive reasoning than the generalist, who must explore possibility, accept uncertainty and marginalize danger. When diagnostic uncertainty is the reason for referral to secondary care, an inductive model is likely to be used, even by an experienced doctor, but many consultations in secondary and tertiary care, particularly in outpatients, are problem orientated and use a hypothetico-deductive base, just like the consultations in primary care.

THE INFLUENCE OF THE CLINICIAN'S PERSONALITY

Dangers lurk: there is an ever-present danger of fitting the evidence to the hypothesis, rather than the other way around – remember Procrustes and his comfortable bed.

> Procrustes lived alone on a busy route between two towns, and there were no hotels nearby. He would invite tired travellers to stay, but he was most particular that they fitted the spare bed exactly. If they were too tall, he cut off their feet, and if too short, he stretched them on a rack.

We are not machines; we have individual personalities and our own foibles, all of which we incorporate into our thinking. It may be useful to consider how we rank the list of our differential diagnoses. Several factors influence how we order the diagnoses we have considered.

- Incidence – age, sex, race, job, lifestyle, etc. This is hard information, not dependent on our individual personalities.
- Expertise – have you heard of it? You cannot diagnose something you have never learned about.
- Seriousness – how threatening is it? We tend to give higher priority to those diseases that cause major harm, e.g. is it carcinoma of the rectum or piles causing this person's rectal bleeding?
- Treatability – do we have any treatment? Conversely, we are sometimes slow to confirm the diagnosis if it is one for which we have no treatment, for instance dementia or one of the degenerative neuromuscular diseases. This is an inevitable corollary of doctors' need to be seen to have a remedy.
- Novelty – 'I read a paper in the *BMJ* last week…'. Things stick in our minds – recent articles, striking cases, or sometimes something we missed once and are determined never to miss again.
- Bias – 'I don't believe that chronic fatigue syndrome exists…'. If so, you cannot diagnose it.

So how should all this influence how you conduct your consultations as a learner in primary care? Take your time; if an idea of a diagnosis occurs to you during the consultation, follow it up, look for supportive or refuting evidence, do the relevant physical examination. If not, follow the inductive model until an idea comes. You should not expect to perform at the same speed as your tutor, and you will almost certainly not have as many well-known 'patterns' in your head as he or she does. Remember, your own personality will colour your choices, so you may have to 'correct' for that, and, above all, remember that when you hear hooves, think of horses, not zebras – that is to say, common things occur commonly.

Practical Exercise

❑ Look at a list of cases you have seen in a morn-ing surgery lately, and consider the diagnoses that you were concerned with. In how many cases did you spend time and order investiga-tions in relation to diagnoses that were not actually the most likely but that you felt obliged to consider for other reasons. What were those reasons?

❑ How often were you able to shorten or tele-scope your consultation because the diagnosis became clear, and how often did you have to perform a classical 'clerking' before you were clear what was going on?

❑ Repeat this exercise after a few weeks, and reflect on the changes, and the reasons for the changes.

❑ Compare your pattern with that of the part-ners in your practice, or with a fellow learner.

DEMONSTRATE GOOD WRITTEN COMMUNICATIONS SKILLS

In writing notes, a report or a referral letter, it is as well to consider what the purpose is, who the reader will be and what they need to know. What should you include, and what leave out? Are there ethical or legal issues that need to be addressed?

THE PURPOSE

This may be to provide information to enable future decision making to be optimized: with-holding sensitive information may prejudice the patient's care in the future if another doctor is unaware or does not think to ask about it, but including it relies on doctors behaving non-judgementally. It may be to record decisions made and actions taken, including postulation of strategies and care plans for the future, with 'if, then' statements, especially if these have been negotiated with the patient. Another purpose may be to enable self-audit and governance.

THE READER

The reader may be another doctor or healthcare worker. General assumptions about confidentiality

and professionalism are beginning to be ques-tioned here, and even now some confidentiality walls occur between, say, psychological/coun-selling services and doctors, or between the genitourinary services and the rest of the National Health Service (NHS). Some tensions occur between disclosure of unnecessary per-sonal details and the desire of some doctors to 'personalize' the patient to the recipient.

Some written documentation is for patients or their non-medical advocates, for instance for applications for support in housing or other social support, or for employment, insurance or other purposes. It is as well to assume that this information will be dealt with by a non-clinician, unless otherwise stated.

Recorded information may be for the use of one of the governance agencies, the Primary Care Organisation (PCO), etc. If uncertain but likely diagnoses are recorded as such, they would then be counted as though they were definite, so it is better to record these as symp-toms, for instance wheezing (instead of asthma) or chest pain (instead of angina), until the diag-nosis is confirmed objectively.

INCLUSION/EXCLUSION

The question of relevance here is all-important. A useful guide is the need-to-know maxim – that is, to do the job requested, what does the reader need to know? The problem here is that you yourself may not be able to answer that, but there are some safety nets. First, if the letter/report is accompanying a clinical situation, the patient can be asked to supplement the informa-tion, but you should ensure that information that the patient may not be clear about is in your communication (e.g. medication history). Second, you can indicate how the reader should contact you for supplementary information.

ETHICAL/LEGAL ISSUES

A few comments here may help to identify the commonest issues, but this list cannot claim to be comprehensive.

■ *Non-judgementalism.* Your language must be non-judgemental, but some doctors believe it is allowable to make 'I statements' if this is materially relevant. An example might be: 'I find it hard to understand what this patient says', rather than 'This patient doesn't speak clearly'. Remember also that you depend on your reader being non-judgemental as well, and if you are not confident about this, you may feel unable to write what is needed.

- *Consent to disclose.* This is particularly important if you are writing to a non-clinician. It has been customary to assume consent, but this is changing, and it might be prudent to obtain consent if you are in any doubt. Alternatively, you can give the letter or report to the patient, allowing them to decide whether or not to pass it on.

- *Third-party interest.* In whose interest is the information to be used? It may not be your patient's. The best example of this is writing to insurance companies. The patient should have consented, but may not be aware of what he or she has consented to. Don't forget that insurance companies are not altruistic; they exist to make money for their shareholders.

- *Honesty and truthfulness.* There is an important but often misunderstood difference between these. You can be honest and untruthful ('I saw you at the pub yesterday' – believing this to be the case, mistakenly) or dishonestly truthful ('I only drink socially' – not mentioning you are in the pub for 4 hours 7 nights a week, that is to say, hiding behind words). You should aim to be both honest and truthful.

- *Governance issues.* Some patients become very anxious about information in their clinical notes being used for governance. Issues about agglomerated and anonymized information are still currently debated; society's unresolved dilemma about individual autonomy claiming superiority over the common good (e.g. 'not in my backyard') is a problem here.

ISSUES ABOUT FORMAT

With much clinical record keeping now computerized, issues about format have become more charged. For some time there has been wide variation in the way notes have been kept – written/typed, 'traditional'/problem orientated (e.g. using 'SOAP' – subjective data, objective data, assessment, plan (Weed, 1969) – headings for your notes), the use of personalized shorthand or cues etc. – and for computer-based records there is the additional problem of free-text computer records being more problematic to search/analyse/audit than formatted or field-based records. Currently it is not possible to know how this debate will unfold, except to say that doctors are not easily corralled into conformity, and so it may be protracted. Perhaps the format is less important than the content, though local policies may have to be adhered to, even if one local policy differs from another.

Thinking and Discussion Point

How do you respond to the question 'Can I tell you something, but I don't want you to write it down in my notes?' What are the advantages/disadvantages to the patient/doctor of agreeing to this request?

Thinking and Discussion Point

Compare notes you have written with those your tutor has written, and consider the advantages and disadvantages of both.

Practical Exercise

Make sure that, if you see a patient who needs a referral, you are the one to write the referral letter, and discuss it with your tutor. Who will sign it?

Practical Exercise

If you have access to a fellow learner, you could each write a referral letter about a case you have recently seen, then swap letters and read the letter as though you were the specialist. Ask yourself, 'What am I being asked to do? Can I do this? What information is missing? Will the patient be able to supply it?'

DEMONSTRATE GOOD WORKING RELATIONSHIPS WITH MEMBERS OF A PRIMARY HEALTHCARE TEAM AND OTHER AGENCIES

You will also find material relevant to this in Chapters 2 and 9. In most disciplines/specialties, most doctors work within a team. Teams provide a mix of knowledge, skills and experience, and differing personalities with differing approaches to care. These attributes may be different but should be complementary to each other, providing holistic care to the patient. Teams are able to share caseload, decision making and the uncertainty of working with patients, often providing a professional safety net.

Working in any team can be challenging for all its members and may be a new experience for pre-registration house officers (PRHOs). Communication and mutual respect are key elements to the success of a team. Teams in primary care will often meet on a weekly basis to discuss and refer patients.

You should know about each member's role and responsibilities and how best to liaise with them. Sitting in and observing them at work is often a valuable way of beginning to understand their work.

As a medical or surgical PRHO, you will find it very useful, when planning a patient's discharge from hospital, to have a working knowledge of members of the primary healthcare team and community professionals – for instance, knowing that a speech therapist can be a vital help for someone with swallowing difficulties after a stroke.

For descriptions of the various posts/roles that members of the primary healthcare team might hold, see Chapter 2.

Practical Exercise

Interview members of your primary healthcare team to find out about their roles and responsibilities. Find out also which patients they feel should be referred to them, and which not. Ask them to give examples of good and poor team working, and consider whether you agree.

Practical Exercise

Looking back on a week's clinical work, which members of the primary healthcare team have you involved in the care of the patients you've seen? How appropriate do you now consider that involvement to be, and did you miss any opportunities with other patients?

SHOW EVIDENCE OF GOOD TIME KEEPING AND ORGANIZATIONAL SKILLS

Clinical work requires using time and resources efficiently. You already know some of how to do this – managing your own time and resources, organizing your own learning – but this section aims to help you improve your skills.

SETTING PRIORITIES

First you should consider how you set priorities. One way is to use a system such as that shown in Fig. 15.5.

You may need to set priorities within a consultation (e.g. the patient who presents a number of issues simultaneously) or within a session's work. The setting of your own priorities needs to take into consideration other people or resources that you wish to engage in the problem, including the patient – everyone has to be meshed in, taking their priorities into consideration too.

	Important	Unimportant
Urgent	(Red)	(Amber)
Not urgent	(Purple)	(Blue)

Figure 15.5 An example of a system for setting priorities.

At the end of a morning surgery, you may find you have a number of activities to juggle – writing letters or e-mails, making phone calls, discussing patients with colleagues, doing house calls, writing repeat prescriptions, having your lunch or going to the loo. (Remember that the last are not the least important, as you may not function very well/quickly, be able to listen or negotiate freely, if you are physically uncomfortable or hungry/thirsty.) Thinking about which tasks to perform when and how long it will take to do them will help you plan the next few hours.

ALLOWING TIME

Time expectations should not necessarily be the same for juniors as for seniors – you should expect to take more time over most consultations, letter writing etc. As with all things, if you find yourself in a real dilemma, it is best to find a colleague to discuss it with or to ask help from. If you run constantly over time, it may be more appropriate to negotiate a different consultation period or insert frequent short breaks than merely to endure (and impose on others) the stress of running late.

MULTI-TASKING

This is the concept of being able to do more than one thing at a time – actually to have more than one activity in process apparently simultaneously (in fact, there is rapid switching of concentration back and forth between activities). Some people find multi-tasking very easy, others less so. If you find it difficult, you should first acknowledge this to yourself and your supervisor, and adapt or find strategies to cope. Such strategies involve taking more care with setting priorities, and also making sure others are aware of your working style.

COPING WITH DISTRACTIONS

Phone calls and other interruptions occur all the time. You may have to have different criteria for allowing these, depending on whether or not you are the doctor on call, but you will need to have strategies for answering or deflecting these requests for your attention that do not offend or alienate the requester.

The other side of the coin is important, too: how to get and hold someone's attention without annoying them. You will discover how useful it is to set ground rules with your tutor/supervisor about how you get their attention when you need it; sometimes the ground rules have to be reviewed if they are not working efficiently.

Thinking and Discussion Point

With your tutor/supervisor, discuss the criteria he or she uses to allow/refuse interruptions, the advantages and disadvantages, and try to develop your own ideal sets of criteria to use in different situations.

Practical Exercise

Write a list at the end of morning surgery of the tasks you have generated, and the other tasks ahead in the day, and consider how you give them priority and whether that priority then remains fixed or continues to change as the tasks unfold.

Practical Exercise

With fellow learners, set up role plays of consultations interrupted by telephone calls or visitors. Practise the communications skills needed to deal with these both during 'ordinary' morning surgery and during a 'duty doctor' session. Get feedback from the people playing the Interrupter and the patient.

IMPLEMENT STRATEGIES FOR MANAGING UNCERTAINTY

WHAT IS 'MANAGING UNCERTAINTY'?

Our consideration of our response to uncertainty has to include both our thinking (the 'decisions') and our behaviour.

Although one might divide uncertainty in the clinical situation into diagnostic and therapeutic uncertainty, it is the former that is commoner. That is to say, although a doctor may be uncertain what to do, it is usually because he or she does not know precisely what the problem is due to; management dilemmas occur less frequently.

DIFFERENTIATION BETWEEN UNCERTAINTY AND IGNORANCE/INCOMPETENCE

Because of the high premium put on knowledge both by society and by traditional medical education (and thus doctors), not knowing is easily equated with incompetence; this is much more in the doctor's mind than in the patient's. However, clinical problems present in a multitude of ways (not least because the person having them is always unique) and at a multitude of points in the natural history of the problem, so it may not be crystal clear to every doctor at every consultation what exactly the problem is. Consequently, handling uncertainty is the stuff of medicine, and general practice is where you can learn about it.

ROLE OF DOCTOR AS OMNISCIENT

The idea of the doctor as an omniscient, where this springs from and who sustains it, is not for this book, but suffice to say that many general practitioners (GPs), and most of their patients, would not recognize it as applying to them. Whilst it may appear at first an attractive and powerful idea, it is a huge and unmanageable burden, one more likely to be dropped than carried successfully. Perhaps partly because of the more personal nature of the relationship of the GP and the patient, expectations are set more realistically on both sides, and the GP is able to express uncertainty without threat to his or her competence.

BEING A JUNIOR

The junior doctor or senior undergraduate medical student is in an even luckier position of 'still learning', so expectations should be lower and asking for help should be easier. However, most juniors have spent most of their time in a hospital context, and have come to expect most clinical situations to be resolved within the time frame of the admission, and may have some difficulty in resisting the temptation to sort out everything in one go and reach a satisfactory conclusion. Many problems in general practice continue to evolve over many consultations; even self-limiting illness, e.g. the presentation of childhood minor illness in a family, will evolve over time as the parents gain experience and confidence. The ability to decide what needs to be dealt with now, and what can be left, depends on the ability to 'manage uncertainty'.

USE OF TIME – AS DIAGNOSTIC AID OR AS THERAPY

Time is one of the major tools in managing uncertainty. Time will permit the problem to evolve, such that either new features appear, making a diagnosis easier, or the problem disappears without our being able to define it. Time may also show the effect of other factors on the problem – self-help, over-the-counter (OTC) remedies or symptomatic treatment – which may illuminate the diagnosis. Indeed, some therapies used in the past depended on the passage of time for their effect – many mixtures and potions, harmless (or intended to be so) in themselves, measuring out 'spoonfuls' of time; we should not need this subterfuge now.

A good example of how time used to manage uncertainty yields many results is the case of possible early appendicitis. A youngster with colicky central abdominal pain, and some nausea, without very marked abdominal tenderness may be seen by the GP, who advises symptomatic relief with fluids and paracetamol, suggesting 'a virus' or 'an upset stomach' as the cause. Indeed, many times this will be the case, the patient will recover none the worse; but the GP will know that, once in a while, one such case will go on to develop the classic history and signs of appendicitis. Does the GP alert the patient and family to this possibility, or does he or she think this is harmful alarmism? If the latter, the patient may turn up in casualty that evening saying, 'My GP told me it was an upset stomach', as the senior house officer (SHO) looks incredulously at a 'barn-door' appendix! Alerting the family involves 'admitting' uncertainty, but is more honest, more likely to enable the family to seek further advice if needed, and more likely to nurture the GP's reputation.

OTHER HELPING HANDS

- *Open door.* The security that the patient can consult again at short notice is a feature of general practice not present in hospital outpatients, where the doctor decides in advance when the patient will next be seen. This allows a sharing of responsibility between the doctor and the patient, relieving some pressure to sort everything out at one go. This placing more of the locus of control with the patient lightens the load of responsibility on the doctor's shoulders.

- *Use of negotiation.* Discussing with the patient the various options available not only also shares some responsibility with the patient, but may also do two other things. First, in many instances, vocalizing the choices available to another person often makes the right choice more obvious. Second, the patient may have views about how acceptable some of the options would be – our advocacy of an option unacceptable to the patient (i.e. lack of concordance between the doctor and patient) will often lead to a poorer outcome.

- *Appropriate goal setting.* To assume that the endpoint of treatment that we have in our minds is the one that the patient shares may be misguided. Some patients will accept some levels of risk that we might not; others might be looking for a goal beyond that which we can achieve with current medicine. Being honest and explicit about these things may help in setting shared, achievable treatment goals; this is another aspect of concordance.

- *Being explicit about expectations.* Distressed or needy people want answers; it is easy to fall into the trap of finding a superficially credible explanation or treatment simply to assuage the distress. Perhaps it might be better to deal with the distress, acknowledge the need for answers, but honestly admit to the uncertainty. Disappointment and disillusionment may occur, but in smaller doses than if an expectation is created that cannot subsequently be met by the healthcare system.

- *Referral.* This could be the GP to the specialist, but the same process occurs (and might be equally useful) in the case of the student asking his/her tutor, the registrar asking his/her trainer, the assistant asking a partner, or one partner asking another. It might also be appropriate to ask a specialist from another discipline – our nursing or therapy colleagues, for example. Saying you need another opinion is not necessarily a sign of intellectual bankruptcy, but more a sign of recognition of your own limits (see below).

DEMONSTRATE AN AWARENESS OF YOUR OWN LIMITATIONS AND AN UNDERSTANDING OF WHEN AND WHERE TO SEEK HELP

Central to the correct response to the awareness of one's own limitations is an honest view of what might reasonably be expected of you, and being open to feedback (see the section 'Accept and utilize constructive criticism...', below). If your competence and the expected level are not in tandem, some more learning is required (see the section 'Adopt strategies for lifelong learning', below).

However, you might be at the level of competence expected of you but be facing a problem that is outside it; this is normal for any clinician, whether generalist or specialist. Learning to respond properly is also covered in the section 'Implement strategies for managing uncertainty' (above), but you need also to be able to seek help.

WHAT KINDS OF HELP ARE THERE?

- Pure information, e.g. in a book or on the Internet.
- Information or a second opinion from a peer/colleague on site.
- Advice from a specialist source on or off site, either instantly or by appointment.

This last source we would recognize as a 'referral', which is easily sanctioned. However, you might consider when making the referral not only the patient's needs, but also your own (can you learn something from this referral?). You should try to understand the needs of the next clinician, too, and provide good referring information and a clear exposition of what the referral is for, why it is necessary, etc.

Checking information should be acceptable, too, but some students or juniors (and some seniors) find it too embarrassing to open the *British National Formulary* in front of a patient. Consider which is more embarrassing, looking, or discovering afterwards that you made an error in prescribing. The manner in which it is done is important: if you feel uncomfortable or embarrassed, it will show (arising from a misplaced internal expectation of 'knowing' lots), and the patient will naturally assume that you are justifiably embarrassed, and his or her expectations of you and your colleagues will simply increase. You are at a stage where it should not be embarrassing to check information, so you have the chance to set healthy behaviours for the future!

Telephoning a specialist registrar may be helpful; they may be flattered that their advice is being sought, particularly if you are seeking advice about how you might handle the problem, and not just handing over the patient to their care, without trying. Not infrequently, an offer of an outpatient appointment may come easily.

Unless one is in single-handed practice, there are almost always fellow clinicians around. As a student in a practice, you may only rarely see your tutor ask a colleague, although you may see him or her being asked. The reason is that while you are there, your tutor already has a colleague on hand – you! Otherwise, it is not that unusual for one doctor to ask another, informally, for a second opinion, either at the time or afterwards. This may be done partly to use a sounding board, checking out what one has decided, or partly to utilize that opinion at the next consultation.

As you are a student, your tutor will almost invariably check the outcome of every consultation, but you may be uncertain about the physical examination or about what a certain part of the history signifies, and so the enquiry ('referral') would be about these things. You should not be too reluctant to ask for this help, as without it you may make an avoidable clinical error (for which the tutor would be responsible), and you would not benefit from the learning that might accrue. It is really important to learn healthy ways of asking for help before you get to your early years as a junior doctor, as a PRHO or registrar, when you may feel you should be able to do more than you actually can – this is a time when you may over-reach yourself unless you have already learned how to ask for help.

PROBLEM AREAS

For some people, asking for help about their skills can be easier than about their knowledge; the techniques are the same, so whichever you find easier, apply the same technique to the other. It is often harder to ask for help if it is one's attitudes that are causing problems, not least because it may be more difficult to see in the first place, and more difficult to admit. Sometimes, people think that their attitudes are private, part of 'them', and therefore not on the agenda for change. However, our attitudes affect our behaviour towards patients and peers, and if our behaviour causes a problem, we must change it, even if we continue to hold our private underlying beliefs.

Asking for help when one is ill is often even harder, particularly if help-seeking behaviour is not well established anyway. Doctors not infrequently work when they should be ill in bed, treat themselves or fail to take time off. Guilt about increasing the workload on their colleagues, and deeper-seated beliefs about showing vulnerability, deny them the time and space they need, that they themselves would advise for their patients. Quite apart from the possibility of clinical mistakes being made, the resulting deep-seated resentment contributes to burnout.

One area where doctors are out of step with other professions is in the matter of supervision. Almost all practitioners of any kind of

---

Practical Exercise

During one session, after each case (or at the end of the morning, reviewing the whole list) look back and ask yourself what, if anything, caused most difficulty in the consultation. Was it something you didn't know? Something you couldn't do? Or something about yourself that 'got in the way' (i.e. your knowledge, skills or attitudes)? Make a note and discuss with your tutor how to deal with these learning needs. Reflect on how you would do this if there were no 'protected' time for supervision in your timetable, and/or how you set this time up.

'talk therapy' (psychotherapy, counselling etc.) have a supervisor; not so the GP. Some GPs join peer-support groups to provide an informal replacement for this function.

ACCEPT AND UTILIZE CONSTRUCTIVE CRITICISM, BE WILLING TO REFLECT ON YOUR OWN STRENGTHS AND WEAKNESSES, AND ACT UPON THEM

CONTEXTUALIZING YOUR OWN PERFORMANCE

As doctors in training, we may confuse capability with 'good/bad'. It is more appropriate to consider whether our performance is above or below expectations, and to consider whose expectations those are and how realistic they are. You may appear to be asked to perform the same task as in previous firms or attachments, and not consider that a higher standard of performance or a greater assumption of responsibility is expected of you. Conversely, a tutor may sometimes overlook the fact that you are not yet a registrar. Being conversant with the standards expected of you at your summative assessment is useful, though not always easy.

The use of methods of self-assessment may also be helpful, and one which has been found applicable to the senior undergraduate years, and may extend further than that, is the RIME model (Pangaro, 1999):

1. reporter – acting as the patient's mouthpiece,
2. investigator – thinking about tests, referrals etc.,
3. manager – thinking about treatments,
4. educator – thinking about explaining to patient/peers.

You can use this model to assess your own role in relation to the patients you are seeing; how, for a series of patients, you may take on several different roles, and how with time the prevailing role changes. You can use it either qualitatively or by totting up your score numerically.

Another method of self-assessment is to notate your learning objectives with confidence ratings, comparing week-on-week or month-on-month improvements in confidence.

OBTAINING AND LISTENING TO FEEDBACK

Direct feedback on your performance can be incredibly helpful, on the process and the outcome. It needs to be useful – that is to say, it needs to be expressed in a way that you can hear, accept and use to change what you have been doing. It might sometimes contain direct suggestions about what you might do instead, although ideally without any element of obligation. It is entirely appropriate for you to ask for this kind of feedback.

One of the things that doctors find hard to do anything with is praise – often it is met with embarrassment and internal disbelief; as such it is not 'useful', though what needs to change here is the attitude of the recipient. It seems to be part of the medical mindset that praise is base currency; perhaps, if punitive criticism were less the norm, praise could be rehabilitated.

Having said that, it is important to accept criticism in a constructive manner. By un-linking criticism from judgementalism, one can 'hear' it, consider its truthfulness, accept it and act on it.

USE OF RECORDING

This can be a most powerful adjunct to another's critique: you yourself are the observer and can see your own performance. It is often very challenging, sometimes disturbing, even embarrassing, but it can also be powerfully affirming. Video is ideal, but audio is not to be ignored and may be technically easier to achieve; consent from the patients is essential. Suitable guidance and a downloadable consent form can be found on http://www.nosa.org.uk/downloads/html/cogped/consent.htm

PERSONAL REFLECTION

The biggest obstacle to personal reflection is the allocation of time, which must be protected time. Since it appears to be entirely selfish, it is often demoted in importance, but it is vital to the preservation of quality.

Some students are still uncertain how to reflect. The process is actually quite simple and unthreatening.

Practical Exercise

Think about something you have experienced.
- ❑ Start by writing down what actually happened; think about what you felt confident about and what you felt uncertain about.
- ❑ What might you have done differently?
- ❑ How did it make you feel?
- ❑ What do you think other people felt?
- ❑ What did you learn?
- ❑ Draw up some action points for you to work on so you can feel more prepared in a similar situation in future.

Aids to reflection may help, by using open question sheets or generating lists or by writing full significant event analyses. The process should embrace honesty, both in the narrative and, ideally, also in the emotional underlay (the reflector's emotions). Examples of more specific types of reflection sheets are given at the end of this section.

There is an important link here with the use of a portfolio, which aids reflection as well as forming a record.

JOHARI WINDOW

Feedback, self-assessment and reflection on our work as professionals can illuminate issues that we wish to develop or change. However, problems can arise if we are unaware of or wish to hide some of our weaknesses, deficiencies or 'black holes'.

The Johari Window shows clearly the various states of self-knowledge (Table 15.1). It was named after its developers, Joseph Luft and Harry Ingham (Luft, 1969). The idea of self-assessment, feedback and reflection is to expand the open box and minimize the other boxes. If you and your

tutors become more aware of your problem areas, you are in a better position to change them. The relationship between student and tutor can play a central role in expanding the open box. A trusting and supportive relationship can provide a safe environment in which to discuss sensitive issues.

NEED FOR CHANGE

There is an active process that precedes change happening: first an acknowledgement that things are not right, and second an acceptance that change is necessary; this is akin to the shift from pre-conceptual to conceptual thinking with which you may be familiar in the context of behaviour modification.

GROUNDING

Key to knowing how much change is necessary is having an understanding of expectations (see the section 'Demonstrate an awareness of your own limitations...', above); being grounded with your peers is of inestimable value. Grounding in this context means having an understanding of what your peers are able to do in similar situations, and having similar expectations of yourself. The best way of being grounded with your peers involves, either formally or informally, some kind of small group activity, such as:
- undergraduate seminars,
- journal club,
- significant event analysis discussion,
- half-day release groups,
- young (or mature) general practice principals groups.

In discussions in such groups, you will quickly gain an idea of where the common standard of competence is, and you will be able to establish whether that standard is sufficient for the expectations of your course/job.

Table 15.1 The Johari Window

	Known to self	Unknown to self
Known to others	Open	Blind
Unknown to others	Hidden	Unknown

Practical Exercise

At the end of the week/course, think back over what you have seen, what you have experienced and what you have learned. Use one of the suggested reflection sheets, or generate your own.

Practical Exercise

Evaluate your RIME score for the last ten patients, and consider how you would have improved your score in each case. Re-evaluate your score a week later.

Reflection sheet

Reflect on the consultations you have undertaken on your own.
☐ Which one has affected your own personal thoughts and feelings most?
☐ Why did it affect you?
☐ What did you learn about yourself from this experience?

Reflection sheet

Reflect on your learning experience in general practice.
☐ What would be the one most important point of feedback you'd like to give to your tutor/ supervisor?
☐ What have you learned in this course that has changed or consolidated your approach to medicine?
☐ What do you perceive are areas of weakness that you have not addressed on this course and would like to build on in the future?

MAINTAIN SOUND PROFESSIONAL CONDUCT

It is is recommendeded that you read the guidance on good medical practice at the General Medical Council's (GMC's) website (http://www.gmc-uk.org/standards/default.htm), in particular; however, you must know the duties of the doctor that the GMC has defined.

> Patients must be able to trust doctors with their lives and well-being. To justify that trust, we as a profession have a duty to maintain a good standard of practice and

care and to show respect for human life. In particular as a doctor you must:

- make the care of your patient your first concern,
- treat every patient politely and considerately,
- respect patients' dignity and privacy,
- listen to patients and respect their views,
- give patients information in a way they can understand,
- respect the rights of patients to be fully involved in decisions about their care,
- keep your professional knowledge and skills up to date,
- recognize the limits of your professional competence,
- be honest and trustworthy,
- respect and protect confidential information,
- make sure that your personal beliefs do not prejudice your patients' care,
- act quickly to protect patients from risk if you have good reason to believe that you or a colleague may not be fit to practise,
- avoid abusing your position as a doctor,
- work with colleagues in the ways that best serve patients' interests.

In all these matters you must never discriminate unfairly against your patients or colleagues, and you must always be prepared to justify your actions to them.

You will already notice how many of these resonate through the subjects of this chapter.

ADOPT STRATEGIES FOR LIFELONG LEARNING

PURPOSE

Why is lifelong learning important? Medicine is changing and developing rapidly and you cannot expect your present knowledge to be up to date for long. As professionals, we have a responsibility to keep up to date to ensure we provide good care to our patients (see also the previous section on the GMC's guidance on good medical practice). We need to be safe practitioners and analyse and learn from our mistakes; to enjoy our work, we need to remain enthusiastic by stimulating our own interest. The public, through our governing body the GMC, needs to be assured that we are maintaining high standards of care: the introduction of annual appraisals with revalidation every 5 years in the UK has already started. Doctors will need to meet an established minimum competence level to be re-licensed to work in the NHS in the UK.

As students and doctors, we need to ensure we continue to learn and we need to develop strategies on how best we learn so that this learning is sustainable throughout our career.

WHAT IS IT?

Incorporating the principles of adult learning is important for lifelong learning and continuing medical education.

Adult learning is about us deciding what we want to learn and using our past experiences. What we learn needs to be relevant to what we do in our everyday practice, so that we improve patient care. It involves the following.

- Identifying your strengths and weaknesses: being able to say, 'I don't know about this'.
- Reflection/Kolb's cycle: it is very powerful if you can put learning into action, confirming the value of what you have learned and stimulating ideas on what else you would like to learn about (see Fig. 15.6; Kolb, 1984). There is more on reflection in the section 'Accept and utilize constructive criticism...', above.
- Setting realistic objectives and goals for yourself.

Lifelong learning is key to our professionalism, and a key part of this is the ability to reflect on our practice and our learning.

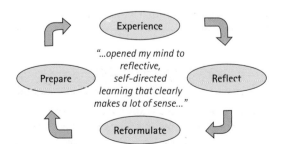

Figure 15.6 Kolb's cycle.

HOW TO DO IT

There are many different ways that we can keep up to date. Some activities will suit you, whereas others will not. Here are a few options.

- Update sessions/courses: these may be useful, but may not always meet your needs.
- Journals and journal clubs: sharing information with peers includes grounding yourself and setting realistic standards of care in your practice or department. This can often be a useful way of providing consistency of care within a team.
- Electronic information: this is available while you consult, and can be shared with the patient. There are now many websites available.
- Developing a special interest or responsibility within a team: this will necessitate you keeping up to date and being a resource to others.
- Keeping a log: we often come across areas of medicine that we are unsure of – everyone has their 'black hole'. By keeping a log of things to look up when seeing patients and following up what we are unsure of, we learn 'on the job'. Try not to be intimidated doing this in front of patients – it is much better to feel sure you are doing the right thing.
- Peer groups: these offer support and an opportunity to reflect on your own practice, and set this in the context of the practice of others at your level (see also the section 'Accept and utilize constructive criticism...', above).
- Correspondence from colleagues: this can be a useful way of learning up-to-date management approaches.
- Informally from colleagues: asking for advice and help from a colleague is a common method used when there is uncertainty in clinical decisions.
- Patients are an invaluable source, particularly since the advent of the Internet.
- Television/media: hearing something on the news or even in a television soap can often be a learning point for us.
- Developing a portfolio (see below).

PORTFOLIOS

These are new in medicine but are common in other professions. Nurses have been using them for a number of years for continuing professional development and accreditation. They originate in graphic arts and consist of a collection of evidence that shows learning has taken place – a portfolio.

You decide what goes into your portfolio. Seeing a patient with a particular illness may spark your interest in finding out more about that illness; when faced with a clinical problem that you are unsure about, you can use the opportunity and include what you learn in your portfolio. As you can see, the portfolio uses your clinical experiences as the starting point for your learning, so that when you next see a patient with a similar problem you will feel more confident managing them. It is very relevant and useable for your future clinical practice.

The success of the portfolio will depend on how much effort and time you put into it. However, be careful not to embark on huge projects that become unmanageable. Try to be specific, e.g. instead of writing about 'ischaemic heart disease', consider focusing on, say, 'the pharmacological treatment of angina'.

Reflecting on experiences is central to developing your portfolio. When thinking about clinical encounters, identify what you feel confident about and what you are unsure about – your strengths and weaknesses. Think of strategies you can use to learn about the areas you do not feel confident in, e.g. read a review article, go to an outpatient clinic, speak to a specialist, read a book. Then write about what you have learnt and how it may affect your clinical practice in the future, e.g. studying the management of urinary tract infections in general practice may increase or decrease your requesting of midstream urines, or your referral rate, etc. Thinking about what you have learnt will often spark ideas of other areas you would like to learn more about, which you could include in your portfolio.

It may also be useful for you to think about how you learnt: did you learn more by reading an article or going to the outpatient department? This can help you identify how best you learn, which should make it easier the next time.

Sharing your portfolio with a tutor or peer may be useful, particularly when discussing what and how you have learnt.

Portfolios can replace formal examinations as a form of assessment. Some medical schools have replaced the traditional final examinations with a portfolio that the student develops in their final year. The advantages of a portfolio as a form of assessment include the following.

- A portfolio can assess areas not easily assessed by other methods, particularly professionalism, because the ability to reflect is a key component of professionalism. This is useful, as there has been a push from the public and the GMC to ensure professional standards are met at graduation and at postgraduate levels.

- Portfolios are authentic; they can chart what the student actually *does* over a period of time. Multiple choice questions (MCQs) are useful for assessing knowledge, and objective structured clinical examinations (OSCEs) assess 'shows how', but this may not be what the student actually does in practice when seeing patients every day.

MAKING A HABIT OF IT

It is our professional responsibility to remain up to date and skilled in our area of medicine. To learn effectively, we need to use strategies that suit us so that we can sustain our learning throughout our career.

Practical Exercise

Set your own learning objectives and start your portfolio; complete a self-assessment exercise or a reflective journal.

Practical Exercise

Write down how you found out about something you were not sure about – books/World Wide Web/asking a colleague etc.

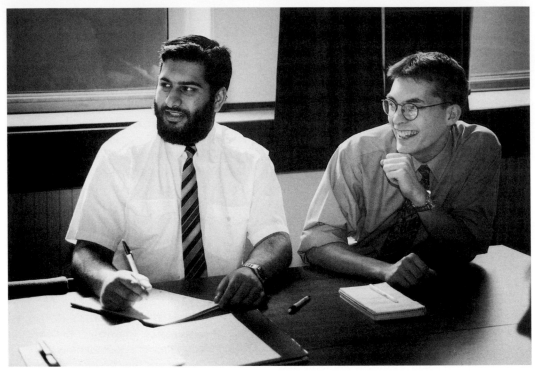

Figure 15.7 Learning can be fun.

SUMMARY POINTS

Things you learn while you are in general practice are useful whatever you do in medicine.

To conclude, the most important messages of this chapter are:

- being aware of how you think and make decisions helps improve how you consult with patients;
- reflective learning is easy and helpful;
- fostering and maintaining relationships with colleagues is crucial to clinical team working;
- organizing your time and resources helps you in your working day;
- being honestly self-aware is healthy and productive;
- feedback from peers, colleagues and patients is a real resource;
- there is a multitude of ways to keep learning;
- productive learning is satisfying and fun (Fig. 15.7).

REFERENCES

Kolb, D. 1984: *Experiential learning: experience as the source of learning and development*, Englewood Cliffs, NJ: Prentice Hall.

Luft, J. 1969: *Of human interaction*. Palo Alto, CA: National Press.

Pangaro, L.N. 1999: A new vocabulary and other innovations for improving descriptive in-training evaluations. *Academic Medicine* 74, 1203–7.

Weed, L.L. 1969: *Medical records, medical education, and patient care. The problem-oriented record as a basic tool.* Cleveland, OH: Case Western Reserve University.

FURTHER READING

Dowie, J. and Elstein, A. 1988: *Professional judgement. A reader in clinical decision making.* Cambridge, Cambridge University Press.

Portfolio-based learning in general practice 1993: Occasional Paper 63. London: Royal College of General Practitioners.

http://www.gmc-uk.org

http://www.nosa.org.uk

http://www.londondeanery.ac.uk

CHAPTER

16

BEING A GENERAL PRACTITIONER

The working life of a general practitioner is largely determined by the structure of general practice and, in the United Kingdom, its position within the National Health Service. Other major determinants include the nature and quality of the relationships between doctors, patients and society at large. At the turn of the twenty-first century, these relationships are in a state of flux. However, as long as general practitioners have a major role in providing primary personal care, a career in general practice will continue to offer variety, choice and many opportunities for personal and professional fulfilment. This chapter explores the variety and richness of the life of a general practitioner.

LEARNING OBJECTIVES

By the end of the chapter, you will be able to:

- define what a general practitioner (GP) is and, in the UK, where general practice fits into the National Health Service (NHS);
- learn about the training and career structure of general practice in the UK;
- describe the main aspects of the work of a GP;
- explore the aspects of general practice life that make it such a uniquely fulfilling career;
- see the pitfalls and potential problems that crop up in the life of a GP;
- discover what it feels like to be a GP, by looking at the day-to-day work of general practice;
- understand why and in which ways general practice is changing and developing;
- see what any doctor, in any branch of medicine, can usefully learn from the life of a GP.

WHAT IS A GENERAL PRACTITIONER?

Approximately one half of all the doctors qualifying in the UK will make their careers in general practice. They will come to this choice through a variety of paths. For some, it will be a decision made very early on, perhaps after a stimulating, thought-provoking or exciting experience of general practice as a medical student.

For others, it may be a second choice after problems experienced along another career path. For some, general practice may be a family tradition, whereas other doctors may discover the joys and opportunities of this unique career at a much later stage in their professional lives.

So, how would one actually define what a GP is? A recent very detailed document produced by the World Organization of Family Doctors (WONCA) defines and explains in detail the key features of the discipline of general practice (WONCA EUROPE, 2002). However, in simple terms, a GP is a doctor who, having gone through the required training process, is available for consultation by members of the public about their health-related needs. As we shall see, these needs are extremely varied, and the members of the public range all the way from completely healthy individuals through to terminally ill patients.

Doctors working in general practice in the UK include:

- those training to be GPs (*GP registrars*),
- those working with a limited commitment and responsibility (*assistants*),
- a small number doing research (*associates*),
- the vast majority, called *GP principals.*

When people talk of GPs in the UK, they are usually referring to GP principals. These are self-employed GPs who have entered into a contract (Department of Health, 1989) with the local primary care trust (PCT). The contract states that the GP will provide 'general medical services' (GMS) to members of the public living in the geographical area of the practice. The NHS makes payments to the GP (via the PCT) for providing these medical services. Thus, as long as the requirements of the GP contract are met, every GP is free to follow his or her own particular approach or interests. Therefore, in theory, every GP could provide a completely unique and individual service. The term used to describe the position of the GP in the UK is that of an 'independent contractor'.

From 1998, an increasing number of GPs have agreed to alter their contracts so that they become Personal Medical Services (Pilot) GPs and practices (NHS Executive, 1997). These are usually known as PMS practices. These practices

negotiate a contract with the PCT in which the practice agrees to provide a level of services for patients, together with additional activities of interest to the GPs and of benefit to the patients of the practice and the health of the local community. In return, the PCT provides the PMS practice with an agreed annual budget to cover the costs of the practice, its staff, its activities and the income of the GPs of the practice. If the agreed budget allows, PMS practices may employ GPs to work for fixed periods of time, for an agreed salary. These GPs are known as PMS-salaried GPs, as opposed to the PMS principals, who are self-employed and are the employers of the practice staff, including the PMS-salaried GPs. The PMS principals are GP principals working within the framework of a PMS contract, as opposed to GMS principals working within a GMS contract (in non-PMS practices).

General practitioner assistants are GPs who are employed long-term by practices and work for the principals of the practice. They have limited responsibilities; in particular they do not have financial responsibility for the practice, as the principals do. A number of new types of GP assistant posts have been developed over the past few years in order to encourage GPs with particular interests. Some may be attached to academic departments of general practice and combine clinical work in practices with research, teaching and personal development projects. These posts are often taken by newly trained GPs who do not yet wish to make a long-term commitment to a particular practice and become a principal. It is likely that, over the years ahead, the variety of GP posts will increase in order to make a career in general practice even more interesting and attractive.

As independent contractors, GPs are in a somewhat unusual position. The vast majority of their work falls within the bounds of the GP contract (GMS or PMS) and so they feel limited and constrained by the policy decisions of the Department of Health or the PCT. On the other hand, as 'independent contractors', GPs are self-employed professionals running their own businesses (the practice), enjoying the freedom to experiment and develop individual ways of working, employing their own staff, and trying out new arrangements and ideas when they wish. As a GP principal, I am aware of a tension between, on the one hand, feeling that I am being told what to do and, on the other hand, a sense of great professional and personal freedom to develop my working life.

From the tension between these two positions emerge the varied patterns of general practice that we see developing in the UK. As political and financial changes have affected health authorities, so the GP contract has been changed radically several times. As well as the many changes in government and health authority policies over the years, the approach of GPs to their own work has also developed and evolved. In addition, it is important to note that the expectations of the public have also gradually developed.

All these changes mean that general practice today is not the same as it was 10, 20 or 30 years ago, and it certainly will look very different in another 10, 20 or 30 years. As discussed in the section covering the main aspects of the work of a GP, an ability to embrace and cope with change is a key personal skill required of all GPs.

General practice, the most common route for the public to obtain medical advice and attention for at least 100 years, has changed in major steps, with the inception of the NHS in the UK in 1948 (Parliament of Great Britain, 1947), and also in a more continuous and evolutionary way. Despite these changes, there remains a consistent pattern, a core, to general practice, that has not altered over the years. This core might be characterized as the consultation between patient and GP, taking place either in the GP's consulting room or in the home of the patient. The consultation has a very special feel, being private, trusting and highly confidential. Discussions take place between GP and patient that might not happen in any other environment, and herein lies much of the thrill and the strength of the GP consultation, a strength that many have likened to that of the confessional in church.

This chapter refers to the work of the GP within the NHS of the UK. However, the information is transferable to systems in other countries. If you are not training in the UK, I urge you to find out from your GP tutor how general or family practice fits into your health system.

HOW DO YOU BECOME A GENERAL PRACTITIONER?

The formal training requirements of a newly qualified doctor vary according to which branch of medicine that doctor chooses to enter. The training requirements for general practice have been very clearly defined and controlled for many years.

In order to be eligible to become a principal in general practice in the UK, a newly qualified doctor must do house officer jobs for 1 year. These usually comprise 6 months in medicine and 6 months in surgery, though there are now also house officer posts in general practice. After house jobs, the doctor must satisfactorily complete a process of vocational training in general practice (Havelock et al., 1995). Vocational training takes a minimum of 3 years, and consists of 2 years of approved hospital doctor posts and 1 year of training in general practice as a GP registrar (formerly called a vocational trainee).

The hospital posts (usually four jobs lasting 2 years in all) must be educationally approved and can cover a wide range of specialties, the most common being general medicine, geriatrics, accident and emergency (casualty), paediatrics, obstetrics and/or gynaecology and psychiatry.

The 1 year of training as a GP registrar takes place in an approved training practice, and the registrar is attached to a GP who is a trainer. In order to be approved as a trainer, a GP must complete a lengthy course and his or her practice must also be approved as a training practice. The GP registrar works in the practice under the supervision of the trainer and has regular tutorial meetings with the trainer. In addition, all GP registrars are expected to attend a day or half-day release course, together with other GP registrars in the area.

Once the GP registrar has satisfactorily completed the vocational training process, he or she is eligible to become a principal in general practice (a GP), either alone (single handed) or in partnership with other GPs as a member of a group practice.

Approximately one half of all GP registrars do their vocational training through organized 3-year vocational training schemes. These can be of great benefit to the registrar, who then does not have to worry about finding and applying for suitable approved hospital jobs and a registrar post in general practice. Other registrars may apply to have some or all of their previous hospital experience approved as part of their training, and then independently organize hospital jobs and GP registrar posts.

Another variant on the basic '3-year plan' of vocational training is that it may be possible to complete some of the training part time (e.g. being a half-time GP registrar for 2 years). This option can be of great benefit to doctors with family or other commitments or interests.

Once a doctor completes training and becomes a GP, the further career path is potentially highly flexible. As mentioned in the section 'Main aspects of the work of a general practitioner' below, there are many different aspects of medical practice in which a GP can choose to take a deeper interest. Some GPs develop great expertise in one or other branch of medicine. Others may develop an interest in medical education, and there are now many academic departments of general practice attached to universities that can help and support GPs in undergraduate teaching, vocational training or other educational activities. Equally, GPs may choose to work on developing the services provided by their practice and take a particular interest in practice management or finance.

The possibilities for career development are endless, and one of the benefits of a career in general practice is that it allows for many changes in path throughout the lifetime of any individual GP.

MAIN ASPECTS OF THE WORK OF A GENERAL PRACTITIONER

As mentioned in the section 'What is a general practitioner?' above, there are number of different ways in which a GP might work, for example as a GMS principal, a PMS (Pilot) principal, a PMS-salaried GP or a GP assistant. The balance and emphasis of the roles and responsibilities of a GP will vary with each of these ways of working, as well as varying according to how different GP practices are organized.

Although the balance may vary, there are a number of major aspects or themes that characterize the working life of all GPs, and these are described below. The list is not exhaustive and, as one might expect, new roles are bound to develop over the years ahead.

- Providing personal medical care to patients and families.
- Providing and managing a service.
- Being part of a team (the primary healthcare team).
- Making decisions and choices.
- Balancing the needs of the individual with those of the wider community.
- Being responsible for personal professional development and standards.
- Additional 'non-basic' work.
- Responding to the developing roles of general practice.

PROVIDING PERSONAL MEDICAL CARE TO PATIENTS AND FAMILIES

This, of course, is the core of what GPs do. They run surgeries in which they can be consulted by patients, either on request or by appointment. They also do house calls to see housebound patients or people who are too ill to leave home and come in to the surgery. Some of these consultations will be generated by the GPs themselves, such as when they see patients for routine review of a chronic clinical condition, but most consultations are at the request of the patient.

In the consultation, the GP has a number of tasks, including:
- identifying the patient's problems, concerns and expectations;
- making a diagnosis of clinical conditions, both physical and psychological;
- distinguishing normal changes from disease processes;
- considering the wider context of the patient – the family and social position of the patient;

- identifying areas of uncertainty in relation to diagnosis;
- clarifying areas of social need;
- identifying areas of appropriate preventive care;
- making appropriate referrals for further investigation or specialist care;
- providing appropriate support for patients in distress;
- considering the need for follow-up care of the patient, especially if the diagnosis is in doubt;
- ensuring that the patient feels satisfied that his or her worries have been addressed.

It will be seen that some of these tasks relate to the medical agenda of the GP (e.g. making diagnoses), whereas other tasks relate to the agenda of the patient (e.g. identifying the patient's concerns and ensuring that they have been addressed). Yet other tasks also relate to a wider public health agenda (e.g. aspects of preventive care).

The GP is often very well placed to assess the influence of the family or social system of the patient on the presentation, diagnosis and management of that patient. This is one reason why 'general practice' is sometimes referred to as 'family medicine'.

Not all of the tasks of the GP in the consultation involve dealing with disease. Sometimes it is part of the role of the GP to support and help patients through life events, both good and bad, such as childbirth, divorce, unemployment, death or bereavement.

Sometimes it is not completely clear who is really the patient, and this may be a very important question to consider; for example the worried mother who repeatedly brings her child to the GP with very minor ailments – which one is the patient?

Practical Exercise

In your time in general practice, try to identify examples where it is not clear who is the 'real' patient.

PROVIDING AND MANAGING A SERVICE

Most GPs (certainly GMS and PMS principals) will be responsible not only for seeing patients in surgery, but also for establishing the context in which the patients can be seen. This means providing adequate premises with consulting and waiting rooms, developing effective patient appointment systems, employing staff (such as receptionists, nurses, counsellors, secretaries, clerks and cleaners, as well as managers to run the service), providing both clinical and IT equipment, and developing clinical and administrative protocols. Many of these aspects of the GP's role can be delegated to practice managers or other healthcare professionals, but ultimately they remain the responsibility of the GP, as long as he or she is a self-employed independent contractor. In effect, the GP, with independent contractor status, is the owner of a small business, the practice.

General practitioners and practices have to make decisions on many matters, ranging from the most mundane to those affecting the whole philosophy or approach of the practice. Most practices hold regular practice staff meetings as well as partners' meetings (for the GPs, sometimes with the practice manager) in which these questions can be discussed. In addition, practices may hold meetings with and for nursing staff and other professional staff working with the practice in order to discuss clinical matters.

Meetings of one sort or another, and working with other members of the practice team, are regular features of general practice life. They serve to guide the provision of the service and also to help the cohesion and effective working of all members of the team (see below).

The role of service provider can be seen as a burden or a challenge. Equally it can be viewed as a superb opportunity for the GP to help develop a service that permits and facilitates the development of his or her professional aspirations. It also allows for the GP to build in flexibility that can make life a great deal easier. For example, as long as the service needs of the patients are catered for, there is no reason why a GP cannot structure the appointment system to make it easier for him or her to deliver or collect children from school.

BEING PART OF A TEAM

It has been recognized for more than 40 years that many of the requirements of general practice can be met well by people other than GPs. Initially, this related to the developing work of receptionists, secretaries and clerks, but soon many GPs realized the benefits of having trained practice nurses working alongside them.

General practices in the UK now have a great variety of different professionals and other healthcare workers, all working together for the benefit of the patients of the practice. These usually include practice managers, receptionists, practice nurses, counsellors, health visitors, district nurses and midwives. In addition, many practices now also have computer and IT specialists, chiropodists, dieticians, specialist nurses and nurse practitioners, physiotherapists, psychologists, osteopaths, acupuncturists and benefits advisers.

Much administrative work can follow on from the clinical decision-making process. Referrals for consultation or admission to hospital require communication of information, sometimes by phone, almost always by letter and/or fax and, nowadays, sometimes by e-mail. Patients may have problems that require a letter to be sent to a housing authority, a solicitor, an insurance company or any of a multitude of other agencies.

Much GP time is spent in writing these letters, and even more time is spent in processing incoming mail, the results of tests and letters from hospitals, solicitors, insurance companies, local authorities, government bodies, and many others, including from patients themselves.

Most practices now employ secretaries and clerks (often receptionists taking on other roles) to help deal with all this paperwork. Nevertheless, this aspect of GP work can be time consuming and is often considered a less attractive part of our job.

The ability to work as part of a team is certainly an advantage, if not a necessity for any competent GP, and understanding how teams work well is useful in getting the best out of all members of the team. It should not be assumed that the GP will always be the leader of these primary healthcare teams. Leading teams is a skill in itself and, although the GP will be an essential core member of the team, it may be that some other member has the required skills to lead the team, or this function may be shared.

MAKING DECISIONS AND CHOICES

This is a key aspect of GP work. During most consultations, a range of questions will arise that involve the ability to make clear and well-balanced choices. These may be clinical decisions. Is the patient seriously ill or suffering from a minor self-limiting condition? Does the patient require referral to hospital, and, if so, with what degree of urgency?

A serious illness may present at an early stage with very minor or non-specific symptoms and signs, and a clear diagnosis may be impossible. The GP must decide the extent to which the problem should be investigated at that stage or whether it should be simply followed up. There immediately follows a tension around the extent to which the patient should be informed of this dilemma. No GP wishes to worry a patient unnecessarily. Equally, patients have an absolute right to know what is happening to them – after all, finding out is often the reason they came to see the GP in the first place. When it is not possible to make a definite diagnosis, the GP has to accept and live with a degree of uncertainty, but it is essential to acknowledge this process and make appropriate arrangements for follow-up.

The decision as to whether to refer a patient for secondary care has traditionally been one of the major roles of GPs in the UK. Much serious illness can be diagnosed, managed and treated in the community, but sometimes specialist help is essential. A good example of this comes with the management of significant mental illness. It has been estimated that GPs diagnose and manage 95 per cent of all mental illness in the UK, with only 5 per cent being treated by specialist psychiatric services. If GPs referred a single additional patient out of every 20 they are treating, the workload of the psychiatric services would be doubled! The process of the GP deciding which patient to refer for secondary care has been often called the 'gatekeeper' role, and it certainly implies that the GP plays an important part in the rationing of scarce health-care resources to the wider community.

The necessity of making decisions in relation to these questions occurs in most consultations. Often there are no easily recognized or obvious 'right' answers as to what needs to be done and, if the truth were told, we do not always get it right. There may well be different approaches or answers to these questions, and they may all be helpful for the patient.

Decisions and choices relating to patient care arise from the consultation between GP and patient. It is often the case that effective decision making can only be achieved if we take the time to discover what the patient thinks or fears about the problem, and what the patient expects. We call this the *patient's agenda*.

Like all other doctors, GPs make many decisions about the management and treatment of patients. These decisions are made on the basis of the training and experience of the GP, guided by his or her knowledge of the patient and the patient's family and social context. Decisions should also be based upon knowledge of the efficacy and toxicity of treatments, and many parts of the UK have developed 'evidence-based' protocols for the management of common conditions such as hypertension, asthma, diabetes and ischaemic heart disease.

Over recent years, the importance of involving patients in the decision-making process has been recognized. Patients generally feel much better when they are actively involved in discussions about, and decisions on, their own treatment. They are then much more likely to be committed to taking treatments that could well be unpleasant or inconvenient. The GP has to consider whether there are any reasons why this principle of sharing decision making with patients should *not* apply, rather than the other way around.

Practical Exercise

Identify contrasting examples of where the GP either has or has not involved the patient in the decision-making process during a consultation.

BALANCING THE NEEDS OF THE INDIVIDUAL WITH THOSE OF THE WIDER COMMUNITY

This role of the GP is a particular example of the decision-making function. Sometimes there is a problem of insufficient financial resources in the NHS to fund treatments that patients might benefit from. A responsible GP will have to address the difficult question of whether or not to prescribe an expensive treatment if that treatment might only give slight or marginal improvement to the patient. This is always an uncomfortable decision. As doctors, all GPs will want to do the best for the patient in front of them, but at the same time they will feel a sense of responsibility towards the health of the whole community.

Sometimes access to a whole service may be subject to restriction, for example plastic surgery or in-vitro fertilization, and the GP must consider if it is appropriate to try to by-pass such restrictions or to attempt to provide an alternative service, at further cost to the NHS.

A frequent dilemma for GPs is how to respond to the parents of young children who do not wish their children to receive immunizations. We recognize the right of parents to make these choices. However, the GP has a separate responsibility to do the best for the child, as well as for the needs of the wider community. The community has a public health need to achieve levels of immunization adequate to provide herd immunity for the whole population, and so prevent epidemics, and the GP has a key role in helping achieve these levels of immunization.

BEING RESPONSIBLE FOR PERSONAL PROFESSIONAL DEVELOPMENT AND STANDARDS

It is the responsibility of any professional person to keep up to date with developing knowledge and practice. GPs maintain their knowledge and skills by reading medical journals (e.g. the *British Medical Journal, Lancet, British Journal of General Practice, Practitioner* etc.). They also attend courses, lectures and other educational events, and may hold educational meetings with other GPs, sometimes in their own practices. Funding is allocated to GPs to enable them to meet this responsibility.

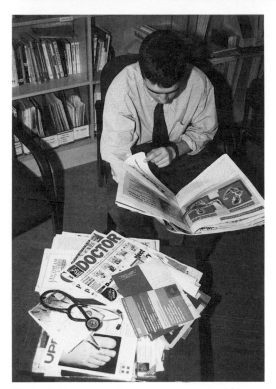

Figure 16.1 Learning to doctor.

dies. Sometimes mistakes are made in the care of patients, and they need to be recognized, rectified if possible, and prevented from recurring. As mentioned elsewhere in this chapter, change and development in primary care are now part of normal working life. Although an ability to cope with change is a very important personal attribute for any GP, repeated changes in the requirements of the NHS and the public can put a lot of pressure on GPs. The ability to recognize all these pressures and the effect they can have on one's morale, personal life and well-being is a very important skill for all GPs. Many GPs now have a support group of colleagues who meet regularly to discuss difficulties and to help each other when there are problems (my own GP support group has been meeting monthly since 1983). One way or another, all GPs have a responsibility to look after themselves in order that they can provide a competent and sensitive service to their patients.

Although this process can be seen as exciting and refreshing, it must also be seen as essential to good professional practice. Scientific knowledge and the practice of medicine are both developing rapidly, and it is important to keep abreast of new developments and to be able to assess these developments critically.

Over recent years, the concept of a 'lifetime of learning' has come to the fore, as well as the appreciation of the importance of reflection as a means of identifying a doctor's personal learning requirements. GPs are increasingly producing and using personal development plans as a way of formalizing their own learning and being able to demonstrate to others that they are keeping up to date.

General practitioners also recognize that they work in an environment that can sometimes be highly stressful. The stress may come from the volume of work or from the nature of the work. A GP will always have patients that he or she knows well who are coming to the end of their life, sometimes prematurely. The GP is bound to feel sad and a sense of loss when that patient

Practical Exercise

Spend a couple of days trying to list all the professional activities of your GP tutor. Identify the three most difficult or stressful events, and then try to work out what made these events difficult. How did (or might) the GP improve things in these three areas?

In addition to being responsible for their own professional and personal standards, it is important that GPs are aware of the needs of their colleagues. In the most extreme circumstances, it may be necessary to involve external authorities when the health or approach of a colleague is giving cause for concern.

ADDITIONAL 'NON-BASIC' WORK

In addition to the basic work of general practice, as outlined above, most GPs undertake other valuable and stimulating activities. These commonly include sessional work in hospitals, either in accident and emergency departments or in a specialist area. Other examples include doing sessions in occupational health departments of large firms, sessional work as a police surgeon, visiting medical officer work for nursing or residential homes for the chronically ill, advising PCTs on health policy for the community, and many others.

Over recent years, many GPs have become involved in teaching undergraduate medical students in their practices or in medical schools. Some GPs work as trainers of GP registrars or in the continuing medical education programmes of established GPs. Quite a number of GPs have become involved in designing and implementing research programmes in the community or in conjunction with hospital colleagues.

These additional activities provide much enjoyment and refreshment for the life of a GP, as well as supplementing the income of the practice.

RESPONDING TO THE DEVELOPING ROLES OF GENERAL PRACTICE

It has already been mentioned that general practice has gone through many major changes over the past 50 years, and this process of development will continue. A number of different factors drive these changes, including:

- changing expectations of the public in terms of what they want from their GPs,
- development of medical knowledge, technology and skills,
- changing attitudes within the medical profession itself,
- the increasing size and age of the population,
- economic and political realities of an increasingly expensive health service.

General practitioners contribute to these developments, and should be seen as experts who are well placed to give good advice to the public and politicians. They have always had a role in advising health authorities on developments in primary care, and continue to be very important in the creation of the policies of PCTs.

However, GPs also have to live through repeated changes, which are sometimes driven more by the needs of politicians to get re-elected than by careful thought about health and the delivery of a service. An ability to cope with change is important for any doctor in any field, and so it is for GPs.

WHY BE A GENERAL PRACTITIONER – WHAT'S GOOD ABOUT IT?

General practice is a branch of medicine that involves long hours, with what can sometimes seem to be endless and limitless demands from patients, staff, health authorities and other official bodies. So why do so many doctors choose to become and remain GPs?

The answer to this question lies in a number of areas that I think of as the 'joy' of general practice. This varies for individual GPs, but for most of us, the aspects of our work that thrill or motivate us fall into one of the four following areas:

- one-to-one work with patients,
- working with other professional staff,
- autonomy in our lives,
- a practical, problem-solving approach to the problems we see.

ONE-TO-ONE WORK WITH PATIENTS

In every surgery, a GP sees patients who choose to come and talk about things that they would not discuss with any other individual. We see patients experiencing the entire range of human emotions, from the excitement of the confirmation of conception through to the sadness and grief at the loss of a loved member of the family. We see patients with an enormous range of concerns, and yet they all share a common feature of trust and hope that we, their GPs, will be able to help.

As time goes by, patients build up trust in their GP, and so feel increasingly able to talk about sensitive or delicate issues, things that may go to the heart of their worries about physical, emotional or personal well-being. Seeing patients repeatedly over the years, sometimes with what may seem relatively minor complaints, is an important tool in developing the strength and usefulness of the doctor–patient relationship.

It is the strength and power of this relationship that is so important in helping patients with their problems, by which I mean both illnesses and worries about health. The power of this relationship produces many consultations that thrill and excite us as GPs and make us feel that our hard work is worthwhile.

CASE STUDY 16.1

In my surgery, I recently saw a 65-year-old single woman who had been injured in a road accident. She had failed to get over this experience as I would have expected. Eventually she found herself telling me about years of repeated abuse she had suffered as a child and teenager, and how these assaults had blighted her life ever since. She had been unable to talk of these events since they occurred, and so the act of disclosure was a major life event in itself. Since then, I have seen the patient again, and arranged for her to get help from our practice psychotherapist. She has joined a group psychotherapy programme, which seems to be helping her. I have a real sense that after 50 or so years, this patient might finally be able to make sense of her appalling experiences and open a new and more positive chapter in her life.

General practitioners will be able to recount lots of similar examples of important and surprising consultations that could only have occurred as a result of the quality of the relationship they have developed with the patient. One should never underestimate the importance of the seemingly trivial consultation in helping patients to develop their side of the doctor–patient relationship.

WORKING WITH OTHER PROFESSIONAL STAFF

As described above, teamwork is one of the major aspects of the work of a GP. GPs now work increasingly closely with other health professionals. Most practices now employ practice nurses to carry out nursing and health-promotion activities such as giving injections, taking blood tests, dressing wounds, immunizing children and adults. Many practice nurses are now trained to work with GPs in looking after patients with chronic illnesses such as diabetes, asthma and epilepsy, and can help patients to think about aspects of their lifestyle that might affect their health, such as smoking, excess alcohol consumption, weight reduction and exercise.

General practitioners also spend time working with their nurses developing programmes of care for individuals and groups of patients, and they are often jointly involved in auditing the work of the practice as a whole, so as to improve the delivery of care to patients.

General practitioners may similarly work with other health professionals such as district nurses, health visitors, community psychiatric nurses, midwives, counsellors, psychotherapists, pharmacists, social workers and hospital consultants working in the community.

All this activity with other professionals, and the building of effective teams, adds greatly to the variety of general practice life. It also helps to support the GP when working with difficult patients. Working with others can be a very effective way of gaining new skills and developing one's knowledge, and so contributes to the continuing learning process for the GP.

Although the creation and nurturing of an effective primary healthcare team can be quite time consuming, the potential benefits are enormous, both for patients and for the members of the team itself.

AUTONOMY IN OUR LIVES

Most doctors enter the medical profession with a great sense of enthusiasm, and are prepared to work long and unsocial hours to help patients and acquire the experience necessary for their own professional development. While working as a junior hospital doctor or a GP registrar, we accept that others often make decisions about the nature and volume of our work. However, as one becomes more experienced, one begins to develop preferences for particular types or styles of work. As the years go by, other non-medical interests may become important, and one may take on other commitments. Doctors, like everyone else, have parents, families, partners and children, not to mention cats, dogs and goldfish.

A GP, as an independent contractor running his or her own practice, is in a good position to be in control and adjust the structure of work to allow for these professional and personal developments. As long as we work within the requirements of the GP contract, we have great flexibility over both the areas of our professional work we might wish to develop and the hours and degree of commitment to the job. This degree of autonomy is relatively rare in a medical career and is one of the big advantages of general practice. It can be very exciting to make decisions about where you want to take your life, and then to be able to achieve those goals.

A PROBLEM-SOLVING APPROACH IN OUR WORK

A brief or superficial look at general practice may sometimes give the impression that the problems dealt with by GPs are relatively minor and straightforward. However, if one spends more time looking at the work of GPs, it becomes apparent that this is not the case. As suggested above, the patient's complaint itself may not be obvious, and sometimes it is difficult or impossible to achieve a clear-cut medical diagnosis. Sometimes such a medical diagnosis is inappropriate or unhelpful.

In the face of these uncertainties, GPs have developed a number of strategies. One of these is to attempt to break down a clinical presentation into a series of problems. These may be problems for the patient and may or may not be of a medical nature. There may also be problems for the family or contacts of the patient (some of whom might also be your patients). It is always helpful to attempt to define any problems for yourself as the GP and for your healthcare team.

Once divided up in this way, it may become much easier to work out what one can do to ameliorate the various different problems, and to be clear with yourself, the patient and others about what can or cannot be done. This problem-solving approach is a very practical way of tackling difficult or vague presentations, and can be both very effective and satisfying to use. It fits neatly into the pragmatic and realistic approach that is so common and necessary in general practice.

WHAT ARE THE NEGATIVE ASPECTS OF BEING A GENERAL PRACTITIONER?

Having talked about some of the exciting and positive aspects of the life of a GP, it is only fair to think about the down side, the problems that sometimes arise in the everyday life and work of general practice. The main areas of difficulty are:

- isolation,
- tensions and anxiety,
- overwork,
- the need to maintain standards and personal learning,
- emotional overload.

ISOLATION

There are many different patterns of general practice in the UK and, over the years, these are constantly changing and developing. In the early years after the Second World War, it was very commonplace to find GPs working on their own in small surgeries with few staff. This pattern of single-handed practice was particularly found in the deprived, run-down central areas of large cities.

It is not hard to imagine how a GP working in this manner might end up feeling cut off, with no other colleagues to talk to, and no sources of help with difficult patients. These GPs would often work long hours, seeing many patients and having to cope with all the worries of the patients as well as their own. Over recent years, this pattern of general practice has become less common, with most GPs working in partnerships, employing a variety of members of staff, and attempting to develop a team approach to the needs of the patients.

Nevertheless, as mentioned earlier, one of the central features of general practice is the closed, confidential consultation between doctor and patient. During consultations, the GP may hear many distressing stories and have to deal with many clinical and psychosocial problems. It has already been mentioned that the GP is frequently faced with vague or non-specific complaints; these may relate to minor self-limiting conditions, but equally may represent the early stages of a more serious illness or be the presentation of another, more deep-seated problem. The GP must inevitably carry a considerable degree of anxiety and uncertainty.

Unless GPs spend time developing ways of sharing their worries about patients, an uncomfortable sense of 'being on your own' can develop, even in large group practices with a well-developed healthcare team. Isolation is always a potential problem for GPs, arising from the close and private one-to-one relationship they have with many of their patients.

TENSIONS AND ANXIETY

As mentioned above, the work of a GP often involves dealing with patients on your own, and so the GP may be left with worries about whether things have gone well with a particular patient, and what might happen if a mistake has been made.

There are a number of other sources of tension and anxiety for GPs. The structure of general practice in the UK is such that the GP, together with his or her partners, has to run the practice and so is responsible for its financial stability. The GP is ultimately responsible for the hiring and firing of all the members of staff, and for attempting to ensure that the staff are able to work together as an effective and happy team.

In the ever-changing environment of the NHS, the GP and the practice need to be able to adapt successfully and still maintain a sense of purpose and identity. There are frequent new demands made on the GP, who has to be able to learn new medical, technological and business techniques and skills.

All of these demands can lead GPs to feel quite tense and anxious, and an important skill to develop is learning how to cope with these worries. This is one of the most important survival skills a GP needs in a changing world.

OVERWORK

In many ways, the work of a GP is very poorly defined. It was mentioned earlier that every UK GP is in contract with the PCT to provide 'general medical services' for the patients, but nobody can really state precisely where these services begin or end. Nor are there clearly defined minimum standards or achievable ideals of practice for GPs to aim towards.

In this environment, there is a tendency for more and more problems to be brought to the GP. Partly because of the vagueness about the limits of their role, and partly because of the close relationship with the patient, GPs are often unable to refuse requests that are probably not part of their role.

If a GP is unable to prioritize and make judgements, it is possible to feel overwhelmed by the sheer volume and intensity of demands that are made. One approach to this problem is for the GP to enter into discussions with the other GPs in the practice and the other members of the primary healthcare team about who does what and where the limits should be placed upon the workload.

Every GP has to learn that there will always be more that could be done for a particular patient, or for the practice, or for the community. However, in the interests of the health of the GP, limits must be set as to the volume of work, anxiety and worry that is taken on.

THE NEED TO MAINTAIN STANDARDS AND LEARNING

Medicine is constantly changing and moving on. Medical knowledge and understanding are increasing, and skills and techniques are developing at a pace that is often remarkable. Over the period of a few years, the pattern of medical care, as well as the pattern of social organization, can change enormously. If I look back over the past 20 years, some diseases, such as smallpox, have actually disappeared (World Health Organization, 1980). Other diseases or conditions have been newly described, such as acquired immunodeficiency syndrome (AIDS), Legionnaire's disease, and the extent of child sexual abuse. International travel is now commonplace and, in many ways, the pressures and stresses of everyday life have increased. New drugs and treatments appear every year, and radical new surgical techniques have been developed over the past few years.

A GP has to keep abreast of these changes and be able to evaluate them critically. The general public is now much more extensively informed about health matters than ever before, and patients frequently ask their GPs for their opinions on new developments. It is therefore a central part of the life of a GP to be able to acquire new knowledge and skills, and to be able to assess and evaluate changes in medicine in all its aspects.

If GPs organize their working life to take account of the need for continuing learning and change, this challenge can be very exciting. However, if inadequate provision is made, the GP can gradually come to feel out of touch and, once again, increasingly isolated from the medical community.

EMOTIONAL OVERLOAD

General practitioners in their practices see many patients on different occasions over a long period of time. As the doctor–patient relationship develops, many patients feel able to bring more difficult and delicate matters to the attention of the doctor. It is therefore not unusual for a GP to see a number of patients every day with distressing stories or deep-seated worries and concerns.

A large number of consultations with GPs (some say more than half) relate to psychological problems or difficulties, and many patients with quite severe mental health problems or psychiatric illnesses are looked after in general practice.

When looked at in this way, it becomes clear that the GP is on the receiving end of a large amount of emotion from patients. Usually this relates to events in the life of the patient, but sometimes the emotions may be directed at the GP. This can be both positive, with patients expressing good feelings such as gratitude towards the doctor, and negative, as when a patient becomes angry with the doctor. In addition, the patient may discuss matters with the GP that touch on aspects of the GP's own life, and sometimes this can be quite taxing for the GP.

General practitioners have to learn to be able to cope with this weight of emotion, and to be able to differentiate between the feelings of the patient and their own feelings. There are many different ways of coping, such as discussing patients with colleagues and advisors, members of the team or family and friends (taking care to maintain patient confidentiality). However, if the emotional load of the GP is not dealt with, it can become very hard for the GP to function normally. This has sometimes resulted in GPs succumbing to anxiety symptoms, depression or alcohol (Allibone et al., 1981) and substance abuse (Morgan, 1992).

Emotional overload is a potential problem for all doctors, but particularly so for GPs, because of the closeness of the relationship with their patients. On the other hand, if GPs are aware of this problem and in control of their own feelings, it may be possible to be even more 'in tune' and helpful to patients suffering distress from any source – another example of how a problem can be turned to your own advantage with a little thought and planning.

Practical Exercise

Mr G is a fit, 80-year-old man who has recently presented to his GP with several months' increasing breathlessness. The GP has known Mr G for 10 years, ever since he cared for Mrs G at home during her terminal illness. Mr G has never really got over his loss, and has often talked to the GP about the sadness and loneliness he feels since the death of his wife. A chest X-ray has revealed Mr G to have an opacity in the lung fields, highly suggestive of a primary bronchial carcinoma.

❑ How do you think the GP might feel when reading the X-ray report?

❑ The GP considers how to proceed with further management of this patient. What are the possible options and the benefits and drawbacks of each option for the GP and for Mr G?

❑ Mr G tells his GP that he does not want any more tests or treatment. He hopes he has cancer so that he can die and join his wife. Do you think the GP should go along with this request and, if so, why?

❑ Several months later, Mr G is deteriorating rapidly and asks his GP to give him drugs to help end his life. He knows this is hard for the GP, but feels he is a real friend who will understand and help him. How might the GP feel being faced with this request?

❑ List the pros and cons of agreeing or declining Mr G's request.

❑ Assuming the GP declines the request, who else might be of help now to the GP and to Mr G, and in what way would they help?

A DAY IN THE LIFE OF A GENERAL PRACTITIONER

What is it really like being a GP? This section is designed to give you an idea of the everyday life of a GP. The best way to learn about this would be to spend time following or shadowing a GP, such as your GP tutor. However, to illustrate some of the things you might witness, I will now describe the timetable of a week in the life of a GP (myself), and then take you through the detail of a fairly typical surgery.

WHAT DOES THE WORKING WEEK OF A GP LOOK LIKE?

In order to describe this, I attempted to note down all my work-related activities during one average November week. This cannot be described as 'typical' because, as discussed above, every GP has a variety of interests and commitments additional to the basic work of providing general medical services. In my case, as you will see, I spend Wednesday and Thursday evenings working for the Department of General Practice and Primary Care of Guy's, King's and St Thomas' School of Medicine, helping to develop the undergraduate medical teaching programme. In addition, I have a variety of personal commitments, including taking my daughter to school in the morning and collecting her on Thursday after school.

Table 16.1 presents an example of one working week in the life of a GP.

WHAT HAPPENS DURING A GP SURGERY?

In order to describe an average or typical GP surgery, I examined one of my Monday morning surgeries in January, noting brief details of each patient I saw, and each other activity I was involved in during the hours of that particular surgery.

The surgery was scheduled to run from 9 a.m. to 12 noon and, as is customary in our surgery, had ten pre-booked appointments and six free appointments that were available for patients to book on that day. Of the 16 appointments, 13 were of 10 minutes' duration, and three were of 15 minutes' duration.

Table 16.2 shows all the activities of that surgery, including the patients seen in surgery and the other activities undertaken during the time of the surgery.

Notes on the morning GP surgery
(see Table 16.2)

1. 9.00 patient. Fairly straightforward review of patient with borderline hypertension. Thought was given to other aspects needing monitoring, such as her renal function, and other risk factors for cardiovascular disease, such as smoking and serum cholesterol level.

2. 9.10 patient. Quite a new patient to our practice. A woman with major upheavals in her personal life, which she is trying to sort out. She has become mildly depressed. At the moment I am seeing her once every 2 weeks, and she is slowly improving.

3. 9.25 patient. Someone whom I know very well. A straightforward upper respiratory tract infection, which is settling. She needed a doctor's certificate for her work.

4. 9.45 patient. A woman, 21 weeks through her first pregnancy, coming for a routine antenatal check. Although all seemed to be well, she was not sure whether she could feel the baby moving, and had become very worried about the baby. I wasn't sure whether I was more worried than the patient by the end of the consultation. I arranged an urgent ultrasound scan to check the health of the baby and pregnancy, and arranged further follow-up with myself.

5. 10.00 patient. A 10-year-old girl having a mild asthma attack. Her mother had stopped all her treatment over a year before. We discussed the need for continuing treatment, as well as how to help settle this attack, and arranged for a follow-up appointment to fully review the management of her asthma.

6. 10.10 patient. The practice nurse had seen a patient with ear and sinus pain and was concerned that she might have an infection requiring antibiotic treatment. It seemed important to support the nurse by seeing the patient straightaway, together with the nurse.

7. 10.20 patient. A man I know well. He is completely deaf, but we communicate by a

Table 16.1 A typical working week in the life of a GP

Monday	Tuesday	Wednesday	Thursday	Friday	Saturday
07.00 On call	08.15 Arrive in practice Paperwork	08.30 Arrive in practice Check the post	07.00 On call	07.00 On call	
08.15 Arrive in practice Paperwork	08.45 Take Miriam to school	08.45 Take Miriam to school	07.30 Call from patient	08.15 Arrive in practice Paperwork	
08.45 Take Miriam to school	09.00 Surgery – 10 patients (including 1 emergency/ urgent case)	09.00 Make 3 phone calls about patients	08.10 Home visit to patient	08.45 Take Miriam to school	
09.00 Surgery – 17 patients (including 6 emergency/ urgent cases)	11.00 2 home visits to patients	10.00 Home – work on medical student feedback on their GP teaching	08.50 Take Miriam to school	09.00 Surgery – 16 patients (including 6 emergency/ urgent cases)	
12.30 Check messages (5) Phone calls (5)	12.00 Check post + paperwork Dictate letters	12.30 Lunch	09.00 Surgery – 15 patients (including 2 emergency/urgent cases) + 1 urgent home visit during surgery	12.30 No home visits today! Dictate letters Repeat prescriptions Phone calls about 2 patients	
13.30 Home visit to 1 patient Sandwich in car	13.30 Practice meeting (including lunch)	13.30 Meeting at medical school on evaluation of teaching programmes	12.30 1 home visit to patient	13.15 Nursing meeting with GPs, practice nurse, health visitor + district nurse	
14.00 Extra/urgent patient in surgery	15.30 Repeat prescriptions Paperwork	15.30 Phone discussion with medical school vice dean about foundation course	13.00 Phone calls to patients (2) Check messages + post Sandwich	14.30 Surgery – 10 patients	
14.30 Meeting with practice manager			13.40 Meeting with new doctor in the practice		

15.30	Repeat prescriptions		
	Dictate letters		
	Chat with new doctor in practice		
	Phone call about a patient		
16.30	Surgery – 11 patients (including 1 emergency/urgent case)		
19.15	Lock up surgery		
19.30	To swimming pool with family		

16.30	Meeting with partner
17.30	Leave for home

16.00	Phone discussion with a GP tutor about problems with a medical student
16.30	Work on practice plans for teaching medical students
17.30	Time at home with children
19.00	Work on plans to accredit new course for GP teachers
21.00	Dinner

14.30	Training meeting with practice nurse
	Repeat prescriptions
15.30	Collect Miriam from school
17.30	Take children to clubs
18.30	Work on new medical school curriculum
20.00	Children home from clubs

16.30	Medical examination for HGV licence
17.00	Medical reports written + other paperwork
19.15	Home
20.00	Read *BMJ* + other journals

19.00	On call with GP co-operative – visiting patients at home and seeing them at the base
01.30	Home to bed

Table 16.2 A morning GP surgery

Patients seen in surgery	Other activities during the surgery
09.00 Woman of 41 for blood pressure check	
09.10 Woman of 48 with depression	
09.25 Woman of 38 with pharyngitis	
09.30 Patient not turned up	09.32 09.30 patient failed to turn up. Phoned a doctor in local hospital to discuss a problem with one of our patients
	09.38 Made a start on doing repeat prescriptions
09.45 Woman of 33 for antenatal check	
10.00 Girl of 10 with flare-up of asthma	
	10.10 Saw a patient with sinus and ear pain together with practice nurse. Nurse concerned about patient
10.20 Deaf man of 45 to review depression	
10.30 Man of 70, a new patient. Very breathless	
10.48 Woman of 75 with arthritis and angina	
11.00 Woman of 70 worried about hospital care	
11.10 Woman of 33 with contraceptive problem	
11.25 Boy of 3, new patient, with ear infection	
11.33 Man of 35 with (a) oesophagitis, and (b) possible ruptured tendon needing hospital treatment	
11.55 Woman of 35 with cough, trying for pregnancy	
12.10 Man of 45 with depression	
12.25 Woman of 24 with sore throat and sore toe	
	12.35 Spent 20 minutes on phone trying to get man from 11.33 above seen by orthopaedic surgeon. He refused, so patient had to be sent to casualty

combination of lip reading and writing notes. Although he has been depressed, he really wanted to discuss difficulties he has been having with his family.

8. 10.30 patient. A man of 70, new to our practice, who is a heavy smoker, and has a past history of chronic obstructive airways disease. He has recently become very breathless, and I am concerned that he may have a malignancy. We have started investigations, and I have also started the process of getting to know him, so as to be able to help him later, if the news turns out to be bad.

9. 10.48 patient. A 75-year-old woman with severe osteoarthritis, whom I have known for

many years. She has recently developed angina, which is coming under control on treatment. Although she is wheelchair bound, she can now see me in surgery, as our new building has ramped wheelchair access.

10. 11.00 patient. A 70-year-old woman with poor circulation and orthopaedic problems affecting her feet. She is very concerned about possible treatment at hospital, and how two different specialists have given her different advice. She doesn't know how to make her mind up.

11. 11.10 patient. A 33-year-old woman needing contraception, who thinks she may have an inherited condition making it more likely

that she will get blood clots when taking the combined contraceptive pill. I don't know enough about this to advise her what to do, but I arrange to get some help over the phone from a specialist, and then speak to her again. We discussed what she could do in the meantime.

12. 11.25 patient. A 3-year-old boy with an otitis media, his second ear infection in a month. I prescribed antibiotics and arranged to review him in 3 weeks.

13. 11.33 patient. A 35-year-old man with two problems. The first was recurrent abdominal pain, which he has had investigated before and was thought to be caused by oesophagitis. The second was pain and difficulty in walking after a footballing injury to his thigh the day before. After examining him, I thought he might have partially ruptured his quadriceps muscle, and wanted an opinion on this from an orthopaedic surgeon. At 12.35 I got little help from the surgeon, who told me to send the patient to casualty!

14. 11.55 patient. A 35-year-old woman with primary infertility who had developed a minor cough and cold. We talked about a number of things, including the possible risks of taking medication if she did manage to fall pregnant. We also discussed the continuing treatment of herself and her husband for infertility.

15. 12.10 patient. A 45-year-old man with depression and alcohol problems. He has come today because of a reduction in his hearing, and having run out of his usual medication.

16. 12.25 patient. A rather over-anxious 24-year-old woman, studying for a degree, who has developed a cold and has pain from an ingrowing toenail. Although I dealt with these problems, I rather felt that I hadn't got to the bottom of what was really bothering her. Perhaps I will another time.

RECENT DEVELOPMENTS IN GENERAL PRACTICE IN THE UK

There are many ways in which general practice has changed over the years, and continues to do so. This is true both in the UK and in other countries, where the pattern of general practice and primary care may be very different. It is important that both students and GPs are aware that the structure of general practice is not fixed, and an ability to understand, influence and cope with change is essential.

The development of general practice has been and continues to be moulded by changes in a number of areas. These include:

■ changes in disease pattern,
■ changes in medical skills, knowledge and technology,
■ changes in society,
■ changes in the structure and organization of general practice,
■ changes in the expectations of patients and the public.

CHANGES IN DISEASE PATTERN

In the early part of the twentieth century, people did not live as long as they do today. If we look around the world today, the average life expectancy varies greatly from country to country. These variations are often due to differences in the standards of public health provision as much as anything else. Worldwide, the provision of clean, fresh drinking water would probably be the single most important contribution to the improvement of health and survival (Espinoza, 1990; World Health Organization, 1996), particularly in babies and children. Factors such as poor housing and sanitation, lack of clean water, poverty and public health education have resulted in changes in disease prevalence (i.e. which diseases are common at any particular time). Developments in worldwide economic and financial activity will have an increasing influence on public health, and this may not always be for the better (Unwin et al., 1998).

In the UK in the early part of the twentieth century, tuberculosis and other infectious diseases were rife, and these were common causes of death. In the latter part of the century, cardiovascular diseases, such as heart attacks and strokes, and cancers were much more important. Since the 1980s, the spread of human immunodeficiency virus (HIV) has become very important, and in some parts of the world AIDS is now a major cause of death. Warfare and civil strife continue to plague many parts of the world, and increasing numbers of people have been displaced within their own countries, or have fled to seek refuge in other, safer countries, including the UK. Refugees have many health problems related to their experiences of persecution, torture, fear and flight, as well as bringing with them some of the health problems that they had in their countries of origin (Burnett and Peel, 2001).

Naturally, the public is also aware of which diseases are common, and this knowledge affects what people worry about – part of their system of health beliefs.

CHANGES IN MEDICAL SKILLS, KNOWLEDGE AND TECHNOLOGY

The ability of society to respond to illness and debility is constantly increasing as a result of research into the causes of disease. New drugs and treatments are developed that can have a major impact on public health. Good examples of this include the development of effective antibiotics to treat diseases such as tuberculosis and pneumonia, or the wide-scale production and use of vaccines to prevent major infectious diseases such as smallpox and diphtheria.

The picture is constantly changing, and it is an important part of the life of any GP to find ways of keeping up to date with developments – part of the idea of 'a lifetime of learning' that has been mentioned previously.

CHANGES IN SOCIETY

As knowledge and awareness of the causes of disease increase, so it becomes possible for society to make changes to reduce the incidence of ill-health. Naturally, improvements may be resisted by cynics, though more often it is people and organizations with vested financial or political interests who prevent change, such as large multi-national corporations. A very good example of this is the dogged persistence with which the tobacco industry fights any changes to reduce the worldwide consumption of tobacco, a known carcinogen and a major factor causing heart, vascular and pulmonary diseases.

Other recent developments have been the rapid increase in the dissemination of information via the Internet. Members of the public are now often much better informed about symptoms, diseases and treatments than they were even 10 years ago. They consult GPs with this knowledge, and they often also carry expectations of treatment that may be hard to meet. One very important job of a GP is to help patients to assess this information. Much of the information found on the Internet is very useful, but sometimes it can be based on poor quality research or personal prejudice, or biased by financial interests.

Not all changes are positive. As mentioned above, the damage to the infrastructure of society caused by warfare or civil strife can have a major negative impact on public health and the prevalence of disease. However, there have been some great successes, such as the worldwide eradication of smallpox as a result of concerted international vaccination programmes.

CHANGES IN THE STRUCTURE AND ORGANIZATION OF GENERAL PRACTICE

Changes in the organization of general practice have occurred throughout its history, and will continue to do so. In part, these changes are the response of society to all the developments mentioned above, bearing in mind the constraint that health care costs money, and the funding of health services will always be finite and limited.

In the UK, there have been major steps forwards, such as the National Insurance Act of 1911 (Parliament of Great Britain, 1911), which provided for health care for the breadwinner of a family, and the National Health Service Act of 1946 (Parliament of Great Britain, 1947), which led to the inception of the NHS in 1948.

All of us have seen changes within our lifetime. When I was a child in the 1950s, general practice was largely conducted by single-handed GPs working from small converted premises, often in their own homes. The GP was usually male, and often the only member of staff was his wife, who functioned as receptionist, message taker and general organizer and support.

The GP charter of the 1960s (British Medical Association, 1965) made it possible for GPs to employ more staff and encouraged them to work in partnerships, in group practices. It became more common for GPs to work from purpose-built surgeries or larger converted premises.

Throughout the 1980s and 1990s, there was an increasing emphasis on the development of teamwork within primary care and in general practice in particular. It is now rare to find a practice without a practice nurse, a reception and clerical team led by a practice manager, and established links with health workers in the community.

The political changes of the 1990s have again altered the nature of relationships between GPs and hospitals, and many GPs are now involved in decisions about the use of NHS funds and how they are spent. There were experiments with some GPs in what were called 'fund-holding practices' controlling a budget to purchase hospital care, drugs and treatments, and to pay the staff working in the practice. These experiments led on to the development of the previously described PMS (Pilot) practices. In these practices, a budget is negotiated with the local PCT, which is used to run the practice, deliver the service and pay the staff and doctors. The practice produces a plan of its proposed medical activities, its priorities and how it will deliver and monitor its activities, which must be agreed with the PCT. The GPs of the PMS practice are then responsible for the good financial management of their budget, though in reality much of this task is delegated to a practice manager. The PCT has its own priorities for raising the standards of health care for the population of the whole area.

In 2002 and 2003, there is much discussion about changing the GP contract again, in other words, changing the way in which the GP service is organized. The talk is about defining basic, core levels of care to be provided by any and all GPs, with agreed levels of enhanced medical practice, which would be funded separately. In addition, there may be the possibility of some GPs developing and practising very specialized skills for patients of their own and other neighbouring practices, and these activities would attract increased pay.

Many GPs are hopeful that these discussions will permit greater variety of commitment and activity in their work. Already, most GPs do not work every night being on-call for their patients. The usual pattern now is that patients requiring medical care out of normal working hours are cared for by a co-operative group of GPs working agreed shifts. The GP now works hard for a few hours each month, rather than being on-call for many nights of each week. In the future it may become easier for GPs to work part-time for some years of their career. It may be easier to spend part of the time as a GP engaged in academic work, or developing particular aspects of the NHS in the local community.

Certainly, general practice in the years ahead will differ in many ways, as will the NHS as a whole, and there is currently a vigorous debate amongst the medical profession, the public, politicians and the media as to how things should develop (Ham and Alberti, 2002).

CHANGES IN THE EXPECTATIONS OF PATIENTS AND THE PUBLIC

Doctors have always been important figures in the mind of the lay public, as have healers in earlier societies. However, what people expect of medicine has changed over the years and is not the same in different cultures. The attitudes and expectations of the public are moulded by the changes discussed above, including the expansion of transfer of information via the Internet. The media play an increasingly important role in setting the agenda for consultations between GPs and their patients.

In line with the greater knowledge and awareness of health issues by the public, there is a noticeable change in the nature of the relationship between doctors, including GPs, and patients. Patients expect to have more control over all aspects of their care and to be advised and helped by their doctor to make their own decisions. They desire much greater autonomy than was the case 20 years ago, and GPs, like all other doctors, are generally in agreement with this trend, although, as ever, some doctors find it hard to make these changes.

Society is becoming increasingly diverse and, given the ease of international travel, it is always important to consider the common health beliefs in other countries and cultures. As a GP, I have been faced several times by patients with what appeared to be bizarre or unusual behaviour that was initially thought to represent symptoms of mental illness. Eventually it transpired that these presentations were the normal reaction to severe stress in people coming from other cultural backgrounds.

Older patients may still carry the health beliefs that were current many years ago, and if these beliefs are not considered, such patients may feel unsatisfied by otherwise perfectly good medical consultations. All the examples of changes in general practice discussed above (and many more could be cited) are raised in order to emphasize how important it is for GPs to be able to understand and cope with new developments in medicine and in the structure of the health service. General practice will inevitably look different in 20 years from now and, in the interests of patients if not of themselves, GPs must be able to influence changes and to work effectively in new situations.

WHAT CAN THE MEDICAL PROFESSION AS A WHOLE LEARN FROM GENERAL PRACTICE?

Medicine is one of the 'caring professions', and perhaps the most important messages to come from general practice relate to care. These cover areas such as:

■ care for patients,
■ care for doctors,
■ care for colleagues and members of the team.

CARE FOR PATIENTS

General practitioners, like other doctors, may become interested in a wide variety of aspects of their work. However, as GPs, if we lose sight of the patient, things happen very quickly to bring us back to our central focus. It is part of the very nature of general practice that we work closely with our patients and staff, and they will not let us drift too far from the needs of our patients before finding some way of letting us know.

It is both a strength and a pressure of general practice that we are unable to hide from our patients, and usually we do not wish to do so.

Doctors working in hospitals and other contexts can sometimes drift away from patients, and the organization and structures of secondary care do not always act to prevent this. General practitioners not infrequently hear stories about hospital doctors who seem more interested in research, clinical trials or impressing their colleagues than in the patient. Our hospital-based colleagues are usually very caring and compassionate people, but the nature of the institutions they work in sometimes leads to the needs of the patient being relegated below other interests and concerns. As GPs, we are fortunate that our patients frequently feel sufficiently empowered to prevent us from doing this.

The *centrality of the patient* is one of the most important features of general practice and the life of the GP.

CARE FOR DOCTORS

As mentioned in the section on the problems associated with being a GP, there are a number of potential pitfalls for GPs arising from the nature of the work. Problems such as isolation, coping with uncertainty and emotional overload have already been discussed. There is another problem that arises directly from the way in which GPs care for patients, and this is the demarcation of the boundary between our professional responsibility and our personal life.

General practitioners work very closely with patients and their families, often over many years. The GPs and their families live in the same community as that of their patients. They frequently bump into patients in the street, in shops, in school playgrounds, at the cinema and in many other places. Unless they can decide clearly where work ends, it is possible to feel completely overwhelmed and overburdened, and this may result in all sorts of personal and relationship problems.

Over recent years, GPs have tried to find ways of dealing with these difficulties. One important step is that many GPs now meet regularly in small groups, a function of which is to facilitate reflection and thought about the pressures coming from work. The sharing of worries, support, practical advice and help often come from these small groups, which many GPs now see as a very important part of their professional practice.

Doctors in all branches of medicine sometimes feel the weight of personal and professional conflicts and responsibilities. General practitioners as a group have provided a model for the whole medical profession in emphasizing the importance of reflecting upon these problems and then creating mechanisms to ameliorate or resolve them.

A doctor who is well meaning and caring, but also exhausted, overwhelmed or sick cannot provide good patient care.

CARE FOR COLLEAGUES AND TEAM MEMBERS

Since the 1960s, general practice has evolved such that most GPs now work closely with other doctors (usually partners in the practice) and with a wide range of members of the practice team. Working with others does not always run smoothly, but most GPs would see part of their job as encouraging the well-being and effective working of their close colleagues and members of staff. In a way, this is not surprising, given the fact that, as independent contractors (see 'What is a general practitioner?' pp. 280–2), GPs are largely responsible for employing their own staff.

With the ever-increasing workload, it has become absolutely clear that the GP cannot do everything alone and must recruit the help of others in the practice and wider primary healthcare team. The successful working of these teams is therefore of prime importance to the GP.

Appreciating the value of medical colleagues and members of our teams, and nurturing and developing their work, are areas in which general practice has shown a lead to other branches of medicine.

Overall, it seems that one of the skills of general practice is the ability to keep all the balls in the air. Ever mindful of the needs of their patients, GPs must ensure the good health and functioning of themselves, the other doctors and all the professional and managerial staff of the practice – a real task, but one that is immensely rewarding and valuable.

SUMMARY POINTS

To conclude, the most important messages of this chapter are:

- general practice is a branch of medicine that allows doctors a great deal of freedom to develop their own professional and personal interests;
- one of the great joys of being a GP lies in having long-term, close working relationships with patients and their families;
- GPs, as independent contractors, can develop and structure their working lives to allow for family and other personal commitments;
- GPs, by having a large degree of control over the work of the surgery, can easily experiment with, and see the effects of, making changes within the practice;
- GPs value the work of other members of the primary healthcare team, and develop ways of working successfully as a part of that team;
- GPs need to guard against isolation, overwork and emotional overload, and have to find ways of dealing with these problems when they occur;
- general practice offers doctors the chance to fulfil their potential by a process of continuing learning and development throughout their career.

REFERENCES

Allibone, A., Oakes, D. and Shannon, H.S. 1981: The health and health care of doctors. *Journal of the Royal College of General Practitioners* 31, 728–34.

British Medical Association 1965: A charter for the family doctor service. *British Medical Journal* (Suppl. 1), 89–91.

Burnett, A. and Peel, M. 2001: Asylum seekers and refugees in Britain: health needs of asylum seekers and refugees. *British Medical Journal* 322, 544–7.

Department of Health (UK) 1989: *General practice in the National Health Service. The 1990 contract.* London: HMSO.

Espinoza, J.O. 1990: *International drinking water supply and sanitation decade. Final evaluation report.* Copenhagen: World Health Organization.

Ham, C. and Alberti, G. 2002: The medical profession, the public and the government. *British Medical Journal* 324, 838–42.

Havelock, P., Hasler, J., Flew, R., McIntyre, D., Schofield, T. and Toby, J. 1995: *Professional education for general practice.* Oxford: Oxford University Press.

Morgan, D.R. (ed.) 1992: *Stress and the medical profession.* London: The Chameleon Press.

NHS Executive 1997: *Personal medical services under the NHS (Primary Care) Act 1997. The contractual framework for PMS provider pilots.* Leeds: NHS Executive.

Parliament of Great Britain 1911: *National Insurance Act of 1911.* London: HMSO.

Parliament of Great Britain 1947: *National Health Service Act of 1946.* London: HMSO.

Unwin, N., Alberti, G., Aspray, T. et al. 1998: Economic globalisation and its effect on health. *British Medical Journal* 316, 1401–2.

WONCA EUROPE 2002: The European definition of general practice/family medicine. WONCA – Europe 2002: http://www.globalfamilydoctor.com/publications/Euro–Def.pdf

World Health Organization 1980: *The global eradication of smallpox. Final report of the Global Commission for the Certification of Smallpox Eradication.* Geneva: World Health Organization.

World Health Organization 1996: *Guidelines for drinking water quality*, 2nd edn. Vienna: World Health Organization.

GLOSSARY

Adult learning An active process, starting with becoming aware of what you need to learn (what you don't yet know, what you can't yet do, etc.) and seeking ways to fill those gaps.

Adverse drug interaction An adverse effect on health as a result of the interaction between two or more medications.

Alcoholism or alcohol dependence An extension of normal behaviour when there is a compulsion to take alcohol. When you suspect such a problem may be present, the CAGE set of questions may be helpful: Have you ever felt you ought to cut down on your drinking? Have people annoyed you by criticizing your drinking? Have you ever felt bad or guilty about your drinking? Have you ever had a drink first thing in the morning to steady your nerves or get rid of a hangover (eye opener)?

Anorexia nervosa Self-induced weight loss, together with an intense desire to be thin, is accompanied by the view that the patient (usually, but not always, a young woman) is still too fat, whereas others clearly think she is now very thin. In its extreme form it is followed by body changes and may be fatal in 10 per cent of cases, although, with treatment, 40–50 per cent return to normal eating.

Argument In ethics this is not about a dispute but is the reasoning that justifies a particular course of action or approach.

Autonomy A person's freedom to make choices about themselves and about issues that concern them is central to the concept of autonomy, which means literally 'self-rule'. Without a justifiable reason to do otherwise, an individual's autonomous choices should be respected by healthcare staff.

Chaperone for intimate examination Someone who accompanies a patient during an examination for the purposes of safeguarding the patient from the possibility of abuse by the examiner and safeguarding the examiner from the possibility of wrongful allegations of abuse from the patient. It usually applies to examination of intimate body areas, and the chaperone is usually a friend or relative of the patient or a member of the healthcare staff.

Chronic illness Illness which, by its impact or its duration, has implications for the health of the patient beyond the immediate presentation and usually for a period of more than 3 months (although this interval is arbitrary). Thirty-three per cent of illness presenting to general practice is chronic.

Classification of drug In the UK, the Medicines Control Agency is responsible for classifying drugs as Prescription only (PoM), Pharmacy only (P: sold only in pharmacies under the supervision of a registered pharmacist but without the need for a prescription) or General Sales List (GSL: available from a wide range of retailers, e.g. supermarkets).

Clinical audit 'Clinical audit is a quality improvement process that seeks to improve patient care and outcomes through systematic review of care against explicit criteria and the implementation of change.' (National Institute for Clinical Excellence, 2002; see p. 247)

Clinical effectiveness Clinical effectiveness and evidence-based medicine comprise a systematic quality improvement process that involves an appraisal of research evidence, the development of protocols and guidelines and their implementation into clinical practice.

Clinical iceberg Only the 'tip of the iceberg' of symptoms experienced by the general population is seen by healthcare professionals. In the UK, 79 per cent of symptoms are dealt with by self-care, 20 per cent by GPs and 1 per cent by hospitals.

Clinical reasoning Process of sorting clinical data (history, physical examination, investigations) to achieve a diagnosis and management plan.

Communication skills Proficiency in the interchange of information between people. In relation to medical practice, communication is between healthcare professionals and patients or members of the healthcare team.

Competence In medicine, this implies the broad ability of patients to make decisions about their own care. A competent person is usually thought of as someone who can be informed about the issue and make a choice, can retain the information and think about it in order to make a decision, and has a reasonably consistent, stable and personal set of values. Ultimately, the law may have to judge, in which case the word 'capacity' is usually used to cover this area.

Compliance The extent to which a patient takes or uses a medicine as intended by the prescriber.

Concordance A partnership between patient and health professional in which an agreement is reached about whether and how medicines are to be taken/used.

Consultation The meeting between a doctor and a patient at which health-related issues are presented and explored and management decisions made.

Computer-based prescribing Tools for computer-based prescribing range from existing general practice systems such as repeat prescriptions, through to computerized textbooks, e.g. the *British National Formulary*, software systems including drug interaction alerts, and sophisticated decision support tools that can extract data from a patient's record and suggest a ranked list of suitable drugs with appropriate doses.

Culture The shared beliefs, values, attitudes and experiences that guide the behaviour of a group of people. Examples relate to age, gender, sexual orientation, physical difference, learning ability, educational background, ethnicity, socio-economic background and health experiences and values.

Disease protocol A set of instructions for the optimal management of a disease from its identification through the range of possible disease trajectories to its eradication or to the demise of the patient.

Disease register A list of all those affected by a particular disease for whom a doctor or an institution has clinical responsibility.

Dispensing practice In the UK, a dispensing practice acts as a pharmacy, buying drugs in, dispensing them and claiming payment from the National Health Service. Practices are allowed to dispense drugs for those patients on their practice list who live more than 1 mile from a pharmacy.

Drug formulary A document containing general information on prescribing, the choice of drugs available to treat particular conditions and detailed information on individual drugs. National formularies exist, such as the *British National Formulary*, and individual hospitals and general practices may develop their own local formularies; these usually specify a limited choice of drugs to use in any particular condition, chosen for their effectiveness, safety and cost.

Ethnic group A group of people who have certain background characteristics, such as language, culture and religion, in common, which provide the group with a distinct identity, as seen by both themselves and others.

Evidence-based medicine A process by which explicit use is made of research evidence in making medical decisions. Evidence-based medicine should integrate best research evidence with clinical expertise and take into account individual patients' circumstances and values.

Formative assessment Assessment of the development of knowledge and skills during training.

General Medical Services (GMS) The contract in the UK National Health Service under which GP principals provide medical care (or services) to patients registered with them. The patients are often referred to as 'being on the list' of the GP. Under a GMS arrangement, an individual GP contracts to deliver care to patients. Payment is through a complex system of fees and allowances aligned to nationally agreed services, without any local flexibility.

General practice An organization, also known as a family practice, providing first-contact, person-centred, comprehensive and continuing care to a patient population. The task of those who work in a general practice is to promote health and well-being and to understand and treat illness in the context of their patients' lives, belief systems and community and work with other professionals in the healthcare setting to co-ordinate care and make efficient use of healthcare resources.

GP co-operatives A formal business arrangement between GPs to share in the provision of services for their patients. In NHS general practice in the UK, GP co-operatives are concerned exclusively with out-of-hours general medical services.

GP principal In the UK, a GP on the list of principals of the primary care trust.

GP registrar In the UK, a qualified doctor going through a period of approved training to be eligible to become a GP principal.

Grounding Having a realistic awareness of what your peers can do, and what you should expect of yourself.

Guidelines Written statements providing 'extensive, critical and well-balanced information on the benefits and limitations of various diagnostic and therapeutic interventions'. Good-quality guidelines should consist of two components:

an evidence section (based on an up-to-date literature review with the level of evidence made explicit) and a detailed instruction section (with grades of recommendations tagged to the level of evidence available).

Health belief model Individuals differ in their perception of their susceptibility and vulnerability to illness, the severity of their symptoms, and the costs and benefits of health-seeking behaviour.

Health promotion A field of study associated with informed and planned interventions to prevent disease and to maintain and improve health. There are many definitions and it is an eclectic and contested field. A working definition for those in medical education could be 'the study of, and the study of the response to, the modifiable determinants of health and disease'. Equally, there are those who advocate health promotion as an ideology, associated with addressing inequalities and poverty, about principles such as autonomy and empowerment.

Health promotion evidence This is usually related to the intervention, its aims and objectives and can relate to both the processes and the outcomes. Evidence can be qualitative and/or quantitative but is rarely conclusive or generalizable.

Health promotion specialist A professional who works in this broad field, often at a strategic level. These specialists are not regulated and come from many different academic and professional backgrounds, but are most likely to have a master's degree in health promotion. It is usually a second or third occupation for those whose previous experiences are relevant to the work area. Many health promotion specialists will be members of one or more professional bodies.

Health promotion theory The body of knowledge that informs health promotion activity is complex and incorporates both sciences and humanities. Theoretical models and approaches to practice are well established but, being a contested field, they are constantly challenged, with new models emerging.

Hospital-at-home A service that provides treatment in the home by healthcare professionals of illnesses that would otherwise require acute treatment in hospital.

Hypochondriasis The persistent preoccupation by the patient that he or she has a serious physical illness in spite of appropriate medical examination with explanation and reassurance to the contrary.

Hypothetico-deductive reasoning Ideas generated by an early phase of information gathering are tested by eliciting further data, and so on in a repeating process until decision making occurs.

Illness behaviour The ways in which given symptoms may be differentially perceived, evaluated and acted upon (or not acted upon) by different people.

Inductive reasoning Information gathering is concluded before decision-making occurs.

Informed consent The process whereby a patient agrees to a procedure, care or treatment after full information has been given by the person seeking that consent.

Major illness Acute and potentially life-threatening illness – 15 per cent of illness presenting to general practice.

Medication review Structured review of the efficacy and continuing appropriateness of a patient's medication. The 'brown bag review' is a particular example of this, where patients are asked to bring in all the medication they have. This allows discussion of both prescribed and over-the-counter (OTC) medications, reveals stockpiles of particular drugs, ancient medications and the patients' degree of understanding about what they take, when and why.

Minor illness Self-limiting illness – 52 per cent of illness presenting to general practice.

Narrative approach An approach used to help people tell their stories.

Negative predictive value This expresses how likely it is that an individual with a negative test is actually clear of the disease and is calculated as the ratio of those who tested negative and do not have the disease to all those who tested negative.

Objective structured clinical examination (OSCE) A standardized method for the assessment of clinical competences in which a candidate is observed and assessed in the demonstration of a range of skills. These may include history-taking and communication skills, physical examination, diagnostic ability, patient management and clinical skills. The observer uses a checklist to record the candidate's competences in the components of the skill under observation.

Out-of-hours care Health care provided outside office hours. In NHS general practice in the UK, out-of-hours care is usually considered to be between 7 p.m. and 9 a.m. Out-of hours organizations such as co-operatives usually only provide cover from 7 p.m. to 7 a.m.

Over-the-counter (OTC) medications Non-prescription medicines purchased from pharmacies and other outlets (including 'alternative' medications).

PACT data In England, detailed information on GPs' prescribing is available in the form of PACT (prescribing analysis and cost) data; similar systems exist in Scotland and Wales. PACT data contain information on prescribing costs, the number of items prescribed and the level of generic prescribing, at individual GP level, health authority and national level.

Paternalism Acting or deciding for someone else, supposedly in their best interests, but without regard to their choice in the matter (as a parent might do for a child) is considered paternalistic. This is not necessarily always wrong, but is to be avoided or minimized wherever possible in medical care.

Pathognomonic 'Specially or decisively characteristic of a disease; indicating with certainty a disease'. In practice, it means a sign or feature so characteristic of a particular disease that after seeing it you would entertain no other diagnosis. An example might be the Koplik's spots of measles that occur in no other situation, but not, paradoxically, the morbilliform (i.e. 'measles-like') rash seen not only in measles but also in many other viral illnesses. From the Greek *pathognomonikos*: *patho-* + *gnomonikos*, able to judge.

Patient centredness Focusing on the patient's story and taking into account the patient's desire for information and for sharing decision making.

Personal Medical Services (PMS) A new type of UK National Health Service contract for GP practices introduced in 1998. Under a PMS arrangement, all GP principals of a general practice contract with their local primary care trust for the clinical services the practice will provide for its patients. In return, the practice is guaranteed a budget to pay for this work and the staff. This is a different contractual arrangement from the General Medical Services. PMS GPs develop their own contract. This contract is with the PCT, not with the Secretary of State for Health; it is local not national. The contract can be tailored to suit the needs of the local population and local medical service provision, focused towards locally agreed priorities. A PMS practice agrees to provide a range of primary care medical services to a defined population for an agreed sum of money.

Polypharmacy Where a patient is prescribed four or more drugs. Prescribing of four or more drugs is not necessarily bad, and indeed may be necessary. However, polypharmacy is a risk factor for potential harm from medication.

Portfolio A collection of evidence of work done, learning achieved, personal reflection, testimonials etc.

Positive predictive value This calculates the likelihood that an individual with a positive test actually has the disease. It is a simple statistic: true positives/(true positives plus false positives) for any test, i.e. it is the ratio of those who tested positive and who genuinely have the disease to all those who have tested positive.

Prescribing budget Budgets set by health authorities or primary care trusts (UK) for prescribing costs for individual general practices.

Primary care trust (PCT) In the UK, primary care trusts are freestanding, legally established statutory NHS bodies that are accountable to the local health authority. They are organizations that integrate primary, secondary and community health services for a locality. They have their own budget for delivering health care in their area; they are able to employ staff (district nurses/health visitors etc.) and to develop new integrated services for patients. They are key NHS partners for local authorities and local voluntary and community organizations. They hold a significant majority of the entire NHS budget and are responsible for GP and community health services and other primary care services such as dental, pharmaceutical and optical. In time, they may also extend to include social care and support services. PCTs commission general and acute services, invest in primary and community care and work to improve the health of their local population. GPs enter into a contract with the PCT (either GMS or PMS) to provide medical services for patients registered at the practice.

Primary health care That which provides health care in the first instance.

Primary healthcare team (PHCT) The primary healthcare team is made up of everyone who works at a general practice or primary healthcare centre: doctors, nurses, health visitors, midwives, physiotherapists, osteopaths, clinical psychologists, counsellors, dieticians, managers, secretarial staff, clerical staff, reception staff, cleaning and maintenance staff and others. The team members may be employed by the practice or by the primary care trust.

Protocol A set way of dealing with a particular condition, often based on a detailed development of existing guidelines, for use by an individual organization, e.g. general practice.

Psychosis The traditional clinical categorization of those (whom lay people might call 'mad') seriously distressed by strange beliefs and abnormal perceptions. These beliefs and perceptions often appear to lead the patients to violence or (self-)destructive behaviour.

Quality improvement A systematic process to manage change within organizations to bring about better patient care. There are many tools and methods used for quality improvement, the most important being clinical audit.

Randomized controlled trial (RCT) A study in which people are allocated at random to receive one of several clinical interventions. Typically, RCTs seek to measure and compare different events that are present or absent after the participants receive the interventions. These events are called outcomes. As the outcomes are quantified (or measured), RCTs are regarded as quantitative studies.

Reflecting Thinking over what has happened and why, what this shows you, and what you need to do differently, or what you need to preserve and strengthen.

Repeat prescribing When a GP makes a decision to continue a drug long term, the patient is allowed to request further supplies without needing to see the doctor each time. Usually the system is computerized.

Research evidence The published results of clinical trials, experiments, evaluations, surveys and other projects. Research aims to answer one or more specific questions and tells us 'what we should be doing'. Research evidence is often thought of as being hierarchical and involving a five-point scale:
1. Strong evidence from at least one systematic review of multiple, well-designed, randomized controlled trials.
2. Strong evidence from at least one properly designed randomized controlled trial of appropriate size.
3. Evidence from well-designed trials such as non-randomized trials, cohort studies, time series or matched case-controlled studies.

4. Evidence from well-designed non-experimental studies from more than one centre or research group.
5. Opinions of respected authorities, based on clinical evidence, descriptive studies or reports of expert committees.

Screening The process of discovering unknown or undisclosed disease risk or actual disease with a view to intervening to prevent the occurrence or the progress of the disease.

Sensitivity A measure of how likely it is that a screening test will correctly identify individuals who really have the disease. With a highly sensitive test, there will be few 'false negatives'.

Significant event analysis A formal type of reflection, important after unusually good or bad outcomes, that is sometimes particularly useful when the event involves several people or a team, as everyone can take part in the reflection.

Skill The ability to perform a task well, usually gained by training or experience.

Skills checklist A list of the components of a specified skill that can be used as a method of ensuring consistency in the performance of a skill.

Skills competence The possession of a satisfactory level in the performance of a skill.

Skills performance The demonstration of a skill in a real-life situation.

Skills proficiency The attainment of a skill to an advanced level. (Practising a skill with adeptness.)

Specificity A measure of how likely it is that a screening test will correctly identify individuals who do not have the disease. With a highly specific test, there will be few 'false positives'.

Structured care A planned approach to disease management based on a register of those affected who can be recalled at set intervals for formal review of the disease in order to maximize the potential to control the disease, treat symptoms and prevent complications.

Suicide The taking of one's own life is still widely considered a tragedy under all circumstances and it remains the doctor's duty to detect suicidal risk and prevent the act if at all possible. In self-harm, there is a spectrum from threats or aggressive cutting/self-poisoning, which does not cause immediate loss of life (typically in the young), to the deliberate planning of a solitary death by the old and ill. However, since the best predictor of completed suicide remains an episode of self-poisoning or self-injury, all such actions should be taken equally seriously.

Summative assessment Assessment of the acquisition of and competence in knowledge, skills and attitudes at the completion of training.

Telephone consultations Consultations with patients that take place by telephone. They may be initiated by the doctor or the patient, and have medico-legal implications and obligations that differ from those of face-to-face consultations. Among these are the security of the communication line and the provision of confidential information when the identity of the other party cannot be assured.

Valuing diversity in health The appreciation of how variations in culture, background and health care may affect health and health care.

INDEX

Page numbers in **bold** type refer to figures; those in *italics* to tables. An asterisk (*) before a page numbers denotes a glossary entry